T0313212

The Statistical Analysis of Multivariate Failure Time Data

A Marginal Modeling Approach

MONOGRAPHS ON STATISTICS AND APPLIED PROBABILITY

Recently Published Titles

Asymptotic Analysis of Mixed Effects Models
Theory, Applications, and Open Problems
Jiming Jiang 155

Missing and Modified Data in Nonparametric Estimation with R Examples
Sam Efromovich 156

Probabilistic Foundations of Statistical Network Analysis
Harry Crane 157

Multistate Models for the Analysis of Life History Data
Richard J. Cook and Jerald F. Lawless 158

Nonparametric Models for Longitudinal Data
with Implementation in R
Colin O. Wu and Xin Tian 159

Multivariate Kernel Smoothing and Its Applications
José E. Chacón and Tarn Duong 160

Sufficient Dimension Reduction
Methods and Applications with R
Bing Li 161

Large Covariance and Autocovariance Matrices
Arup Bose and Monika Bhattacharjee 162

The Statistical Analysis of Multivariate Failure Time Data: A Marginal Modeling Approach
Ross L. Prentice and Shanshan Zhao 163

For more information about this series please visit: *http://crcpress.com/go/monographs*

The Statistical Analysis of Multivariate Failure Time Data

A Marginal Modeling Approach

Ross L. Prentice
Shanshan Zhao

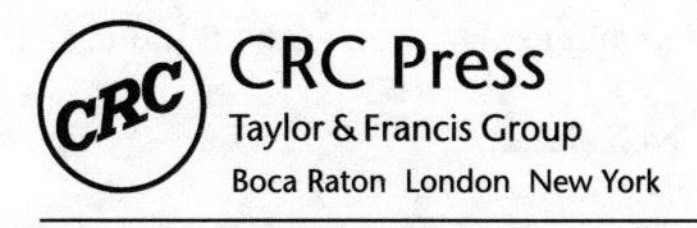

CRC Press is an imprint of the
Taylor & Francis Group, an **informa** business

CRC Press
Taylor & Francis Group
6000 Broken Sound Parkway NW, Suite 300
Boca Raton, FL 33487-2742

Printed on acid-free paper
Version Date: 20190416

International Standard Book Number-13: 978-1-482-25657-4 (Hardback)

Visit the Taylor & Francis Web site at
http://www.taylorandfrancis.com

and the CRC Press Web site at
http://www.crcpress.com

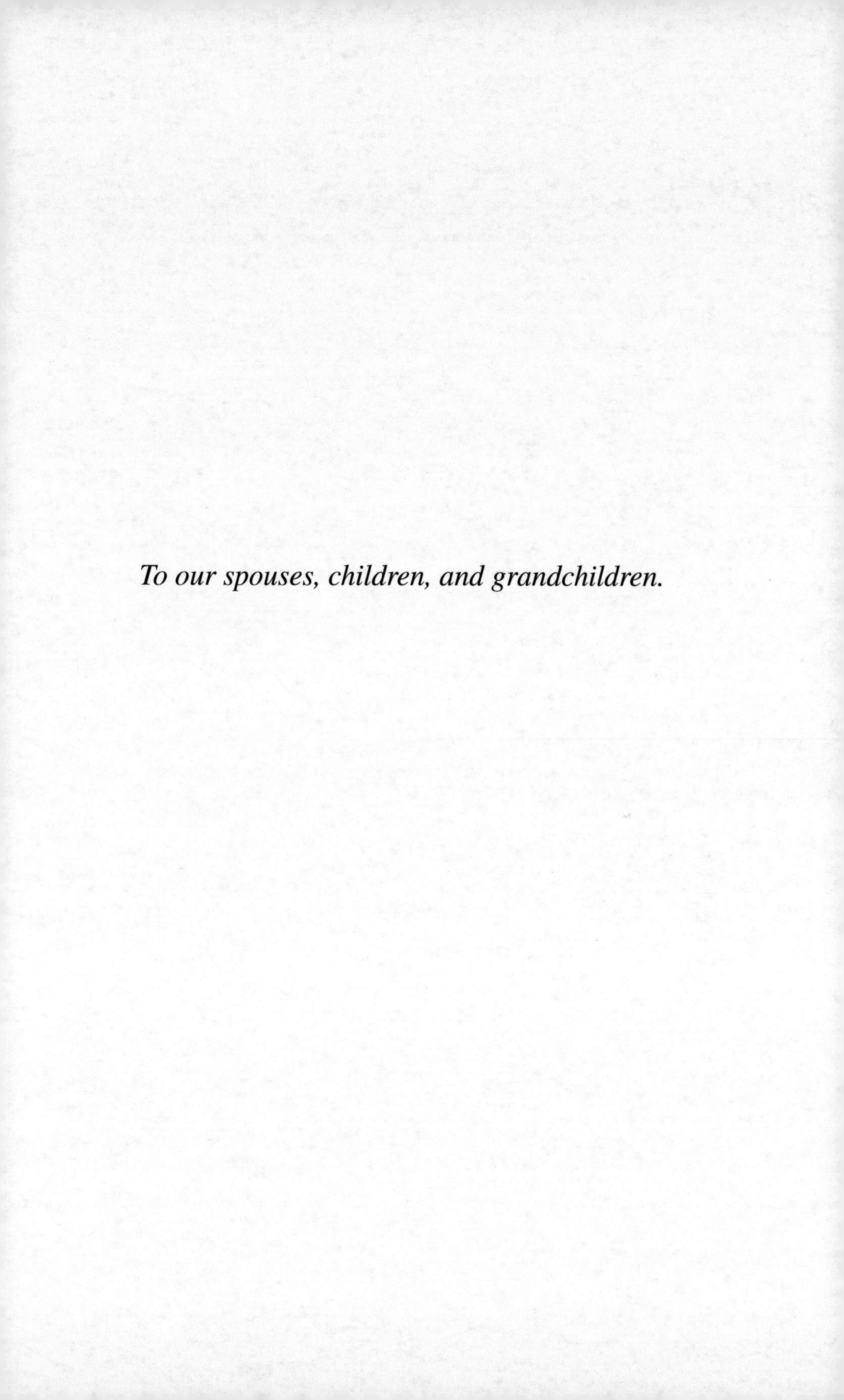

To our spouses, children, and grandchildren.

Contents

Preface

Over the past several decades statistical methods for the analysis of univariate failure time data have become well established, with Kaplan–Meier (KM) curves, censored data rank tests, and especially Cox regression, as core analytic tools. These tools arise substantially from nonparametric and semiparametric likelihood considerations. The likelihood developments have mostly started with a focus on the survivor function F, defined by $F(t) = P(T > t)$, for a random failure time variate $T > 0$; or, in conjunction with a corresponding covariate p-vector $z = (z_1, z_2, \ldots, z_p)$, on the survivor function given z, defined by $F(t;z) = P(T > t;z)$.

Because of the usual presence of right censoring, the hazard function λ, defined with absolutely continuous failure times by $\lambda(t : z) = f(t;z)/F(t;z)$, where $f(t;z) = -dF(t;z)/dt$ is the failure time density (given z) at follow-up time t, plays a key role in the likelihood-based developments. In fact, a focus on hazard rates over time allows considerable modeling flexibility compared to that for F given z, since hazard rates can be allowed to depend, not just on a set of "baseline" covariates, but also on covariate changes and on the occurrence of events of various types arising during the follow-up of study subjects. As a result, hazard, and more specifically intensity, rate regression analyses are sometimes referred to as event history analyses. The Cox (1972) model stands as the major tool for univariate failure time regression analysis. Under this model $\lambda(t;z)$ is written as a product of a baseline rate $\lambda\{t; z = (0, \ldots, 0)\}$, hereafter $\lambda(t;0)$, and a hazard ratio factor that is usually expressed in exponential form as $\exp(z\beta)$, with column vector $\beta = (\beta_1, \ldots, \beta_p)'$. The hazard ratio parameter β is often the principal target of estimation in univariate failure time analysis, and efficient and reliable procedures are available for its estimation, via Cox's (1975) partial likelihood method. There are other classes of hazard rate regression models, including accelerated failure time models that allow covariates to affect the "speed" at which an individual traverses the failure time axis, and transformation models that combine these and other classes of regression models, but the vast majority of applications in various disciplines and settings focus on the Cox model. This model is quite comprehensive when the time-dependent covariate feature is fully exercised. While it is clearly useful to have more than a single framework for failure time regression analysis, other classes of semiparametric regression models typically do not enjoy the same utility of parameter interpretation, ease of modeling, and computational efficiency as does the Cox model. There are a number of books that provide excellent accounts of many of these univariate failure time analysis developments, including early books by Kalbfleisch and Prentice (1980, 2002), Breslow and Day (1980, 1987), Lawless (1983, 2002), Cox and Oakes

(1984), Fleming and Harrington (1991), and Andersen, Borgan, Gill, and Keiding (1993), among several others. These books vary in the extent of their coverage and in their degree of technical formality. Some of them provide a rather thorough account of asymptotic distribution theory via counting process and martingale methods. For example, Andersen et al. (1993) present comprehensive distribution theory using martingale and counting process convergence theory for a fairly broad range of topics, from an event history analysis perspective.

The methods just alluded to can be obtained alternatively by plugging empirical hazard rate estimators into a representation for F given Z, where Z is a possibly evolving covariate history, or by using a mean parameter estimating equation approach (e.g., Liang & Zeger, 1986) for parameter estimation. The utility of each of these approaches can be considered for the analysis of multivariate failure time data.

A mature theory for the analysis of multivariate failure time data has been slow to develop. Most of the books just mentioned include some account of analysis methods for select types of multivariate failure time data; for example, Kalbfleisch and Prentice (2002) include chapters on correlated failure time methods and on recurrent event methods. However, consensus is still lacking on such basic topics as the preferred means of estimating the joint survivor function F, defined by $F(t_1,t_2) = P(T_1 > t_1, T_2 > t_2)$, for a pair of failure time variates (T_1,T_2), even in the homogeneous (non-regression) situation. Also, a compelling semiparametric approach to the conceptualization and modeling of dependency among failure time variates, that is suited to right censored data, has yet to be established.

In more recent times, specialized books have been devoted to multivariate failure time data analysis. Hougaard (2000) provides a thorough account of multivariate failure time methods proposed up to that point in time, with considerable emphasis on the use of frailty models to induce dependencies, and on the use of transformation models for marginal distributions in conjunction with copula models for dependency. Crowder (2012) provides an update on these same approaches along with a detailed account of parametric methods for multivariate failure time data analysis. Cook and Lawless (2007) provide an excellent account of the more specialized topic of recurrent event data analysis methods.

The frailty approach has also been the subject of specialized books (Duchateau & Janssen, 2010; Wienke, 2011) on data modeling and analysis. Frailty models are usually formulated by multiplying univariate hazard rate models by a positive random effect, or frailty, variate that is shared by failure time outcomes that may be dependent. These methods are well suited to assessing comparative hazard rates for individuals in predefined clusters, which could be an important application goal. Frailty models, on the other hand are not so well suited to estimating population-averaged regression effects. Regression coefficients in frailty models have an interpretation that is conditional on the random effect for the correlated outcomes, while corresponding marginal regression associations typically have a complex form. Additionally, frailty factors may need to be allowed to vary over the follow-up period of the study to span a broad range of dependencies among failure times, adding further complexity. Nevertheless, much useful information can often be extracted by the careful application of frailty models. Therneau and Grambsch (2000), provide a valuable account of

Cox model extensions using frailty models with emphasis on model testing and the adaptation of existing software.

The copula approach to multivariate failure time data analysis has also received considerable attention. This approach embraces univariate survivor function models, including those incorporating time-dependent covariates, for marginal survivor functions, and brings these together using a parametric copula model to yield a joint survivor function for a multivariate failure time variate given covariates. As such marginal regression parameters retain the usual population averaged interpretation that attends corresponding univariate data analyses. The models are typically applied in a two-stage fashion (e.g., Shih & Louis, 1995) so that dependency assumptions imposed through the choice of copula neither bias or enhance the efficiency of marginal hazard rate regression analyses compared to univariate failure time data analyses. With a choice of copula function that is in good agreement with the data, this analytic approach can lead to useful summary measures of dependence between dependent failure times, as is a major goal in some application settings, such as family studies in genetic epidemiology. As typically applied, however, copula models tend to impose strong assumptions on the nature of dependencies among failure times, and are not convenient for allowing such dependencies to depend on covariates that may be evolving over the study follow-up period(s).

Counting process intensity modeling provides an important approach to the regression analysis of multivariate failure time data, with Andersen and Gill's (1982) development of distribution theory for semiparametric intensity models of multiplicative (Cox model) form standing out as a major development. When individual study subjects have multiple failure times, of the same or different types, on the same failure time axis, intensity modeling can lead to valuable insights into how failure rates at a given follow-up time depend on the preceding covariates and failure histories for the individual. Often, however, primary interest resides in the dependence of hazard rates on preceding covariate, but not preceding "counting process" history, requiring a different regression methodology. Also the counting process intensity modeling is not suited to multiple failure types for an individual with failure types each having different potential censoring times, as may occur if failure types have their own outcome ascertainment processes. Furthermore, the nice martingale convergence results that attend multivariate failures on a single failure time axis have not been extended to multiple time axis (see Andersen et al., 1993 for discussion). Also see Aalen, Borgan, and Gjessing (2010) for an account of the various modeling approaches mentioned above, with a major emphasis on counting process intensity modeling, as well as the comprehensive recent book by Cook and Lawless (2018) on multistate models for life history data analysis.

A marginal modeling approach can substantially fill the gap left by the previously mentioned modeling approaches. This approach, championed by Danyu Lin, L. J. Wei and colleagues considers semiparametric models for the single failure hazard rates for a multivariate failure time response (e.g., Spiekerman & Lin, 1998; Lin, Wei, Yang, & Ying, 2000). Estimating equations have been developed for hazard rate parameters, and empirical process convergence results lead to corresponding distribution theory. The present authors have recently proposed an extension of these methods using semiparametric models for both single and dual outcome hazard rates for correlated failure time outcomes. This extension leads to novel survivor function estimators for pairs of failure time outcomes that may be accompanied by evolving covariates, and to semiparametric estimates of dependency between pairs of failure time variates. Importantly, these dual outcome hazard rate methods can provide additional insight into the effects of the treatments or exposures under study, beyond single outcome analyses. A primary aim of the presentation here is to provide a summary of these marginal methods. The frailty, copula and counting process intensity approaches have been well covered in other venues, but we provide sufficient coverage here to offer the reader an introduction to these methods, and to provide some comparisons and contrasts with the marginal modeling approach.

While it is not feasible to provide a thorough account of asymptotic distribution theory for the estimators presented, we sketch the main elements of such theory development, based mainly on empirical process theory, and make some use also of martingale convergence results. While our account does not provide a complete and rigorous development, we hope to provide enough detail to provide insight into associated distributional results, and to provide a useful linkage to sources that provide such rigor and completeness. Also, our presentation emphasizes the modeling of observable quantities, with little attention given, for example, to the counterfactual approach to causal inference with observational data, the latent failure time approach to competing risks, or even to random effects models generally. These approaches each involve assumptions about unobservable quantities. As such they may be best thought of as adjuncts to observable data modeling methods that may be considered to address further data analytic questions, but typically do so under additional untestable model assumptions.

The present effort is essentially a research monograph. We do not attempt to present a compendium of the rather voluminous set of methods that have been proposed for some aspect of multivariate failure time data analysis, and we apologize to other authors if their methodologic contributions are not discussed comprehensively, or even at all. Furthermore, the data analysis methods emphasized require moderately large numbers of pairs of outcome events during cohort follow-up, precluding useful illustrations using classroom-type data sets. Partly for this reason we have chosen to illustrate these multivariate methods using data from large cohorts in the national Women's Health Initiative in which we are engaged. The methods emphasized may require novel software. We provide a description of, and link to, the software used in most of our illustrations in appendix materials.

This book is intended primarily for statistical and biostatistical researchers as a source of useful and interpretable data analysis methods, and as a basis for ideas for further methodology development. The book could also serve as a text for a graduate-level course in statistics or biostatistics among students having a reasonable command of calculus and probability theory. Prior exposure to univariate failure time methods for such students would also be helpful, though a presentation of the "core" univariate methods mentioned above is included here. A set of exercises is included with each chapter to enhance the usefulness of the presentation as a graduate text. Many of the examples used to illustrate the methods described are drawn from epidemiologic cohort studies or from randomized controlled clinical trials, and this book may also serve as a useful reference source for quantitative epidemiologists, and for biomedical scientists more generally, who are working with data of the type discussed here. Statistical and biostatistical practitioners can derive utility from our presentation, since we attempt to describe the analytic procedures and underlying concepts in terms that are mostly not highly technical.

The authors would like to thank Aaron Aragaki for help with Women's Health Initiative illustrations, including creation of the platter plots shown on the front cover; and to thank Noelle Noble for tremendous help with manuscript preparation.

Ross L. Prentice and Shanshan Zhao

Chapter 1

Introduction and Characterization of Multivariate Failure Time Distributions

1.1 Failure Time Data and Distributions

This book is concerned with methods for the analysis of time-to-event data, with events generically referred to as failures. Typically there is an underlying study population from which a cohort of individuals is selected and followed forward to observe the times to occurrences of events of interest. Data analysis goals may include estimation of the failure time distribution, and study of dependencies of failure times on study subject characteristics, exposures, or treatments, generically referred to as covariates. The nature and strength of dependencies among the failure times themselves may be also of interest in some settings. The types of mean and covariance models used for the analysis of multivariate quantitative response data more generally can be considered for multivariate failure time data analyses, but there are some important features of multivariate time to response data that need to be acknowledged, as is elaborated below.

Failure time methods have application in many subject matter and research areas, including biomedical, behavioral, physical, and engineering sciences, and various industrial settings. Most of the illustrations in this book will be drawn from the biomedical research area in which the authors are engaged.

A major reason for specialized statistical methods for failure time data analysis is the usual presence of right censoring since some, or perhaps most, study subjects will not have experienced the event or events of interest at the cutoff date for data analysis, and some may have discontinued participation in study follow-up procedures used to ascertain failures prior to such cutoff date. The usual assumption about censoring is that of independence, which requires the set of subjects who are uncensored and continuing to be monitored for failures at any follow-up time to be representative of individuals at risk for failure in the study population in terms of their failure rates, conditional on a specified set of covariates.

Most failure time methods have focused on a single failure time variate $T > 0$. The distribution of T can be characterized by its survivor function F, where $F(t) = P(T > t)$ and P denotes probability, which can be thought of in terms of frequencies in the underlying, typically conceptual, study population. To accommodate continuous, discrete and mixed failure times, F is usually assumed to be continuous from the right with left-hand limits, whence the probability function corresponding to F is defined at time t by $-F(dt)$ where

$$-F(dt) = \begin{cases} \lim_{\Delta t \downarrow 0}[\{F(t) - F(t+\Delta t)\}/\Delta t]dt & \text{if } t \text{ is a continuity point of } F \\ F(\Delta t) & \text{if } t \text{ is a mass point of } F, \end{cases}$$

and where $F(\Delta t) = F(t^-) - F(t)$, with $F(t^-) = \lim_{s \uparrow t} F(s)$.

The need to accommodate right censoring in data analysis leads naturally to a focus on the corresponding (cumulative) hazard function Λ, specified by

$$\Lambda(dt) = -F(dt)/F(t^-).$$

$\Lambda(dt)$ is referred to as the hazard rate at follow-up time t. It is the failure probability, or failure probability element if t is a continuity point of F, at time t conditional on lack of failure prior to t. The absolutely continuous, discrete and mixed special cases can be combined using Stieltjes integrals so that, for example, the probability distribution function $\underline{F}$ and the (cumulative) hazard function at time t are given, respectively, by

$$\underline{F}(t) = 1 - F(t) = 1 + \int_0^t F(ds) \text{ and } \Lambda(t) = \int_0^t \Lambda(ds).$$

Also F can be written in product integral notation as

$$F(t) = \prod_0^t \{1 - \Lambda(ds)\} \tag{1.1}$$

where $\prod_a^b$ denotes the product integral over $(a,b]$. Expression (1.1) reduces to

$$F(t) = \exp\left\{-\int_0^t \Lambda(ds)\right\} \tag{1.2}$$

if T is absolutely continuous. Product integrals are quite useful for likelihood construction, and for data analysis more generally, with failure time data. In part this utility arises because product integration allows discrete and continuous components of the distribution of F to be included in a single notation. Appendix A provides some background on the definition and properties of Stieltjes integrals and product integration.

One could speculate that failure time data would be analyzed mostly using linear models, or generalized linear models, or other standard statistical procedures, were it not for the presence of right censoring. This would be an oversimplification, however, since a focus on hazard functions is helpful for statistical modeling and leads to useful parameter interpretation regardless of the presence of censoring. Importantly, hazard rate modeling allows inference to be made on failure rates that evolve over the cohort follow-up period in a manner that may depend on covariates that are also changing over time, or on other types of events that are experienced by individuals during the study follow-up period. Also, in some contexts the inclusion of time-varying covariates may be necessary for an independent censoring assumption to be plausible. The simplest type of covariate is a fixed vector $z = (z_1, \ldots, z_q)$ ascertained at time zero (e.g., at or before the date of enrollment in a cohort study) for each study subject. Such a "baseline" covariate q-vector can include various aspects of the individual's preceding history that may be of interest in relation to subsequent survival probabilities or hazard rates. In an observational epidemiology context, for example, z may include exposures or characteristics that may be associated with the risk of occurrence of a study disease. In an industrial accelerated lifetime product testing situation z may include the temperature, or stress level, applied to a product to produce early breakdowns of various types. In a randomized controlled trial (RCT) z would typically include indicator variables for treatment assignments, possibly along with product terms between these indicator variables and other factors that may influence the magnitude of any treatment effect on a failure time outcome.

In general there may be a covariate process, Z, that evolves over the study follow-up period. For notation, one can denote by $z(s) = \{z_1(s), z_2(s), \ldots\}$ the covariate value at follow-up time $s \geq 0$ and write $Z(t) = z(0) \vee \{z(s); 0 < s < t\}$ to denote the collection of an individual's covariate data up to time t, including baseline covariates that can include exposures and characteristics that pertain to the time period prior to study enrollment. Here $Z(t)$ is usually defined to involve sample paths that are continuous from the left; that is $Z(t) = \lim_{s \uparrow t} Z(s)$ when $t > 0$, so that the history $Z(t)$ does not include covariate "process" jumps occurring at time t. It is often useful to specify a statistical model for Λ given Z. In fact many, perhaps most, univariate failure time data analysis applications involve the modeling and estimation of hazard rates of this type. This statistical approach, and the use of the Cox (1972) regression model specifically with its nonparametric "baseline" hazard function, will be described in Chapter 2. There are many variants of the simple cohort study design in which data are ascertained on a random sample of a study population conditional on $Z(0)$; for example, study subjects may enter the cohort late ($t > 0$), or be ascertained with varying selection probabilities according to their covariate histories, or according to their failure experience during study follow-up; there may be variations in how and when covariates are measured, and in the reliability of those measurements. Also subjects may cease continued study participation, censoring their failure times, for complex reasons, possibly including their experiences during the study follow-up period. These and other study features necessitate a corresponding rich class of statistical models and methods for data analysis. Hazard rate models provide a major unifying concept, and related methods have come to be known as event history analysis methods. The usual presence of right censoring has implications for the types of statistical models that can be reliably applied, even if the covariates are time-independent. For example linear regression models and maximum likelihood-based regression parameter estimators have valuable robustness properties in that consistent estimators of regression parameters typically arise even if the parametric form for the linear model error variable is misspecified, in the absence of censoring or other forms of missing or incomplete data. Unfortunately, this robustness is not retained in the presence of right censoring, motivating the application of nonparametric or semiparametric models, and estimation procedures that will have good behavior regardless of the value of a nonparametric model component. This topic, too, will be elaborated in Chapter 2 for univariate failure time data.

1.2 Bivariate Failure Time Data and Distributions

Multivariate failure time data arise when univariate failure times for individuals in the study cohort need not be statistically independent, or when multiple events of the same or of different types are recorded for the same individual in a study cohort. Noteworthy special cases include RCTs where the treatment(s) may affect two or more failure time outcomes; epidemiologic follow-up studies of family members in an attempt to learn about inherited and shared environment in relation to the risk of a disease; studies of the timing of multiple disease recurrences among treated patients; or studies of the sequence of breakdown times for a manufactured product. While univariate failure time data analysis methods can be regarded as well-established and mature, the same cannot be said for multivariate failure time analysis methods. Even such basic topics as nonparametric estimation of the bivariate survivor function remain the topic of continuing statistical research.

Let $T_1 > 0$ and $T_2 > 0$ denote a pair of failure time variates that may be dependent. Their joint survivor function F is given by $F(t_1,t_2) = P(T_1 > t_1, T_2 > t_2)$. The two variates may be subject to the same, or different, censoring patterns complicating the estimation of F. F can be characterized by its marginal survivor functions, given by $F(t_1,0)$ and $F(0,t_2)$, and its so-called double failure hazard function Λ_{11}, where

$$\Lambda_{11}(dt_1,dt_2) = F(dt_1,dt_2)/F(t_1^-,t_2^-). \tag{1.3}$$

Here the bivariate probability element $F(dt_1, dt_2)$ can be written

$$F(dt_1,dt_2) = \begin{cases} \{\partial^2 F(t_1,t_2)/\partial t_1, \partial t_2\} dt_1 dt_2 \text{ if } (t_1,t_2) \text{ is a continuity point of } F \\ \{-\partial F(t_1,\Delta t_2)/\partial t_1\} dt_1 \text{ if } F \text{ is continuous in } t_1 \text{ but not in } t_2 \text{ at } (t_1,t_2) \\ \{-\partial F(\Delta t_1,t_2)/\partial t_2\} dt_2 \text{ if } F \text{ is continuous in } t_2 \text{ but not in } t_1 \text{ at } (t_1,t_2) \\ F(\Delta t_1,\Delta t_2) = F(t_1^-,t_2^-) - F(t_1,t_2^-) - F(t_1^-,t_2) + F(t_1,t_2) \\ \qquad \text{if } F \text{ is discontinuous in both components at } (t_1,t_2), \end{cases}$$

where ∂ denotes partial derivative.

Specifically, since $F(t_1,t_2) = 1 - P(T_1 \leq t_1) - P(T_2 \leq t_2) + P(T_1 \leq t_1, T_2 \leq t_2)$, one can write

$$F(t_1,t_2) = F(t_1,0) + F(0,t_2) - 1 + \int_0^{t_1}\int_0^{t_2} F(s_1^-,s_2^-)\Lambda_{11}(ds_1,ds_2), \tag{1.4}$$

defining a Volterra integral equation for F, in terms of $F(\cdot,0), F(0,\cdot)$ and Λ_{11}, that has a unique solution. That solution is in a rather inconvenient Péano series form. Nevertheless, the fact that F is determined by its marginal hazard rates, and its double failure hazard rate provides useful background for bivariate failure time data modeling. See Appendix A for the definition of two-dimensional Stieltjes integrals. The Péano series solution to (1.4) is given in §3.2.1.

It is natural to consider the joint probability distribution for (T_1, T_2) as comprised of its marginal survivor functions, or equivalently its marginal hazard functions, and a component that measures dependency between T_1 and T_2 given the marginal distributions. In fact, the copula approach to bivariate distribution modeling uses this conceptualization through specification of a parametric model that brings together the marginal survivor functions for T_1 and T_2 to form their joint survivor function.

Dependency between T_1 and T_2 at follow-up time (t_1,t_2) can also be characterized by comparing the double failure hazard rate $\Lambda_{11}(dt_1,dt_2)$ to the product of corresponding single failure hazard rates at (t_1,t_2). The single failure hazard rate functions Λ_{10} and Λ_{01} are defined respectively by $\Lambda_{10}(dt_1,t_2^-) = -F(dt_1,t_2^-)/F(t_1^-,t_2^-)$ and $\Lambda_{01}(t_1^-,dt_2) = -F(t_1^-,dt_2)/F(t_1^-,t_2^-)$ for $t_1 \geq 0$ and $t_2 \geq 0$; and by $\Lambda_{10}(t_1,t_2) = \int_0^{t_1} \Lambda_{10}(ds_1,t_2)$ and $\Lambda_{01}(t_1,t_2) = \int_0^{t_2} \Lambda_{01}(t_1,ds_2)$. In particular one can compare $\Lambda_{11}(dt_1,dt_2)$ to $\Lambda_{10}(dt_1,t_2^-)\Lambda_{01}(t_1^-,dt_2)$ at any $t_1 > 0$, $t_2 > 0$ through the ratio

$$\alpha(t_1,t_2) = \Lambda_{11}(dt_1,dt_2)/\{\Lambda_{10}(dt_1,t_2^-)\Lambda_{01}(t_1^-,dt_2)\}, \tag{1.5}$$

which expresses double failure rate departure from local independence on a relative scale. The function α is referred to as the cross ratio function, terminology that reflects the expression $\alpha(t_1,t_2) = \frac{F(dt_1,dt_2)F(t_1^-,t_2^-)}{F(dt_1,t_2^-)F(t_1^-,dt_2)}$. It provides a possible means of characterizing dependency between T_1 and T_2 in that its set of possible values is essentially unrestricted by the corresponding marginal hazard rates $\Lambda_{10}(dt_1,0)$ and $\Lambda_{01}(0,dt_2)$. In fact $\alpha(t_1,t_2)$ may take any value in $[0,\infty)$ for absolutely continuous failure times.

It turns out that the bivariate survivor function F is completely determined also by its marginal hazard rate $\Lambda_{10}(\cdot,0)$ and $\Lambda_{01}(0,\cdot)$ and its cross ratio functions. The joint modeling and estimation of marginal hazard rates and cross ratios, however, is complicated by the lack of a closed form expression for F in terms of these distributional components.

There is, however, a closed form expression for the survivor function in terms of its single failure hazard rates more generally and its cross ratio function. Specifically F is given, in product integral notation (see Appendix A), by

$$\begin{aligned} F(t_1,t_2) &= \prod_0^{t_1}\{1-\Lambda_{10}(ds_1,0)\}\prod_0^{t_2}\{1-\Lambda_{01}(0,ds_2)\} \\ &\quad \prod_0^{t_1}\prod_0^{t_2}\left[1+\frac{\Lambda_{11}(ds_1,ds_2)-\Lambda_{10}(ds_1,s_2^-)\Lambda_{01}(s_1^-,ds_2)}{\{1-\Lambda_{10}(\Delta s_1,s_2^-)\}\{1-\Lambda_{01}(s_1^-,\Delta s_2)\}}\right] \\ &= \prod_0^{t_1}\{1-\Lambda_{10}(ds_1,0)\}\prod_0^{t_2}\{1-\Lambda_{01}(0,ds_2)\} \\ &\quad \prod_0^{t_1}\prod_0^{t_2}\left[1+\frac{\{\alpha(s_1,s_2)-1\}\Lambda_{10}(ds_1,s_2^-)\Lambda_{01}(s_1^-,ds_2)}{\{1-\Lambda_{10}(\Delta s_1,s_2^-)\}\{1-\Lambda_{01}(s_1^-,\Delta s_2)\}}\right]. \end{aligned} \tag{1.6}$$

The first expression is Dabrowska's (1988) representation of the bivariate survivor function in terms of single and double failure hazard rates, while the second simply substitutes (1.5). The first two product integrals in (1.6) are the marginal survivor functions, while the third involves the cross ratios α, but also the single failure hazard rates away from the coordinate axes. However, straightforward calculations give

$$\Lambda_{10}(dt_1,t_2) = 1-\{1-\Lambda_{10}(dt_1,0)\}\prod_0^{t_2}\left[1+\frac{\{\alpha(t_1,s_2)-1\}\Lambda_{10}(dt_1,s_2^-)\Lambda_{01}(t_1^-,ds_2)}{\{1-\Lambda_{10}(\Delta t_1,s_2^-)\}\{1-\Lambda_{01}(t_1^-,\Delta s_2)\}}\right]$$

from which one sees that $\Lambda_{10}(dt_1,t_2)$ is determined by the marginal hazard rate $\Lambda_{10}(dt_1,0)$, the cross ratios $\alpha(t_1,s_2)$ for $0 < s_2 \leq t_2$, the single failure hazard rates $\Lambda_{10}(dt_1,s_2)$ for $0 < s_2 < t_2$, and single failure hazard rates $\Lambda_{01}(t_1^-,ds_2)$ for $0 < s_2 \leq t_2$. Note that the right side of this expression does not involve single failure hazard rates $\Lambda_{10}(ds_1,s_2)$ or $\Lambda_{01}(s_1,ds_2)$ at $(s_1,s_2) = (t_1,t_2)$. This, and a corresponding expression for $\Lambda_{01}(t_1,dt_2)$, support an inductive proof that F is determined by its marginal hazard rate and cross ratio functions for discrete failure times (T_1,T_2). The induction hypothesis specifies this to be true for all points $\{(s_1,s_2); 0 \leq s_1 \leq t_1, 0 \leq s_2 \leq t_2, (s_1,s_2) \neq (t_1,t_2)\}$. The single failure hazard rate expressions at (t_1,t_2) then show the hypothesis to hold also at (t_1,t_2). Since the induction hypothesis holds trivially along the coordinate axes, it follows that it holds also throughout the set of grid points (t_1,t_2), where $P(T_1 = t_1) > 0$ and $P(T_2 = t_2) > 0$, and hence for the discrete failure time survivor function as a whole.

If the distribution of (T_1,T_2) includes continuity points then the T_1 and T_2 axes can each be partitioned with F, by definition of the product integrals in (1.6), given by the limit of discrete distributions formed by these partitions as the mesh of the grid decreases to zero. Each such approximating discrete distribution can be characterized by its marginal hazard rate and cross ratio functions, and these functions converge to those from F as the partition mesh becomes small. It follows that F is uniquely determined generally by its marginal hazard rate and cross ratio functions. In fact, one could regard marginal hazard rates and cross ratios as key building blocks for bivariate survival data modeling. Note that if F is absolutely continuous (1.6) simplifies to

$$\begin{aligned} F(t_1,t_2) &= \exp\Bigg[-\int_0^{t_1}\Lambda_{10}(ds_1,0)-\int_0^{t_2}\Lambda_{01}(0,ds_2)+ \\ &\qquad \int_0^{t}\int_0^{t_2}\{\Lambda_{11}(ds_1,ds_2)-\Lambda_{10}(ds_1,s_2)\Lambda_{01}(s_1,ds_2)\}\Bigg] \\ &= \exp\Bigg[-\int_0^{t_1}\Lambda_{10}(ds_1,0)-\int_0^{t_2}\Lambda_{01}(0,ds_2)+ \\ &\qquad \int_0^{t_1}\int_0^{t_2}\{\alpha(s_1,s_2)-1\}\Lambda_{10}(ds_1,s_2)\Lambda_{01}(s_1,ds_2)\Bigg]. \end{aligned}$$

The survivor function F can be characterized also in terms of its marginal hazard rate functions $\Lambda_{10}(\cdot,0)$ and $\Lambda_{01}(0,\cdot)$ and its "covariance rate" function Ω_{11}, defined by $\Omega_{11}(t_1,t_2)=\int_0^{t_1}\int_0^{t_2}\Omega_{11}(ds_1,ds_2)$ where

$$\Omega_{11}(ds_1,ds_2)=\frac{\Lambda_{11}(ds_1,ds_2)-\Lambda_{10}(ds_1,s_2^-)\Lambda_{01}(s_1^-,ds_2)}{\{1-\Lambda_{10}(\Delta s_1,s_2^-)\}\{1-\Lambda_{01}(s_1^-,\Delta s_2)\}}.$$

This characterization, from (1.6), expresses $F(t_1,t_2)$ as a product of its marginal survival probabilities $F(t_1,0)$ and $F(0,t_2)$ and a factor reflecting dependency between T_1 and T_2 over $(0,t_1]\times(0,t_2]$. With absolutely continuous failure times the denominator terms in Ω_{11} equal one, and $\Omega_{11}(dt_1,dt_2)$ is simply the difference between the double failure hazard element at (t_1,t_2) and the "local independence" product of the corresponding single failure hazard elements.

Often with bivariate failure time data, primary interest will focus on marginal hazard rates and their dependence on covariates. The reader might logically ask, why not simply apply the well-established univariate failure time methods that were previously mentioned for inference on marginal hazard rates, while bringing in a complementary dependency function only if there is additional interest in the nature of any dependency between T_1 and T_2. In fact, much of the available literature on copula models uses this type of two-stage modeling with a parametric "copula" model for F given its marginal hazard rates. This same approach will be considered in Chapter 4, but with semiparametric and parametric regression models for marginal hazard rates and for cross ratios, respectively.

A simple, but important, special case of a bivariate survivor function is provided by the Clayton–Oakes model

$$F(t_1,t_2)=\{F(t_1,0)^{-\theta}+F(0,t_2)^{-\theta}-1\}^{-1/\theta}\vee 0,\ \text{for } \theta\geq -1. \tag{1.7}$$

This joint survivor function (Exercise 1.1) has marginal survivor functions given by $F(t_1,0)$ and $F(0,t_2)$ and is an example of a copula model, wherein the marginal survival probabilities are brought together through a copula function C, here $C(u_1,u_2) = \{u^{-\theta} + u_2^{-\theta} - 1\}^{-1/\theta} \vee 0$, to give the joint survivor function. The parameter θ measures dependence between T_1 and T_2 with (1.7) approaching the independence special case, $F(t_1,t_2) = F(t_1,0)F(0,t_2)$, as $\theta \to 0$, and the so-called upper Fréchet bound of $F(t_1,0) \wedge F(0,t_2)$ as $\theta \to \infty$. Also the distribution for (T_1,T_2) is everywhere absolutely continuous for $\theta > -0.5$. For $\theta \leq 0.5$ probability begins to accumulate along the lower Fréchet bound $F(t_1,0) + F(0,t_2) - 1 \vee 0$, but with each (t_1,t_2) a continuity point away from this lower bound. As $\theta \to -1$ all probability is eventually assigned to the Fréchet lower bound, and the probability density converges to zero away from this bound. In these expressions, $\wedge$ and $\vee$ refer to minimum and maximum, respectively.

At any continuity point (t_1,t_2) the cross ratio from (1.7) is simply $\alpha(t_1,t_2) = 1+\theta$. Hence the cross ratio function from (1.7) is assumed to take a constant value, independently of t_1 or t_2. This illustrates a potential limitation in using a copula model with dependencies between T_1 and T_2 characterized by one or a few parameters: Such models may make efficient use of data, for example for marginal hazard rate estimation, but in doing so they may introduce biases if the dependency modeling assumptions are not in agreement with available data. For example, if cross ratios tend to be relatively larger at small compared to large follow-up times, then use of (1.7) may lead to biased estimates of marginal hazard rates. A modeling challenge then is to avoid unduly strong assumptions on cross ratios, and on other dependency functions, in the estimation of F. Nonparametric estimation of F will be discussed in Chapter 3.

1.3 Bivariate Failure Time Regression Modeling

Suppose now that the failure times (T_1,T_2) are accompanied by a covariate $z = (z_1,z_2,\ldots)$ available at $t_1 = 0, t_2 = 0$. The arguments of the preceding section generalize directly to show that the survivor function F given z defined by $F(t_1,t_2;z) = P(T_1 > t_1, T_2 > t_2; z)$, is uniquely determined by its marginal hazard rate functions given z and its cross ratio function given z. For example, the marginal hazard rates are defined by

$$\Lambda_{10}(dt_1,0;z) = -F(dt_1,0;z)/F(t_1^-,0;z) \text{ and } \Lambda_{01}(0,dt_2;z) = -F(0,dt_2;z)/F(0,t_2^-;z).$$

More generally (T_1,T_2) may be accompanied by an evolving covariate process Z. Let $z(t_1,t_2) = \{z_1(t_1,t_2), z_2(t_1,t_2),\ldots\}$ denote the covariate value at time (t_1,t_2) for $t_1 \geq 0$ and $t_2 \geq 0$ and denote by

$$Z(t_1,t_2) = \{z(s_1,s_2); s_1 = 0 \text{ if } t_1 = 0,\ s_1 < t_1 \text{ if } t_1 > 0; \text{ and } s_2 = 0 \text{ if } t_2 = 0,\ s_2 < t_2 \text{ if } t_2 > 0\}$$

the covariate history up to (t_1,t_2). One can define single and double failure hazard rates at (t_1,t_2) given $Z(t_1,t_2)$, respectively, by

$$\begin{aligned}
\Lambda_{10}\{dt_1,t_2^-;Z(t_1,t_2)\} &= P\{T_1\in[t_1,t_1+dt_1);T_1\geq t_1,T_2\geq t_2,Z(t_1,t_2)\},\\
\Lambda_{01}\{t_1^-,dt_2;Z(t_1,t_2)\} &= P\{T_2\in[t_2,t_2+dt_2);T_1\geq t_1,T_2\geq t_2,Z(t_1,t_2)\}, \text{ and}\\
\Lambda_{11}\{dt_1,dt_2;Z(t_1,t_2)\} &= P\{T_1\in[t_1,t_1+dt_1),T_2\in[t_2,t_2+dt_2);\\
&\qquad T_1\geq t_1,T_2\geq t_2,Z(t_1,t_2)\},
\end{aligned}$$

and corresponding single and double failure hazard processes $\Lambda_{10},\Lambda_{01}$ and Λ_{11} by

$$\begin{aligned}
\Lambda_{10}\{t_1,t_2^-;Z(t_1,t_2)\} &= \int_0^{t_1}\Lambda_{10}\{ds_1,t_2^-;Z(s_1,t_2)\},\\
\Lambda_{01}\{t_1^-,t_2;Z(t_1,t_2)\} &= \int_0^{t_2}\Lambda_{01}\{t_1^-,ds_2;Z(t_1,s_2)\}, \text{ and}\\
\Lambda_{11}\{t_1,t_2;Z(t_1,t_2)\} &= \int_0^{t_1}\int_0^{t_2}\Lambda_{11}\{ds_1,ds_2;Z(s_1,s_2)\}.
\end{aligned}$$

Regression modeling can focus, for example, on marginal hazard rates $\Lambda_{10}\{dt_1,0;Z(t_1,0)\}$ for $t_1\geq 0$ and $\Lambda_{01}\{0,dt_2;Z(0,t_2)\}$ for $t_2\geq 0$, and cross ratios $\alpha\{t_1,t_2;Z(t_1,t_2)\} = \Lambda_{11}\{dt_1,dt_2;Z(t_1,t_2)\}/\ [\Lambda_{10}\{dt_1,t_2^-;Z(t_1,t_2)\}\Lambda_{01}\{t_1^-,dt_2;Z(t_1,t_2)\}]$ for $t_1>0$ and $t_2>0$. Given the common focus on mean and covariance parameter modeling with uncensored data a focus on marginal hazard rates and a complementary dependency function seems natural for bivariate failure time modeling. A conceptualization based on a marginal hazard rates and the double failure hazard rate pattern of co-occurrence for the two failure time events is also very natural. For example, in a clinical trial context there may be interest in whether a treatment influences the rate of development of two important clinical outcomes jointly. The joint modeling of marginal single and double failure hazard rates is useful for these types of applications, and will be a major focus of the presentation in this book beginning in Chapter 3, with regression extensions in Chapter 4 and in later chapters.

1.4 Higher Dimensional Failure Time Data and Distributions

The concepts of the preceding sections can be generalized to more than two failure time variates, as will be elaborated in Chapters 5 and 6. For the present, consider three absolutely continuous failure time variates T_1,T_2 and T_3. The survivor function F, defined by $F(t_1,t_2,t_3)=P(T_1>t_1,T_2>t_2,T_3>t_3)$ for $t_i\geq 0, i=1,2,3$ can be written using concepts given in Dabrowska (1988) as

$$\begin{aligned}
F(t_1,t_2,t_3) = \exp\{&-\int_0^{t_1}\Lambda_{100}(ds_1,0,0)-\int_0^{t_2}\Lambda_{010}(0,ds_2,0)-\int_0^{t_3}\Lambda_{001}(0,0,ds_3)\\
&+\int_0^{t_1}\int_0^{t_2}\Omega_{110}(ds_1,ds_2,0)+\int_0^{t_1}\int_0^{t_3}\Omega_{101}(ds_1,0,ts_3)+\int_0^{t_2}\int_0^{t_3}\Omega_{011}(0,ds_2,ds_3)\\
&-\int_0^{t_1}\int_0^{t_2}\int_0^{t_3}\Omega_{111}(ds_1,ds_2,ds_3)\},
\end{aligned}\qquad(1.8)$$

where, for example, $\Omega_{110}(ds_1,ds_2,s_3) = \{\partial^2 \log F(s_1,s_2,s_3)/\partial s_1 \partial s_2\}ds_1,ds_2$ is the covariance rate for (T_1,T_2) at (s_1,s_2,s_3) and

$$\begin{aligned}\Omega_{111}(ds_1,ds_2,ds_3) =&\{-\partial^3 \log F(s_1,s_2,s_3)/\partial s_1 \partial s_2 \partial s_3\}ds_1 ds_2 ds_3\\ =&\Lambda_{111}(ds_1,ds_2,ds_3) - \Omega_{110}(ds_1,ds_2,s_3)\Lambda_{001}(s_1,s_2,ds_3)\\ &- \Omega_{101}(ds_1,s_2,ds_3)\Lambda_{010}(s_1,ds_2,s_3)\\ &- \Omega_{011}(s_1,ds_2,ds_3)\Lambda_{100}(ds_1,s_2,s_3)\\ &- \Lambda_{100}(ds_1,s_2,s_3)\Lambda_{010}(s_1,ds_2,s_3)\Lambda_{001}(s_1,s_2,ds_3).\end{aligned}$$

In this expression Λ_{111} is the triple failure hazard rate function given by

$$\Lambda_{111}(ds_1,ds_2,ds_3) = [\{-\partial^3 F(s_1,s_2,s_3)/\partial s_1 \partial s_2 \partial s_3\}/F(s_1,s_2,s_3)]ds_1 ds_2 ds_3.$$

Note that $\Omega_{111}(ds_1,ds_2,ds_3)$ contrasts the triple failure hazard rate at (s_1,s_2,s_3) with that under local independence after allowing for dependencies at (s_1,s_2,s_3) that emanate from the pairwise marginal covariance rates.

In Chapter 5 we will consider modeling the trivariate survivor function, and regression extensions thereof. As a specific survivor function consider

$$\begin{aligned}F(t_1,t_2,t_3) =&\{F(t_1,t_2,0)^{-\theta} + F(t_1,0,t_3)^{-\theta} + F(0,t_2,t_3)^{-\theta}\\ &- F(t_1,0,0)^{-\theta} - F(0,t_2,0)^{-\theta} - F(0,0,t_3)^{-\theta} + 1\}^{-1/\theta} \vee 0 \qquad (1.9)\end{aligned}$$

for $-1 \leq \theta < \infty$, which is a trivariate generalization of (1.7). Expression (1.9) has marginal survivor functions given by $F(t_1,0,0), F(0,t_2,0), F(0,0,t_3)$ and corresponding pairwise marginal survivor functions given by $F(t_1,t_2,0), F(t_1,0,t_3)$ and $F(0,t_2,t_3)$. For example, Clayton–Oakes models (1.7) could be specified for these pairwise marginal survivor functions, each with its own cross ratio parameter. The parameter θ in (1.9) governs dependencies among the three failure times beyond those attributable to the pairwise dependencies. As $\theta \to 0$, (1.9) approaches

$$F(t_1,t_2,0)F(t_1,0,t_3)F(0,t_2,t_3)/\{F(t_1,0,0)F(0,t_2,0)F(0,0,t_3)\}.$$

Also (1.9) approaches the upper Fréchet bound $F(t_1,t_2,0) \wedge F(t_1,0,t_3) \wedge F(0,t_2,t_3)$ as $\theta \to \infty$, and the lower Fréchet bound

$$\{F(t_1,t_2,0) + F(t_1,0,t_3) + F(0,t_2,t_3) - F(t_1,0,0) - F(0,t_2,0) - F(0,0,t_3) + 1\} \vee 0$$

as $\theta \to -1$. All (t_1,t_2,t_3) values away from this lower bound are continuity points for (T_1,T_2,T_3) for any $\theta \in [-1,\infty)$.

Straightforward calculations from (1.9), at continuity points, show

$$\begin{aligned}\Omega_{111}(dt_1,dt_2,dt_3) = \theta\{&\Omega_{110}(dt_1,dt_2,t_3)\Lambda_{001}(t_1,t_2,dt_3)\\ &+ \Omega_{101}(dt_1,t_2,dt_3)\Lambda_{010}(t_1,dt_2,t_3)\\ &+ \Omega_{011}(t_1,dt_2,dt_3)\Lambda_{100}(dt_1,t_2,t_3)\}\\ &- \theta^2\Lambda_{100}(dt_1,t_2,t_3)\Lambda_{010}(t_1,dt_2,t_3)\Lambda_{001}(t_1,t_2,dt_3) \qquad (1.10)\end{aligned}$$

under (1.9), so that the parameter θ governs the magnitude of any trivariate dependency among the three variates.

In the very special case in which each of the three pairwise marginal survivor functions adheres to (1.7) with the same θ value as in (1.9), this trivariate survivor function reduces to

$$F(t_1,t_2,t_3) = \{F(t_1,0,0)^{-\theta} + F(0,t_2,0)^{-\theta} + F(0,0,t_3)^{-\theta} - 2\}^{-1/\theta} \vee 0,$$

which some authors have considered as the trivariate generalization of (1.7). However, this survivor function may be too specialized for many applications: not only are the pairwise cross ratios independent of their respective time arguments, but these marginal cross ratios take the identical value $(1+\theta)$ for each pair of failure times. Generalization of (1.9) to an arbitrary number of failure time variates will be given in Chapter 6, along with estimation procedures for trivariate and higher dimensional failure time data analysis more generally.

1.5 Multivariate Response Data: Modeling and Analysis

Historically multivariate response data analysis methods have relied on a multivariate normal modeling assumption. Estimation procedures focusing on parameters in the response mean vector and covariance matrix have long ago been derived using multivariate t-distributions and Wishart distributions. Many problems of scientific interest can be formulated in terms of multivariate mean regression parameters, or covariance matrix patterns. Many of these developments are summarized in the classic book by Anderson (1984). Because many response variables are decidedly nonnormal in distribution, estimating equations for mean parameters, and for mean and covariance parameters, subsequently came to provide a central approach to the modeling and analysis of multivariate response data, with major stimulus from the work of Liang and Zeger (1986) and Zeger and Liang (1986). By construing censored failure time data as a set of binary variates, "generalized estimating equations" may be considered also for the analysis of univariate and multivariate failure time data, as will be illustrated in subsequent chapters. Appendix A provides a brief account of generalized estimating equations for mean parameter estimation.

Analysis methods based on multivariate normal theory, on more general parametric maximum likelihood theory or M-estimation, or based on generalized estimating equations enjoy some valuable robustness to departure from distributional form working model assumptions. With right censoring however, or with other forms of censoring or missing data, this robustness is typically lost, providing a reason to emphasize nonparametric and semiparametric models and estimation procedures. Also, as with generalized estimating equations for mean and covariance parameters, with censored data it is valuable to consider models and estimation procedures for dependency parameters that do not compromise the properties of marginal distribution parameter estimates. Hence the approach emphasized in subsequent chapters will estimate marginal distribution parameters using the associated univariate data, with additional estimating procedures for multivariate parameter estimation. Related procedures using dependency parameter estimates to weight unbiased marginal distribution parameter estimating functions will also be mentioned.

The discussion of this section focuses on marginal, or population-averaged, quantities. There is also a substantial multivariate failure time literature on the modeling and estimation of evolving failure rates that include each study subject's prior failure time history in the failure rate specification. Such rates are referred to as intensities, and the associated modeling and estimation procedures play a major role in recurrent event methods and in more general multistate modeling methods.

1.6 Recurrent Event Characterization and Modeling

In an important subclass of applications there is a single failure time axis with individuals experiencing a failure continuing to be followed for second and subsequent failures. Such recurrent failure time process data $T_1, T_2, \ldots$ may be subject to a single censoring process that discontinues the follow-up for the study subject. In many respects the modeling and analysis of this type of recurrent event data is more like the univariate failure time data modeling mentioned in §1.1 than the correlated failure time modeling discussed in §§1.2–1.4. For example, recurrent event modeling can focus on failure rates

$$\Lambda\{dt; \mathscr{H}(t)\} = P\{\text{failure in } [t, t+dt); \mathscr{H}(t)\} \tag{1.11}$$

where the conditioning event $\mathscr{H}(t)$ includes not only the covariate history $Z(t)$ prior to time t, but also the failure history for the individual prior to time t. This latter history is conveniently described by the counting process N, where $N(dt)$ equals the number of failures experienced by the individual at time t and $N(t) = \int_0^t N(ds)$. Recurrent event data frequently involve a large number of failures on individual study subjects, and the modeling of (1.11) sometimes involves simplifying assumptions as to how the intensity at time t depends on the preceding failure history $\{N(s), s < t\}$ for the individual, with Markov and semi-Markov assumptions commonly imposed. Of course, there may be recurrent events for several types of failure time variates in which case the concepts of this and the preceding sections can be combined leading to the modeling of marginal failure rate processes (1.11), along with corresponding cross ratio processes for example, in each case with the conditioning event including not only the covariate, but also the preceding failure history for each event type. The modeling and analysis of recurrent event data will be discussed in Chapter 7. Importantly, marginal modeling approaches in which one models failure rates at follow-up time t as a function of the preceding failure, but not the preceding counting process history, will also be considered in Chapter 7, along with generalizations to include failures of various types on the same or different failure time axes.

Chapter 8 considers a variety of additional important topics in the modeling and analysis of multivariate failure time data, including censoring schemes that are "dependent;" cohort sampling procedures where some components of covariate histories are assembled only for failing individuals and a subcohort of individuals who are without failure during certain follow-up periods; data analysis procedures when covariate values are subject to measurement error or missing values, and joint models for covariate histories and failure times, among other topics.

We end this chapter by describing a few application areas encountered in our applied work. These settings will be used to illustrate modeling and analysis methods in subsequent chapters.

1.7 Some Application Settings

1.7.1 Aplastic anemia clinical trial

Table 1.1 shows failure time data for 64 patients having severe aplastic anemia. These data are from Storb et al. (1986) as presented in Kalbfleisch and Prentice (2002, Table 1.2). Patients were conditioned with high-dose cyclophosphamide followed by bone marrow cell infusion from a human lymphocyte antigen (HLA)–matched family member. Patients were then randomly assigned to receive either cyclosporine plus methotrexate (CSP + MTX) or methotrexate alone (MTX) with time from assignment to the diagnosis of stage 2 or greater acute graft versus host disease (A-GVHD) as a key outcome. Table 1.1 also shows whether (LAF $= 1$) or not (LAF $= 0$) each patient was assigned to a laminar air flow isolation room, and the patient's age in years, both at baseline ($t = 0$). Note that 44 of the 64 patients had right censored times to A-GVHD, with censored times indicated by an asterisk. A principal study goal was to assess whether the addition of CSP to the MTX regimen reduced the A-GVHD risk. An independent censoring assumption requires patients who are still alive without A-GVHD at the cutoff date for data analysis to be representative of patients who are without an A-GVHD diagnosis at this censoring time, conditional on treatment, LAF assignments and age (assuming that these variables are included and well modeled in the data analysis). This independent censoring assumption is satisfied for patients alive and without A-GVHD at the time of data analysis. Many of the asterisks in Table 1.1, however, attend the days from randomization to death for patients who died without having an A-GVHD diagnosis. It may seem like Table 1.1 provides censored bivariate failure time data on time (T_1) from randomization to A-GVHD and time from randomization to death (T_2), but the table only gives times to the smaller of T_1 and T_2. Competing risk methods (e.g., Kalbfleisch & Prentice, 2002, Chapter 8) indicate that A-GVHD hazard rates (among surviving patients) can be estimated simply by regarding death times as additional censored observations. Hence these data can be analyzed as censored univariate failure time data to relate treatment assignment and other study subject characteristics to A-GVHD incidence, as will be illustrated in Chapter 2. Genuinely bivariate data could be obtained in this application by recording also the time to death for patients experiencing A-GVHD. These more comprehensive data would support estimation of double failure hazard rates (for A-GVHD followed by death) and their comparison among randomization groups, as well as analyses of dependency between time to A-GVHD and time to death at specified values of randomization assignment and other covariates.

Table 1.1 *Time in days to severe (stage ≥ 2) acute graft versus host disease (A-GVHD), death, or last contact for bone marrow transplant patients treated with cyclosporine and methotrexate (CSP + MTX) or with MTX only*[a]

CSP+MTX						MTX					
Time	LAF	Age	Time	LAF	Age	Time	LAF	Age	Time	LAF	Age
3*	0	40	324*	0	23	9	1	35	104*	1	27
8	1	21	356*	1	13	11	1	27	106*	1	19
10	1	18	378*	1	34	12	0	22	156*	1	15
12*	0	42	408*	1	27	20	1	21	218*	1	26
16	0	23	411*	1	5	20	1	30	230*	0	11
17	0	21	420*	1	23	22	0	7	231*	1	14
22	1	13	449*	1	37	25	1	36	316*	1	15
64*	0	20	490*	1	37	25	1	38	393*	7	27
65*	1	15	528*	1	32	25*	0	20	395*	0	2
77*	1	34	547*	1	32	28	0	25	428*	0	3
82*	1	14	691*	1	38	28	0	28	469*	1	14
98*	1	10	769*	0	18	31	1	17	602*	1	18
155*	0	27	1111*	0	20	35	1	21	681*	0	23
189*	1	9	1173*	0	12	35	1	25	690*	1	9
199*	1	19	1213*	0	12	46	1	35	1112*	1	11
247*	1	14	1357*	0	29	49	0	19	1180*	0	11

Source: Kalbfleisch and Prentice (2002, Table 1.2)

[a]Asterisks indicate that time to severe A-GVHD is right censored; that is, the patient died without severe A-GVHD or was without severe A-GVHD at last contact.

1.7.2 *Australian twin data*

Duffy, Martin, and Mathews (1990) present analyses of ages at appendectomy for twin pairs in Australia. This study was conducted, in part, to compare monozygotic (MZ) and dizygotic (DZ) twins with respect to the strength of dependency in ages of occurrence between pair members for various outcomes, including vermiform appendectomy. Twin pairs over the age of 17 years were asked to provide information on the occurrence, and age at occurrence, of appendectomy and other outcomes. Respondents not undergoing appendectomy prior to survey, or suspected of undergoing prophylactic appendectomy, give rise to right-censored ages at appendectomy. There were 1953 twin pairs, comprised of 1218 MZ and 735 DZ pairs. Among MZ pairs there were 144 pairs in which both members, 304 pairs in which one member, and 770 in which neither member underwent appendectomy. The corresponding numbers for DZ twins were 63, 208 and 464, respectively.

Comparison of strength of dependency between MZ and DZ twins may provide insight into the importance of genetic factors for the outcome under consideration, though the possibility that environmental factors (e.g., diet, physical activity patterns) are more closely shared by MZ than by DZ twins also needs to be entertained. Also, the twin pair ascertainment process may need to be modeled for some analytic purposes. Here, for purposes of illustration (Chapter 3), as in Prentice and Hsu (1997), we will regard these data as a simple cohort study of twin pairs without allowing for the possible analytic impact of ascertainment criteria, continued survival, and willingness (of both pair members) to respond to the study survey.

1.7.3 Women's Health Initiative hormone therapy trial

A setting that we will use for illustration in various chapters is the Women's Health Initiative (WHI) hormone therapy trials. The WHI, in which the authors are engaged, is a National Institutes of Health–sponsored disease prevention and population science research program among post-menopausal women in the United States. It includes a multifaceted randomized controlled trial (RCT) of four different preventive interventions (treatments) in a partial factorial design, and a prospective observational cohort study. The RCT included 68,132 women, each of whom enrolled either in a postmenopausal hormone therapy (HT) trial (27,347 women) or a low-fat dietary pattern intervention trial (48,835 women), or both, while the observational study enrolled 93,676 women from essentially the same catchment populations in proximity to 40 clinical centers across the United States. The HT trials included two separate randomized, placebo controlled comparisons: conjugated equine estrogen (CEE-alone; 0.625 mg/d continuous) among women who were post-hysterectomy (10,739 women), or the same estrogen preparation plus medroxyprogesterone acetate (CEE + MPA; 2.5 mg/d MPA continuous) among women having a uterus (16,608 women). Postmenopausal estrogens became widely used in the 1960s as an effective means of controlling vasomotor symptoms associated with the menopause. Progestational agents were added starting in the late 1970s to protect the uterus, when a 5- to 10-fold increase in uterine cancer risk was observed among CEE-alone users. By the time the WHI trials began in 1993, about 8 million women were using the precise CEE-alone regimen studied and about 6 million women were using the precise CEE + MPA regimen studied, in the United States alone. These potent hormonal preparations lead to approximate doubling of blood estrogens (estradiol, estrone, estrone sulfate) and an approximate doubling of their offsetting sex-hormone binding globulin, whether or not progestin is included. In a mass spectrometry-based serum proteomic profiling study, evidence emerged that CEE-alone and/or CEE + MPA changed circulating protein concentrations for nearly half of the 350 proteins quantified, including proteins involved in growth factors, inflammation, immune response, metabolism and osteogenesis, among other biological pathways. Hence it may not be surprising that the use of these preparations has implications of the risk of important chronic diseases. The CEE + MPA trial intervention (active treatment or placebo) was stopped early, in 2002, on the recommendation of the external Data and Safety Monitoring Committee for the WHI, when an increase in breast cancer risk was observed, and a designated global index, defined as the time to the earliest of coronary heart disease (CHD), stroke, pulmonary embolism, (invasive) breast cancer, colorectal cancer, endometrial cancer, hip fracture or death from any other cause, was also in the unfavorable direction. These results were quite a shock to researchers and practitioners, especially concerning CHD, for which an early hazard ratio (HR) elevation was observed. In fact CHD was the designated primary outcome in the

HT trials, and a major risk reduction was hypothesized for both regimens, primarily based on an extensive observational epidemiology literature. A more sustained HR elevation in stroke risk was also observed, as was a substantial early HR elevation in pulmonary embolism, and in venous thromboembolism more generally. On the other side of the ledger, the rate of colorectal cancer diagnosis was lower in the active treatment compared to the placebo group, and the incidence of hip fracture, and of bone fractures more generally, were lower with active treatment. Nevertheless, the global index mentioned above was decidedly in the unfavorable direction, contributing to the early trial stoppage decision.

The CEE-alone trial intervention was also stopped early, in 2004, about a year before the planned completion of its intervention phase, substantially because a stroke risk elevation of similar magnitude to that for CEE + MPA was observed. However, the global index was essentially null for this trial, due to a balancing of health benefits and risks. In particular breast cancer risk was somewhat lower in the CEE-alone treatment versus the placebo group, and fracture risk reduction of similar magnitude to that with CEE + MPA was observed. Follow-up continues, to explore the long-term effects of an average 5.6 years of CEE + MPA treatment, or an average of 7.1 years of CEE-alone treatment, more than 14 years after the conclusion of the HT trial's intervention phase.

In these controlled trials it is natural to define failure times for each woman as the time from trial enrollment to disease event occurrence. Individual women can be followed to observe the time to occurrence of CHD (T_1), breast cancer (T_2), stroke (T_3), hip fracture (T_4), among other clinical outcomes. Even though these are among the most common chronic diseases among postmenopausal women, only a few percent of trial enrollees experienced any one of these types of failures during trial follow-up, with other women having censored times, as determined by death, loss to follow-up, or alive and under active follow-up without the study disease at the cutoff time for data analysis. Analyses to date have mostly looked at hazard rates for clinical outcomes one at a time, with follow-up continuing even after the occurrence of nonfatal events of other disease types. Some univariate failure time data analyses from the HT trials will be described in Chapter 2 and multivariate analyses will be considered in Chapters 5 and 6.

The availability of multivariate failure time data $(T_1, T_2, \ldots)$ opens up some additional data analytic opportunities: Women at elevated risk for stroke also tend to be at elevated risk for other cardiovascular diseases, including CHD. One can ask whether the incidence data on CHD can be used to increase the precision of hazard-based treatment evaluation for stroke, or whether some composite CHD and stroke outcomes may be informative. This type of "strength borrowing" is commonplace in other data analytic contexts, for example, using generalized estimating equations, but is it of practical importance for failure time data and, if so, how should analyses be carried out? Any such strength borrowing would require, for example, continued follow-up for T_1 following a T_2 event, and events of a particular disease type may then need to distinguish fatal from non-fatal disease events. The nature and strength of dependencies between non-fatal disease occurrences could be of some interest itself in this type of setting, particularly if the study treatment had an influence on such dependencies.

Some of the diseases relevant to hormone therapy may occur on more than one occasion during the follow-up of a particular woman as for venous thromboembolic events, fractures, or even cancers of certain types either through recurrence or a new primary diagnosis. One can ask whether treatment assessments can be more informative if the total event history during follow-up, rather than time to the first event of each specific type, is included for each woman; and whether data summaries, such as comparisons of estimated mean numbers of events over a follow-up period of a certain duration may be helpful.

An additional goal of multivariate failure time data analysis in some contexts may be a summary of the effects of a treatment or an exposure across a range of health-related outcomes, or across a set of failure-types more generally. While the construction of summaries of this type may require data beyond that available in a given study, or judgments by subject matter specialists concerning the severity or impact of each failure type, the value of suitable summary measures, or indices, is quite evident for study monitoring and reporting purposes, and it is useful to examine methodologic approaches to addressing statistical aspects of such data summaries. See Anderson et al. (2007) for further detail on statistical aspects of the monitoring and reporting on the WHI hormone therapy trials.

The multivariate failure time variables $T_1, T_2, \ldots$ defined above can be considered in this context as correlated failure times on the same time from randomization axis. The potential censoring times for failures of different types may vary however, since outcome ascertainment procedures and outcome data sources may vary by failure type.

1.7.4 Bladder tumor recurrence data

Table 1.2, obtained from Table 9.2 of Kalbfleisch and Prentice (2002), shows data from a randomized trial of patient recurrences of superficial bladder tumor recurrence as conducted by the Veterans Administration Cooperative Urological Group. As discussed in Byar (1980) these data were used to compare the frequency of recurrences among 48 patients assigned to placebo, among whom there were a total of 87 post-randomization recurrences, and 38 patients assigned to treatment with a drug called thiotepa, among whom there were 45 recurrences during the trial follow-up period, which averaged about 31 months. Tumors present at baseline were removed transurethrally prior to randomization. In addition to studying the influence of thiotepa on recurrence frequency, there was interest in the dependence of such recurrence rates on the number and size of prerandomization tumors. Note that some patients experience multiple recurrences during the study follow-up period, and useful data analyses may focus on the mean number of recurrences during a specified follow-up period. However, care may be needed in the modeling of data of this type since patients experiencing recurrences could be more likely to cease trial participation prematurely, giving rise to censoring rates that could depend on the preceding failure time history for the patient. Also note in Table 1.2 that recurrence times have

Table 1.2 *Bladder tumor recurrence data*

Initial Tumors[a]		Censoring[b]	Recurrence Times[b]	Initial Tumors		Censoring	Recurrence Times
Number	Size	Time	$T_1, T_2 \ldots$	Number	Size	Time	$T_1, T_2 \ldots$
Placebo Group							
1	1	0		1	5	30	2,17,22
1	3	1		2	1	30	3, 6, 8, 12, 26
2	1	4		1	3	31	12, 15, 24
1	1	7		1	2	32	
5	1	10		2	1	34	
4	1	10	6	2	1	36	
1	1	14		3	1	36	29
1	1	18		1	2	37	
1	3	18	5	4	1	40	9, 17, 22, 24
1	1	18	12, 16	5	1	40	16, 19, 23, 29, 34, 40
3	3	23		1	2	41	
1	3	23	10, 15	1	1	43	3
1	1	23	3, 16, 23	2	6	43	6
3	1	23	3, 9, 21	2	1	44	3, 6, 9
2	3	24	7, 10, 16, 24	1	1	45	9, 11, 20, 26, 30
1	1	25	3, 15, 25	1	1	48	18
1	2	26		1	3	49	
8	1	26	1	3	1	51	35
1	4	26	2, 26	1	7	53	17
1	2	28	25	3	1	53	3, 15, 46, 51, 53
1	4	29		1	1	59	
1	2	29		3	2	61	2, 15, 24, 30, 34, 39, 43, 49, 52
4	1	29		1	3	64	5, 14, 19, 27, 41
1	6	30	28, 30	2	3	64	2, 8, 12, 13, 17, 21, 33, 49
Thiotepa Group							
1	3	1		8	3	36	26, 35
1	1	1		1	1	38	
8	1	5	5	1	1	39	22, 23, 27, 32
1	2	9		6	1	39	4, 16, 23, 27, 33, 36, 37
1	1	10		3	1	40	24, 26, 29, 40
1	1	13		3	2	41	
2	6	14	3	1	1	41	
5	3	17	1, 3, 5, 7, 10	1	1	43	1, 27
5	1	18		1	1	44	
1	3	18	17	6	1	44	22, 20, 23, 27, 38
5	1	19	2	1	2	45	
1	1	21	17, 19	1	4	46	2
1	1	22		1	4	46	
1	3	25		3	3	49	
1	5	25		1	1	50	
1	1	25		4	1	50	4, 24, 47
1	1	26	6, 12, 13	3	4	54	
1	1	27	6	2	1	54	38
2	1	29	2	1	3	59	

Source: Kalbfleisch and Prentice (2002, p. 292)
[a]Initial number of tumors of 8 denotes 8 or more; Size denotes size of largest such tumor in centimeters.
[b]Censoring and recurrence times are measured in months.

been grouped into months, giving a moderate number of tied recurrence times. Data analysis methods that can accommodate these types of tied times without incurring appreciable bias are needed for this and other applications.

1.7.5 Women's Health Initiative dietary modification trial

As introduced in §1.7.3 a total of 48,835 post-menopausal US women were assigned to either a low-fat dietary pattern intervention (40%) or to a usual diet comparison group (60%) as a part of the multifaceted Women's Health Initiative clinical trial. Intervention group women were taught nutritional and behavioral approaches to making a major dietary change, in groups of size 10–15 led by nutritionists. The dietary goals included fat reduction to 20% of energy (calories), fruit and vegetable increase to 5 servings/day, and grains increase to 6 servings/day. The comparison group received printed health-related materials only. Breast and colorectal cancer incidence were designated primary outcomes for disease risk reduction, and coronary heart disease (CHD) and total cardiovascular disease (CVD) incidence were designated secondary trial outcomes.

The trial proceeded to its planned termination (March 31, 2005) at which time breast cancer incidence results were in the favorable direction for intervention versus comparison-group women, but not statistically significant ($p = 0.09$) at conventional levels. There was no evidence of an intervention influence on colorectal cancer incidence; and CHD and overall CVD results were also neutral in spite of evidence of favorable change in low-density lipoprotein cholesterol among intervention, but not comparison group, women.

These findings were somewhat disappointing, given the magnitude of effort required to mount such a large, complex trial. However, the adherence of intervention women to dietary fat goals was only about 70% of that anticipated in the trial design resulting in loss of power for trial outcomes, and the differential breast cancer incidence in the intervention versus the comparison group was also about 70% of that projected in the trial design. Also, this nutritional and behavioral intervention can be projected to favorably influence a range of other important outcomes, including disease-specific and total mortality. This opens the possibility of more definitive results for composite outcomes, such as breast cancer followed by death from any cause. In spite of much reduced incidence rates for composite outcomes (double failures) of this type, randomization comparisons may have greater power than either of the marginal hazard rate comparisons, depending on the strength or relationship between the double failure hazard rates and the randomization indicator variable. HI investigators have recently conducted further trial analyses of this type, finding nominally significant intention-to-treat effects on breast cancer followed by death, and on diabetes requiring insulin injections. The related bivariate failure time analyses will provide illustration in Chapters 4 and 7. Another valuable development in a recent round of data analysis was the identification of post-randomization confounding by differential use of statins between randomization groups among women who were hypertensive at baseline or who had prior cardiovascular disease. Statin use in the trial cohort increased markedly during the trial follow-up period, and these potent preparations are known to have a strong influence on low-density lipoprotein cholesterol concentrations in the blood, and on coronary heart disease incidence. In contrast there was no evidence of such confounding among baseline healthy (normotensive, without prior CVD) women, and in this stratum intervention group, women experienced a Bonferroni–adjusted significantly lower CHD incidence compared to comparison group women. Trial women have continued to be followed for clinical outcomes during the post-intervention period, and new information is still emerging on the effects of this low-fat intervention program on clinical outcomes during the combined intervention and post-intervention follow-up periods. Statistical methods are needed to take full advantage of the wealth of data obtained in this type of enterprise, including analyses of single and double hazard failure rates in relation to randomization indicator variables and in relation to other study subject characteristics and exposures over the trial follow-up period.

BIBLIOGRAPHIC NOTES

There is a long history of modeling failure time data using survivor and hazard functions. The preface lists a number of books that describe these functions, and their estimation under independent censorship, in some detail, including early books by Kalbfleisch and Prentice (1980, 2002), Breslow and Day (1980, 1987), Lawless (1983, 2002), Cox and Oakes (1984), Fleming and Harrington (1991), and Andersen et al. (1993). A thorough account of product integration, as in (1.1), is given by Gill and Johansen (1990) with applications to failure time data (see Appendix A). Dabrowska (1988) provided the nice representation (1.6), which expresses the survivor function in terms of its marginal hazard rates and dependency rates that contrast the double failure hazard rate to the product of corresponding single failure hazard rates locally. Dabrowska (1988) also alludes to higher dimensional representation from which (1.8) derives. See also Gill and Johansen (1990) and Prentice and Zhao (2018) for such higher dimensional representation. Clayton (1978) introduced the bivariate survivor function model (1.7) with $\theta > 0$, which was further developed by Oakes (1982, 1986, 1989). This model was generalized to higher dimensions in Prentice (2016). The focus here on modeling marginal hazard rates, and on marginal single and double failure hazard rates, will be used in an attempt to provide a unified presentation throughout this book. Key references for marginal hazard rate analyses for single failure hazard rates include Wei, Lin, and Weissfeld (1989), Spiekerman and Lin (1998), and Lin et al. (2000). The literature on the modeling and analysis of recurrent events is described in some detail in Cook and Lawless (2007) while the same authors have recently provided (Cook & Lawless, 2018) a detailed account of multistate models for event history analyses more generally. Anderson (1984) provides a unified record of multivariate normal-based modeling and estimation procedures. Key references for mean and covariance estimation with (uncensored) discrete and continuous data include Liang and Zeger (1986), Zeger and Liang (1986), and Prentice and Zhao (1991).

EXERCISES AND COMPLEMENTS

Exercise 1.1

Show that the Clayton–Oakes bivariate survivor function (1.7) for failure time variates T_1, and T_2 given by

$$F(t_1,t_2) = \{F(t_1,0)^{-\theta} + F(0,t_2)^{-\theta} - 1\}^{-1/\theta},$$

for $\theta > 0$ has marginal survivor functions given by $F(t_1,0)$ and $F(0,t_2)$ and a time-independent cross ratio function equal to $1+\theta$. Also, by considering $\log F(t_1,t_2)$, show this survivor function converges to the independence special case $F(t_1,t_2) = F(t_1,0)F(0,t_2)$ as $\theta \downarrow 0$. Further show that this survivor function can be extended to

$$F(t_1,t_2) = \{F(t_1,0)^{-\theta} + F(0,t_2)^{\theta} - 1\}^{-1/\theta} \vee 0$$

to allow negative dependencies ($\theta < 0$), that this distribution approaches the upper Fréchet bound of $F(t_1,0) \wedge F(0,t_2)$ for maximal positive dependency as $\theta \to \infty$, and approaches the lower Fréchet bound of $\{F(t_1,0)+F(0,t_2)-1\} \vee 0$ for maximal negative dependency as $\theta \to -1$. Comment on the extent to which absolute continuity is retained as θ becomes increasingly negative.

Exercise 1.2

The trivariate survivor function, for failure time variates T_1, T_2 and T_3 given by

$$F(t_1,t_2,t_3) = \{F(t_1,0,0)^{-\theta} + F(0,t_2,0)^{-\theta} + F(0,0,t_3)^{-\theta} - 2\}^{-1/\theta} \vee 0$$

$\theta \geq -1$ is sometimes considered as the trivariate generalization of the Clayton and Oakes model (1.7). Show that the pairwise marginal cross ratio functions are each constant and equal to $1+\theta$ at all continuity points. Discuss whether this model would be suited to the analysis of a family breast cancer data set in which T_1, T_2, and T_3 denote ages of breast cancer occurrence for an index case (T_1), her sister (T_2) and her daughter (T_3).

Consider the more general trivariate survivor function (1.9). Show that the pairwise marginal survivor functions are given by $F(t_1,t_2,0)$, $F(t_1,0,t_3)$ and $F(0,t_2,t_3)$. Suppose that these marginal distributions have time-independent cross ratios of $1+\theta_{110}$, $1+\theta_{101}$ and $1+\theta_{011}$ respectively at continuity points for the three variates. Derive the trivariate hazard rate function Λ_{111} and show that Λ_{111} approaches zero at all continuity points as $\theta \to -1$. From this calculate the trivariate dependency function Ω_{111} given in (1.10). Discuss any implications for modeling the distribution of (T_1, T_2, T_3).

Exercise 1.3

For absolutely continuous failure time variates T_1, T_2 and T_3 show that

$$\int_0^{t_1}\int_0^{t_2}\int_0^{t_3}\{d^3 \log F(s_1,s_2,s_3)/ds_1,ds_2,ds_3\}ds_1,ds_2,ds_3$$
$$= \log F(t_1,t_2,t_3) - \log F(t_1,t_2,0) - \log F(t_1,0,t_3) - \log F(0,t_2,t_3)$$
$$+ \log F(t_1,0,0) + \log F(0,t_2,0) + \log F(0,0,t_3).$$

Also show that

$$\frac{d^3F(s_1,s_2,s_3)}{ds_1ds_2ds_3}\Big/F(s_1,s_2,s_3) = \frac{d^3 \log F(s_1,s_2,s_3)}{ds_1ds_2ds_3}$$
$$+\frac{d^2 \log F(s_1,s_2,s_3)}{ds_1ds_2}\frac{d \log F(s_1,s_2,s_3)}{ds_3}$$
$$+\frac{d^2 \log F(s_1,s_2,s_3)}{ds_1ds_3}\frac{d \log F(s_1,s_2,s_3)}{ds_2}$$
$$+\frac{d_2 \log F(s_1,s_2,s_3)}{ds_2ds_3}\frac{d \log F(s_1,s_2,s_3)}{ds_1}$$
$$+\frac{d \log F(s_1,s_2,s_3)}{ds_1}\frac{d \log F(s_1,s_2,s_3)}{ds_2}\frac{d \log F(s_1,s_2,s_3)}{ds_3}.$$

Integrate this latter expression over $(0,t_1] \times (0,t_2] \times (0,t_3]$ and combine with the former expression to yield the absolutely continuous survivor function representation (1.8).

Exercise 1.4

Derive a test for whether the censoring times in Table 1.2, in a given treatment group, depend on the preceding bladder tumor recurrence pattern for each patient as observed during trial follow-up.

Exercise 1.5

Consider discrete failure time variates (T_1,T_2). Show that the quantity in square brackets in the double product integral on the right side of (1.6) can be expressed as $F(s_1^-,s_2^-)F(s_1,s_2)/\{F(s_1^-,s_2)F(s_1,s_2^-)\}$ and thereby show through massive cancellation that this double product integral reduces to $F(t_1,t_2)/\{F(t_1,0)F(0,t_2)\}$, so that the right side of (1.6) equals $F(t_1,t_2)$.

Exercise 1.6

Consider $m > 2$ failure time variates $T_1,\ldots,T_m$ having joint survivor function ($\theta \geq -1$) (Prentice, 2016) given by

$$
\begin{aligned}
F(t_1,\ldots,t_m) = \{&F(t_1,\ldots,t_{m-1},0)^{-\theta} \\
&+F(t_1,\ldots,t_{m-2},0,t_m)^{-\theta} + \cdots + F(0,t_2,\ldots,t_m)^{-\theta} \\
&-F(t_1,\ldots,t_{m-2},0,0)^{-\theta} - F(t_1,\ldots,t_{m-3},0,t_{m-1},0)^{-\theta} - \cdots - \\
&F(0,t_2,\ldots,t_{m-1},0)^{-\theta} - \cdots - F(0,0,t_3,\ldots,t_m)^{-\theta} \\
&+F(t_1,\ldots,t_{m-3},0,0,0)^{-\theta} + \cdots + F(0,0,0,t_4,\ldots,t_m)^{-\theta} - \cdots - \\
&+(-1)^{m-2}F(t_1,0\ldots,0)^{-\theta} + (-1)^{m-2}F(0,t_2,0\ldots,0)^{-\theta} + \cdots + \\
&(-1)^{m-2}F(0,\ldots,0,t_m)^{-\theta} + (-1)^{m-1}\}^{-1/\theta} \vee 0
\end{aligned}
$$

where, for example, the second component of this expression consists of all $m(m-1)/2$ pairs with two arguments equal to zero and the third component is composed of all $m(m-1)(m-2)/6$ triplets with three arguments equal to zero. Show that the upper bound for this survival probability given by $F(t_1,\ldots,t_{m-1},0) \wedge F(t_1,\ldots,t_{m-2},0,t_m) \wedge \ldots F(0,t_2,\ldots,t_m)$ is approached as $\theta \to \infty$, and that the lower bound is given by the expression above evaluated at $\theta = -1$. Also show that as $\theta \to 0$ this survival probability approaches the product of marginal survival probabilities having a positive coefficient divided by the product of all survival probabilities having a negative coefficient on the right side of the above expression. Can you develop an expression for $F(t_1,\ldots,t_m)$ in terms of marginal survival probabilities of dimension q or less, where $1 \leq q < m$ upon assuming that all marginal probabilities of dimension more than q have a survivor function of this same form, with the same θ value?

Exercise 1.7

Suppose that failure time variates T_1 and T_2 are statistically independent given the value of a shared random effect W, where W is a gamma variate rescaled to have mean one and variance $\theta > 0$ that acts multiplicatively on the hazard rate. Show that the Clayton (1978) model

$$F(t_1,t_2) = \{F(t_1,0)^{-\theta} + F(0,t_2)^{-\theta} - 1\}^{1/\theta}$$

then arises by integrating over the joint distribution of the random effect, which is often referred to as a “frailty” variate in this context. Generalize this result to $m > 2$ failure time variates and derive pairwise marginal cross ratio functions for each pair of the m variates.

Exercise 1.8

Consider the WHI hormone therapy trial context of §1.7.3 with T_1 defined as time from randomization to CHD and T_2 time from randomization to stroke. Describe the difference in interpretation between the marginal T_1 hazard process Λ_{10} given by $\Lambda_{10}\{dt_1,0;Z(t_1,0)\}$ and the recurrent event intensity process for T_1, given by $\Lambda_1\{dt_1;\mathscr{H}_t\} = P\{\text{CHD event in } [t,t+dt);\mathscr{H}_t\}$ as in (1.11).

Exercise 1.9

In the same WHI hormone therapy trial context (§1.7.3) define T_1 as time from randomization to breast cancer diagnosis, and T_2 as time from breast cancer diagnosis to death following breast cancer. Write down expressions for hazard rate processes for T_1 and for T_2 given $T_1 \leq t_1$. Can you develop an expression for the hazard rate for the composite time from randomization to death following breast cancer outcome $T_3 = T_1 + T_2$ in terms of these component hazard functions. Discuss the advantages and disadvantages of comparing randomization groups in terms of T_3 hazard rates versus separate analyses for T_1 and T_2 hazard rates.

Chapter 2

Univariate Failure Time Data Analysis Methods

2.1 Overview

There is an extensive literature on statistical modeling and estimation for a univariate failure time variate $T > 0$. In this chapter some core methods, which we will build upon in subsequent multivariate failure time methods presentations, will be described. The core methods include Kaplan–Meier survivor function estimation, Cox model hazard ratio parameter estimation with its associated logrank test, as well as other censored data rank tests. The presentation will focus on nonparametric and semiparametric likelihood formulations for estimator development for reasons mentioned in Chapter 1. A brief account of asymptotic distribution theory for these testing and estimation procedures will also be given.

2.2 Nonparametric Survivor Function Estimation

Consider a failure time variate with $T > 0$ having survivor function F, so that $F(t) = P(T > t)$ for any $t \geq 0$. Suppose that n individuals are chosen at random from a study population, and are followed forward from $t = 0$ to observe individual failure times, subject to independent right censoring. Here, independent right censoring means that the set of individuals without prior failure or censoring has a hazard rate equal to that for the study population, at any follow-up time $t > 0$. Denote by $t_1 < t_2 < \cdots < t_I$ the ordered distinct failure times in the sample, and suppose that d_i individuals fail at t_i, out of the r_i individuals who are without failure or censoring prior to time $t_i, i = 1, \ldots, I$. A nonparametric likelihood function for F can be written

$$L = \prod_{k=1}^{n} \left[\{-F(ds_k)\}^{\delta_k} F(s_k)^{1-\delta_k} \right], \tag{2.1}$$

where s_k is observed and is the smaller of the failure or censoring time for the kth individual in the sample and δ_k takes a value of 1 if s_k is uncensored and a value 0 if s_k is censored. Expression (2.1) can be maximized within the class of discrete, continuous and mixed survivor functions by placing mass (probability) only at the observed uncensored failure times, or on the half line beyond the largest s_k value if uncensored. Doing so yields a discrete, step function estimator of F, starting with $F(0) = 1$. Substituting

$$F(t_i) = \prod_{\ell \leq i} \{1 - \Lambda(dt_\ell)\} \text{ and } -F(dt_i) = \prod_{\ell < i} \{1 - \Lambda(dt_\ell)\} \Lambda(dt_i)$$

using the discrete special case of (1.1) and collecting terms, then gives a partially maximized likelihood of

$$L = \prod_{i=1}^{I} [\Lambda(dt_i)^{d_i} \{1 - \Lambda(dt_i)\}^{r_i - d_i}], \tag{2.2}$$

which is maximized at $\Lambda(dt_i) = d_i/r_i, i = 1, \ldots, I$, yielding the well-known Kaplan–Meier (1958) product limit survivor function estimator

$$\hat{F}(t) = \prod_{t_i \leq t} \{1 - d_i/r_i\}. \tag{2.3}$$

Of course F is not identifiable at times where no individuals are "at risk" for failure, so $\hat{F}$ is undefined beyond the largest follow-up time (i.e., the largest s_k value) observed in the sample. The corresponding hazard function estimator $\hat{\Lambda}$ is given by

$$\hat{\Lambda}(t) = \sum_{t_i \leq t} d_i/r_i,$$

which is often referred to as the Nelson–Aalen estimator. Note that, in keeping with (1.1)

$$\hat{F}(t) = \prod_{0}^{t} \{1 - \hat{\Lambda}(ds)\}.$$

Informally, the ith factor in (2.2) can be recognized as a binomial likelihood for $\Lambda(dt_i)$. Conditioning on all failure and censoring information prior to t_i, thereby fixing r_i, shows $\hat{\Lambda}(dt_i) = d_i r_i^{-1}$ to have a conditional, and hence an unconditional, mean of $\Lambda(dt_i)$. Similarly, for $i < j$, conditioning on all failure and censoring information prior to t_j fixes $\hat{\Lambda}(dt_i)$ and shows $\hat{\Lambda}(dt_i)$ and $\hat{\Lambda}(dt_j)$ to be conditionally, and hence unconditionally, uncorrelated. Application of the delta method then leads to

$$\hat{\text{var}}\hat{F}(t) = \hat{F}(t)^2 \sum_{t_i \le t} \{d_i/(r_i - d_i)\}$$

as a variance estimator for $\hat{F}(t)$, referred to as the Greenwood formula. To avoid influences from the range restrictions, $0 \le F(t) \le 1$, one can apply a normal distribution approximation to the unconstrained function given by $\log\{-\log F(t)\}$ leading, for example, to an approximate 95% confidence interval for $F(t)$ of

$$\hat{F}(t)\exp\{\pm 1.96\hat{v}(t)\} \tag{2.4}$$

where $\hat{v}(t)^2 = \hat{\text{var}}\hat{F}(t)/\{\log\hat{F}(t)\}^2$ at times where $\hat{F}(t) > 0$.

One can also obtain the Kaplan–Meier estimator using mean parameter estimating equations as follows: Reconstrue the censored failure time data (s_k, δ_k) as a sequence of uncorrelated binary variates

$$W_{ki} = \begin{cases} 1 & \text{if } s_k = t_i \text{ and } \delta_k = 1 \\ 0 & \text{otherwise} \end{cases}$$

and also define "at-risk" indicator variables

$$Y_{ki} = \begin{cases} 1 & \text{if } s_k \ge t_i \\ 0 & \text{otherwise} \end{cases}$$

for $i = 1, \ldots, I$, for each $k = 1, \ldots, n$. Under a discrete failure time model with hazard rate $\Lambda(dt_i)$ at $T = t_i, i = 1, \ldots, I$ one has

$$\mu_{ki} = E(W_{ki}) = Y_{ki}\Lambda(dt_i), \text{ partial derivatives } \partial\mu_{ki}/\partial\Lambda(dt_i) = Y_{ki},$$
$$\text{and } \text{cov}\{(W_{ki} - \mu_{ki})(W_{kj} - \mu_{kj})\} = \begin{cases} \mu_{ki}(1 - \mu_{ki}) & \text{if } i = j \\ 0 & \text{otherwise.} \end{cases}$$

This leads to mean parameter estimating equations (see Appendix A, expression A.5)

$$\sum_{k=1}^{n} Y_{ki}(W_{ki} - \mu_{ki}) = 0, \textit{ for } i = 1, \ldots, I$$

and to the Kaplan–Meier (KM) estimator. Hence the nonparametric maximum likelihood, the survivor function or hazard function representation plug-in, and the mean parameter estimating equation approaches each lead to the same nonparametric survivor function estimator (2.3). $\hat{F}$ has been shown to be strongly consistent for F, and $n^{1/2}(\hat{F} - F)$ has been shown to be weakly convergent to a mean zero Gaussian process over a time period $[0, \tau]$, where τ is in the support of the observed follow-up times. Moreover, in keeping with its nonparametric maximum likelihood development, $\hat{F}$ has also been shown to be nonparametric efficient as an estimator of F over $[0, \tau]$. Some detail on these asymptotic results will be given in §2.9.

2.3 Hazard Ratio Regression Estimation Using the Cox Model

Suppose now that a covariate history $\{Z(t), t \geq 0\}$ is recorded for each individual in the study sample. The hazard rate regression model introduced by Sir David Cox revolutionized the analysis of censored failure time data, and Cox (1972) is one of the most highly cited statistical papers of all time. The Cox model, for an absolutely continuous failure time variable T, specifies a hazard rate at time t given the preceding covariate history $Z(t)$, having the multiplicative form

$$\lambda\{t;Z(t)\} = \lambda_0(t)\exp\{x(t)\beta\}, \tag{2.5}$$

where $x(t) = \{x_1(t), \dots, x_p(t)\}$ is a modeled covariate p-vector comprised of data-analyst-defined functions of $Z(t)$ and possibly product terms between such functions and t. This modeled regression variable, with sample paths that are continuous from the left with limits from the right, is intended to "capture" the dependence of the hazard rate at time t on the preceding covariate history, through the value of the hazard ratio parameter $\beta' = (\beta_1, \dots, \beta_p)$, where a prime ($'$) denotes vector transpose. The function λ_0 in (2.5) is referred to as the baseline hazard function, and $\lambda_0(t)$ is the hazard rate at a reference covariate history $Z_0(t)$ for which the modeled covariate is $x(t) \equiv 0$, a zero vector for all t. The hazard process model given Z is semiparametric with the p-vector β and the nonparametric function Λ_0, where $\Lambda_0(t) = \int_0^t \lambda_0(s)ds$, as parameters to be estimated.

Denote by $T_1, \dots, T_n$ the underlying failure times for a random sample of size n from a study population followed forward in time from $t = 0$. Suppose that T_k is subject to right censoring by a variate C_k, so that one observes $S_k = T_k \wedge C_k$ and non-censoring indicator variable $\delta_k = I[S_k = T_k]$. Suppose also that covariate histories $Z_k(S_k)$ are recorded, $k = 1, \dots, n$. An independent censoring assumption requires the hazard rate $\lambda\{t;Z(t)\}$ in (2.5) to equal the same hazard rate, but with $C_k \geq t$ added to the conditioning event. That is, independent censorship implies that the subset of individuals who are without prior failure or censoring at any follow-up time t, referred to as the "risk set" at time t and denoted $R(t)$, is representative of the study population in terms of hazard rate at t given $Z(t)$. This assumption needs to be carefully considered in the context of specific applications, and may be able to be relaxed as necessary.

A semiparametric likelihood function, analogous to (2.1), can be written

$$L = \prod_{k=1}^{n} \left[\left\{ \lambda_0(s_k) e^{x_k(s_k)\beta} \right\}^{\delta_k} \exp\left\{ - \int_0^{s_k} e^{x_k(u)\beta} \lambda_0(u) du \right\} \right],$$

where (s_k, δ_k) and $Z_k(s_k), k = 1, \dots, n$ are the observed data in the study sample.

Several approaches have been considered for dealing with the nonparametric aspect of this model, including partial likelihood (Cox, 1972, 1975), marginal likelihood (Kalbfleisch & Prentice, 1973), and approximate likelihood (Breslow, 1974) methods.

The Breslow (1974) approach begins by noting that the above likelihood can be maximized by placing all failure probability within the risk region of the data, defined by $R = \{t; s_k \geq t \text{ for some } k \in (1, \dots, n)\}$, on the observed uncensored failure times $t_1 < t_2 < \cdots < t_I$ in the sample. This implies that censored s_k values can be replaced by censored values at the immediately preceding uncensored failure time in the sample without diminishing the likelihood. Now if one approximates the baseline rate function by $\lambda_0(t) = \lambda_i$ whenever $t \in (t_{i-1}, t_i], i = 1, \ldots, I$ one can write the likelihood, following the censored data shifting just mentioned, as

$$L = \prod_{i=1}^{I} \left[\prod_{k \in D(t_i)} \lambda_i e^{x_i(t_i)\beta} \prod_{k \in R(t_i)} \exp\left\{ -e^{x_k(t_i)\beta} \lambda_i \Delta t_i \right\} \right] \tag{2.6}$$

where $D(t_i)$ denotes the set of d_i individuals having uncensored failures at $T = t_i$, and $\Delta t_i = t_i - t_{i-1}, i = 1, \ldots, I$, with $t_0 = 0$. In this form L can be recognized as having the form of a parametric likelihood to which application of standard likelihood methods can be considered.

Specifically, one can solve the equations $\partial \log L / \partial \lambda_i = 0, i = 1, \ldots I$ explicitly giving

$$\hat{\lambda}_i(\beta) = d_i \Big/ \left\{ \Delta t_i \sum_{k \in R(t_i)} e^{x_k(t_i)\beta} \right\}, i = 1, \ldots, I,$$

which can be inserted into (2.6) to give the profile likelihood

$$L(\beta) = \prod_{i=1}^{I} \left[\prod_{k \in D(t_i)} e^{x_k(t_i)\beta} \Big/ \left\{ \sum_{k \in R(t_i)} e^{x_k(t_i)\beta} \right\}^{d_i} \right], \tag{2.7}$$

which is Breslow's tied data approximation to the Cox partial likelihood.

The corresponding estimating function for β is

$$\begin{aligned} U(\beta) &= \partial \log L(\beta) / \partial \beta \\ &= \sum_{i=1}^{I} U_i(\beta) \\ &= \sum_{i=1}^{I} \left[\sum_{k \in D(t_i)} x_k(t_i)' - d_i \sum_{k \in R(t_i)} x_k(t_i)' \exp\{x_k(t_i)\beta\} \Big/ \sum_{k \in R(t_i)} \exp\{x_k(t_i)\beta\} \right]. \end{aligned} \tag{2.8}$$

Conditional on all failure, censoring and covariate information up to t_i, one can see, under (2.5), that the conditional, and hence also the unconditional, expectation of $U_i(\beta)$ is zero for all, $i = 1, \ldots I$, so $U(\beta) = 0$ provides an unbiased estimating equation for β. Similarly for $i < j$ conditioning on all failure, censoring and covariate information up to t_j fixes $U_i(\beta)$ and gives a conditional, and hence unconditional expectation of zero for $U_i(\beta)U_j(\beta)$, all (i, j). Hence $I(\beta) = -\partial^2 \log L / \partial \beta \partial \beta'$ has expectation equal to the variance matrix for $U(\beta)$. Direct calculation gives

$$\begin{aligned} I(\beta) = \sum_{i=1}^{I} d_i \Bigg[& \frac{\sum_{k \in R(t_i)} x_k(t_i)' x_k(t_i) e^{x_k(t_i)\beta}}{\sum_{k \in R(t_i)} e^{x_k(t_i)\beta}} \\ & - \frac{\sum_{k \in R(t_i)} x_k(t_i)' e^{x_k(t_i)\beta} \sum_{k \in R(t_i)} x_k(t_i) e^{x_k(t_i)\beta}}{\{\sum_{k \in R(t_i)} e^{x_k(t_i)\beta}\}^2} \Bigg]. \end{aligned} \tag{2.9}$$

Under mild conditions $\hat{\beta}$ that maximizes (2.7), which is sometimes referred to as the maximum partial likelihood estimate of β, has an asymptotic distribution, with consistent variance matrix estimator, given by

$$n^{\frac{1}{2}}(\hat{\beta}-\beta) \sim \mathscr{N}\{0, nI(\hat{\beta})^{-1}\}$$

where $\mathscr{N}$ denotes a normal distribution. Also, the corresponding baseline hazard estimator $\hat{\Lambda}_0$, where

$$\hat{\Lambda}_0(t) = \hat{\Lambda}_0(t,\hat{\beta}) = \sum_{t_i \le t} \left[d_i \Big/ \sum_{k \in R(t_i)} \exp\{x_k(t_i)\hat{\beta}\} \right] \tag{2.10}$$

is such that $n^{\frac{1}{2}}\{\hat{\Lambda}_0(\cdot) - \Lambda_0(\cdot)\}$ converges jointly with $n^{\frac{1}{2}}(\hat{\beta}-\beta)$ to a zero mean Gaussian process over a time period $[0,\tau]$, where τ is in the support of the follow-up times (S values). The estimator $\hat{\beta}$ has also been shown to be semiparametric efficient under (2.5) in the special case of time-independent covariates.

The Cox likelihood can be derived similarly by setting the overall sample empirical hazard rates d_i/r_i equal to the model-based average $\sum_{\ell \in R(t_i)} \lambda_0(t_i) e^{x_\ell(t_i)\beta}/r_i$ and solving for $\lambda_0(t_i)$ at each $i = 1,\ldots,I$. Plugging these values into the semiparametric likelihood gives (2.7).

A mean parameter estimating equation development can also be considered: As above set

$$W_{ki} = \begin{cases} 1 & S_k = t_i, \text{ and } \delta_k = 1 \\ 0 & \text{otherwise} \end{cases}, \text{ and } Y_{ki} = \begin{cases} 1 & S_k \ge t_i \\ 0 & \text{otherwise} \end{cases}, \text{ for all } (k,i).$$

Under a model of the form (2.5) one has $\mu_{ki} = E(W_{ki}) = Y_{ki} e^{\alpha_i + x_k(t_i)\beta}$, where $\alpha_i = \log \Lambda_0(dt_i)$, the uncorrelatedness of $W_{ki}, i = 1,\ldots,I$ for each k, and mean parameter estimating equations (Appendix A, A.5) for $(\alpha_1,\ldots,\alpha_I)$ that solve

$$\sum_{k=1}^{n} (W_{ki} - \mu_{ki}) = 0, \text{ for } i = 1,\ldots,I.$$

Solving these equations gives

$$e^{\alpha_i} = d_i \Big/ \sum_{k=1}^{n} Y_{ki} e^{x_k(t_i)\beta}, i = 1,\ldots,I,$$

which can be inserted into the estimating equation for β giving $\sum_{i=1}^{I} W_{ki} x_{ki}(t_i)' - d_i \sum_{i=1}^{I} \{\sum_{k=1}^{n} Y_{ki} x_k(t_i)' e^{x_k(t_i)\beta} / \sum_{k=1}^{n} Y_{ki} e^{x_k(t_i)\beta}\} = 0$, yielding (2.8) and (2.10). Also the model-based variance estimator, using the notation of Appendix A, is

$$\left(\sum_{k=1}^{n} \sum_{i=1}^{I} Y_{ki} \hat{D}_{ki}' \hat{V}_{ki}^{-1} \hat{D}_{ki} \right)^{-1},$$

where ˆ denotes evaluation at $(\hat{\alpha}_1, \ldots, \hat{\alpha}_I, \hat{\beta})$ solving these equations, which equals $I(\hat{\beta})^{-1}$ from (2.9).

It follows that maximum likelihood, empirical hazard plug-in, and mean parameter estimating functions again agree for this rather general regression estimation problem. Generalizations of these approaches will be considered in later chapters to manage nonparametric aspects of models specified for multivariate failure time regression estimation.

The asymptotic developments mentioned above assume absolutely continuous failure times, so that technically we should have $d_i = 1, i = 1, \ldots, I$. However $(\hat{\beta}, \hat{\Lambda}_0)$ as described above can tolerate some tied failure times without incurring appreciable asymptotic bias. A rule of thumb may be that the number of ties d_i should not be more than a few percent (e.g., 5%) of the size, r_i, of the corresponding risk set at uncensored failure times. Nearly all available computer software for the Cox model allows tied failure times, and applies the expressions given above, even though more sophisticated approximations have been proposed for handling tied failure times.

2.4 Cox Model Properties and Generalizations

A few points can be made about the Cox model estimation procedure described above. First, it is easy to see that the hazard ratio function comparing covariate histories Z_1 and Z_2 is given by

$$\lambda\{t; Z_1(t)\}/\lambda\{t; Z_2(t)\} = \exp\{x_1(t) - x_2(t)\}\beta$$

at time t, and does not depend on the choice of baseline covariate history Z_0.

Also, it is worth commenting that the time-varying feature of (2.5) can be quite powerful. This feature allows hazard ratios for a specific covariate to vary in a user-defined fashion as a function of follow-up time, and it allows hazard rates to be defined that condition on stochastic covariates that are recorded during study follow-up.

From (2.10) one can specify

$$\hat{F}\{t; Z(t)\} = \prod_{t_i \leq t} \left\{ 1 - d_i \exp\{x_i(t)\hat{\beta}\} \Big/ \sum_{k \in R(t_i)} e^{x_k(t_i)\hat{\beta}} \right\},$$

which has a survivor function interpretation with time-independent covariates $Z(t) \equiv z$, or with evolving covariates that are external to the failure process in the sense that the covariate paths are unaffected by the failure time process under study. Note that $\hat{F}$ reduces to the Kaplan–Meier estimator at $\hat{\beta} = 0$.

A simple, but very useful, relaxation of the Cox model (2.5) allows the baseline hazard function to vary among strata, which also may be time-dependent. Specifically, one can write

$$\lambda\{t; Z(t)\} = \lambda_{0u}(t) \exp\{x(t)\beta\}, \tag{2.11}$$

where stratum $u = u\{t, Z(t)\} \in \{1, \ldots, m\}$, has sample paths that are continuous from the left with limits from the right. Under (2.11) the study population is partitioned into m mutually exclusive strata at each follow-up time t. For example, this stratification feature can allow the baseline hazard rate at time t to vary in an unrestricted manner for some variables defined by $\{t, Z(t)\}$, while imposing a parametric hazard ratio model on variables of principal interest that are used to define $x(t)$. The hazard ratio parameter β can be estimated under (2.11) using a product of factors (2.7), one from each stratum, while $U(\beta)$ and $I(\beta)$ are given by sums over the strata of (2.8) and (2.9). For example, in large epidemiologic cohort studies with most observed times censored it is often possible to incorporate extensive baseline stratification, thereby enhancing confounding control, with little effect on the efficiency with which hazard ratio parameters of primary interest are estimated.

In some settings a univariate failure time variate $T > 0$ may be accompanied by a failure type $J \in \{1, \ldots, q\}$, sometimes referred to as a "mark." The hazard ratio methods of the preceding section extend readily to failure type–specific hazard models

$$\lambda_j\{t; Z(t)\} = \lambda_{0j}(t)\exp\{x(t)\beta_j\}, j = 1, \ldots, q \tag{2.12}$$

simply by applying a (partial) likelihood function that is a product of terms (2.7) for each type-specific hazard ratio parameter, following the imposition of additional censorship wherein follow-up times for estimating β_j are additionally censored at the time of failure of any type other than j. Data of this type are sometimes formulated in terms of potential failure times, say $U_1, \ldots, U_q$ with $T = \min(U_1, \ldots, U_q)$, and the estimation of marginal hazard rates, or other distributional characteristics, for these latent failure times is referred to as the competing risk problem. However, the joint distribution of $(U_1, \ldots, U_q)$ given Z, for a time-independent covariate, is not identifiable without strong additional assumptions, such as independence among such times, unless genuinely multivariate failure time data are available. Genuinely multivariate failure time data arise when individuals continue to be followed beyond the time of their first failure to observe second and subsequent failure times for the individual. The analysis of such multivariate failure time data is a major focus of this book.

If the failure time variate, T, includes discrete elements then some care may be needed in applying (2.5) since the hazard rates at a mass point cannot exceed one. Depending on the distribution of the modeled covariate $x(t)$, a different regression model form, such as a logistic hazard rate model, may be preferable if T has some large point masses. This topic will be elaborated in §2.11.

2.5 Censored Data Rank Tests

In addition to Kaplan–Meier survival curves and Cox regression, censored data rank tests that are used to test equality of two or more survival curves, can be included among core univariate failure time methods.

The score test

$$U(0) = \sum_{i=1}^{I}\left[\sum_{k \in D(t_i)} x_k(t_i)' - \frac{d_i}{r_i}\sum_{k \in R(t_i)} x_k(t_i)'\right] \tag{2.13}$$

from (2.8) can be used to test $\beta = 0$, by comparing

$$U(0)'V(0)^{-1}U(0)$$

to an asymptotic chi-square distribution on p degrees of freedom where $V(0)$ is a variance estimator for $U(0)$ with $x(t)$ is composed of indicator variables for p of $p+1$ samples whose failure rates are being compared. This $p+1$ sample comparison test is referred to as the logrank test. The corresponding hazard rates under (2.5) are proportional to each other, so it should not be surprising that the logrank test has attractive power properties for testing the null hypothesis against proportional hazards alternatives. This class of null hypothesis tests can be broadened to

$$\sum_{i=1}^{I}\left\{\sum_{k\in D(t_i)} h(t_i)x_k(t_i)' - \frac{d_i}{r_i}\sum_{k\in R(t_i)} h(t_i)x_k(t_i)'\right\} \tag{2.14}$$

by introducing a weight function h, where $h(t)$ can depend on failure and censoring information prior to t, in order to provide, for example, greater sensitivity to hazard rate differences early versus late in the follow-up period, or vice versa. A corresponding variance estimator under $\beta = 0$ is given by

$$V(0) = \sum_{i=1}^{I} h(t_i)^2 V_i$$

where $(V_i)_{jj} = r_{ij}(r_i - r_{ij})d_i(r_i - d_i)r_i^{-2}(r_i-1)^{-1}, j = 1,\ldots,p$ and $(V_i)_{jk} = -r_{ij}r_{ik}d_i(r_i-d_i)r_i^{-2}(r_i-1)^{-1}$, $j \neq k$, where, for example, r_{ij} is the size of the risk set in the jth sample at t_i. Tests of the form (2.14) are known as weighted logrank tests. In addition to $h(t) \equiv 1$, another commonly used test specifies $h(t) = \hat{F}(t)$, with $\hat{F}$ a survivor function estimator under the null hypothesis. This generalized Wilcoxon test applies greater weight to early failures, compared to the logrank test. Weight functions h that may depend on failure, but not censoring, distribution estimates are preferable for test interpretation.

2.6 Cohort Sampling and Dependent Censoring

There are many variations in the criteria for study subject selection and follow-up with univariate failure time data. For example, if T is defined to be age at disease occurrence in an epidemiologic cohort study with a minimum age criterion, there would typically be late entry into the cohort as study subjects are enrolled at ages beyond the specified minimum. The hazard rate methods described above readily adapt to such late entries by adjusting the risk sets $R(t)$ to include only subjects who are under active follow-up at time t.

Since some cohort studies involve very heavy censorship, with only a few percent of study subjects experiencing the failure time outcome under study, it may be inefficient or impractical to assemble cohort histories on the entire study cohort. Such assembly, for example, may involve expensive laboratory analysis of stored biospecimens. Cohort sampling methods, such as matched case–control or case–cohort methods are often applied. Hazard ratio parameter estimates under sampling in which each failing individual (a case) is matched to one or more cohort members (controls) who are without failure at the time of case failure occurrence (t) can be derived by applying (2.7) with $D(t)$ and $R(t)$ respectively the case and the combined case and its matched controls. Similarly if cases arising in a cohort are ascertained along with a random subsample of the cohort, hazard ratio parameters can be estimated by applying (2.7) with $R(t)$ comprised of the case(s) occurring at time t and the subcohort members at risk at time t, though a refinements of (2.9) is needed for variance estimation to acknowledge dependencies among the scores $U_i(\beta), i = 1,\ldots,I$. Missing data methods, which make fuller use of the available data, including covariate data subsets that are available for the entire cohort, can provide efficiency improvements for hazard ratio parameter estimation, and the subcohort can be selected in a more refined fashion so that cases and their comparison group align closely for some important potential confounding variables.

Other sampling variations include interval censorship, rather than right censorship only, and observation only of whether or not failure has occurred prior to an individual-specific assessment time (current status data). Many of these variations have a substantial corresponding statistical literature and are of considerable applied importance.

Covariate measurement error is another important aspect of many univariate failure time data sets, particularly in such areas as nutritional or physical activity epidemiology where covariates (e.g., exposures) of interest may be poorly measured. In many such settings failure probabilities during the study follow-up period are small, and a simple regression calibration approach that replaces $x(t)$ in (2.5) by an estimate of the conditional expectation $E\{x(t)|Z^*(t)\}$, where $Z^*(t)$ is equal to $Z(t)$ aside from the substitution of error-prone versions of the variables used to form $x(t)$. For example, if a biomarker assessment $w(t)$ that equals $x(t)$ aside from classical mean zero measurement error is available on a random biomarker subsample of the cohort, this expectation can typically be estimated by linear regression of $w(t)$ on an error-prone assessment of $x(t)$ that is available on the entire cohort along with other components of $Z^*(t)$ as needed. Though technically inconsistent, such regression calibration estimators of β in (2.5) typically exhibit little bias and tend to be more efficient than available nonparametric measurement error correction alternatives. A sandwich, or bootstrap, variance estimator is needed to acknowledge uncertainty in calibration equation parameter estimates.

Scientific interest may focus on hazard rate dependencies on a specific covariate, with low-dimensional modeled covariates. However, an independent censoring assumption may be justified only if Z includes additional covariates that may be related to censoring rates. The methods described above will then require Z to include these additional variables, and for their association with hazard rates to be accommodated by regression modeling or stratification. This can sometimes be accomplished without requiring undue model complexity and without materially affecting hazard ratio parameter interpretation.

More generally consider Z_1 and Z_2, where $Z_1(t)$ is composed of the covariates at time t (e.g., treatments, exposures) of primary interest and variables needed to control confounding, $Z_2(t)$ is composed of additional variables needed to justify an independent censoring assumption. The type of Cox model application just described would examine hazard rate dependencies on $Z = (Z_1, Z_2)$. An alternate analytic approach would define $Z = Z_1$ and would modify the estimating function (2.10) by weighting each $x_1(t_i)$ in $U_i(\beta)$ by the inverse of the estimated probability of not being censored prior to $t_i, i = 1,\ldots,I$. This inverse probability weighting aims to recover a representative risk set in terms of their modeled covariate values, at each uncensored failure time. For example, a Cox model of the form (2.5) could be applied to the censoring, rather than the failure hazard, to produce estimates of the non-censoring probability at each follow-up time. Since these estimates at time t will depends only on information prior to t, needed modifications of (2.8) and (2.9), simply replace each $x_k(t)$ by the ratio of $x_k(t)$ to the inverse of the estimated non-censoring probability at follow-up time t. Sampling variation in estimating the non-censoring probabilities may affect the estimation procedure, so it is wise to avoid weights that are unnecessarily grainy or noisy, as these could reduce the efficiency of the resulting estimates of β and Λ_0, at least with a moderate sample size n. Estimation procedures of the type just described, with inverse non-missingness probability weighting, are sometimes referred to as marginal structural modeling procedures (e.g., Robins, Hernan, & Brumback, 2000).

The topics of this subsection will be considered further in Chapter 8, with emphasis on multivariate failure time generalizations.

2.7 Aplastic Anemia Clinical Trial Application

Figure 2.1 shows Kaplan–Meier survivor function estimates (2.3) separately for the CSP and CSP + MTX arms of the randomized trial data given in Table 1.1 with times from randomization for patients who are alive without A-GVHD at the time of data closure, or for patients who died without an A-GVHD diagnosis regarded as censored. Application of the Cox model (2.5) to these data with a simple modeled covariate $x = 0$ for CSP + MTX and $x = 1$ for MTX gives $\hat{\beta} = 1.143$, with an estimated standard error of $I(\hat{\beta})^{-1/2} = 0.517$. Hence under this simple model the hazard ratio for severe A-GVHD is estimated by $\exp(1.143) = 3.14$, with approximate 95% confidence interval of $\exp\{1.143 \pm 1.96 \times 0.517\} = (1.14, 8.64)$, supporting a benefit for the addition of CSP to the severe A-GVHD prevention regimen. The addition of indicator variables for the age categories 16–25 and ≥ 26 years at randomization, along with a treatment $\times$ follow-up time interaction variable provides evidence (likelihood ratio test significance level of $P = 0.05$) based on (2.7) for a treatment hazard ratio that increases with follow-up time, as is suggested by Figure 2.1, and also shows higher A-GVHD incidence among patients in the older two age categories compared to the youngest category of age ≤ 15 years. See Kalbfleisch and Prentice (2002, p 112–114) for additional detail on the analysis of these data. Note that the number of failures here is only 20, so asymptotic distributional approximations may be somewhat inaccurate. Because of their invariance under 1-1 parameter transformations, likelihood ratio procedures can be expected to provide better approximations compared to those (i.e., Wald procedures) based on an asymptotic normal approximation for the distribution of $\hat{\beta}$. Also note that the interpretation of the hazard ratio comparing treatments could be affected by treatment effects on death without A-GVHD in this application, pointing to the value of bringing data on time of death following A-GVHD into the data analysis.

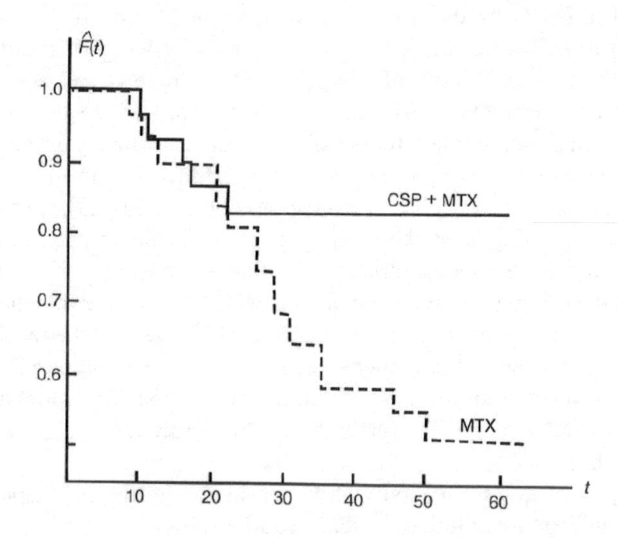

Figure 2.1 *Kaplan–Meier survivor function estimates for time to severe acute graft-versus-host disease for patients randomized to cyclosporine and methotrexate (CSP + MTX) or methotrexate only (MTX). From Kalbfleisch and Prentice (2002).*

2.8 Women's Health Initiative Postmenopausal Hormone Therapy Application

Now consider the application of the univariate failure time regression methods described above to the analysis of the two WHI hormone therapy trials described in §1.7.3. A major advantage of the randomized, double blind, placebo controlled design of these trials is the absence of confounding by pre-randomization factors. The comparability of active treatment and placebo groups at baseline carries through to the comparison of failure time outcomes between the randomized groups in so-called intention-to-treat (ITT) analyses, in which $x(t) = x$ in model (2.5) is defined as an indicator variable for assignment the active hormone therapy group. The validity of ITT tests of the null hypothesis (e.g., $\beta = 0$ in (2.5)) requires only that failure time outcome data be obtained accurately obtained or, at least, be obtained in an identical manner between randomized groups. The incorporation of masking (or blindedness) is often crucial to ensuring equal outcome ascertainment between groups. The baseline stratification feature of the Cox model (2.5) is quite valuable in this setting, since risks for outcomes of interest vary considerably among women according to age at randomization and other factors. The application of (2.5) to the WHI hormone therapy trial data described below stratified baseline disease rates on age at randomization in 5-year age groups, prior history of the outcome in question, and on randomization status (intervention group, control group, not randomized) in the companion WHI Dietary Modification trial (see §1.7.5).

Figures 2.2–2.4 present some Cox model analyses for several important disease

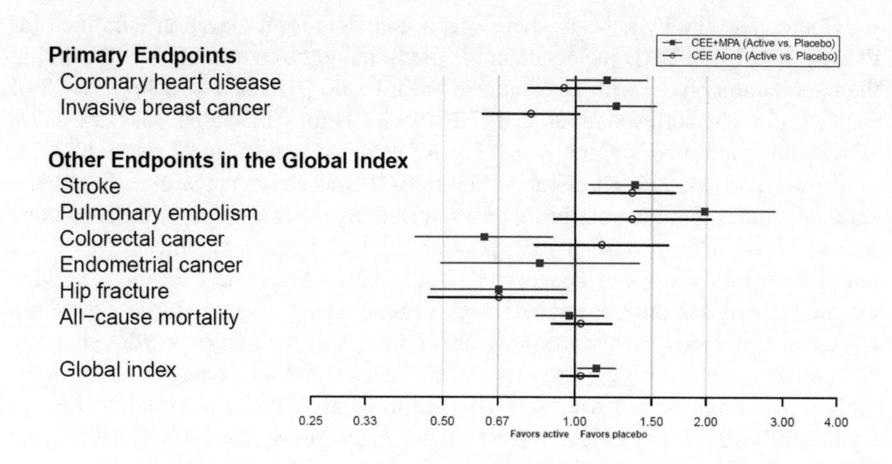

Figure 2.2 *Intention-to-treat hazard ratio parameter estimates and (asymptotic) 95% confidence intervals for various clinical outcomes, during the intervention phase of the Women's Health Initiative CEE + MPA and CEE-Alone postmenopausal hormone therapy randomized, placebo controlled trial. Adapted from a pre-publication version of Manson et al. (2013).*

outcomes in both the estrogen plus progestin (CEE + MPA) and estrogen-alone (CEE-alone) trials. These figures were adapted from a pre-publication version of Manson et al. (2013) that describes results over the intervention phase (5.6 years on average, ended July 7, 2002 for CEE + MPA trial; 7.2 years on average, ended February 29, 2004 for the CEE-alone trial) and post-intervention phase (additional 8.2 years of follow-up on average for CEE + MPA trial; additional 6.6 years on average for the CEE-alone trial) data through September 30, 2010. Participating women were re-consented following the planned intervention phase with 81.1% of surviving women agreeing to additional non-intervention follow-up. See Manson et al. (2013) for additional detail, including the number of disease events, for each outcome listed, by randomization group and trial phase.

Figure 2.2 shows intervention phase estimated active versus placebo hazard ratios and (asymptotic) 95% nominal confidence intervals (CIs) for the trials primary outcome coronary heart disease, for the primary "safety" outcome invasive breast cancer, and for other major outcomes (stroke, pulmonary embolism, colorectal cancer, endometrial cancer, hip fracture and all-cause mortality), that were included along with the two primary outcomes in defining a "global index." The global index aimed to provide a useful single health benefit versus risk index for trial monitoring and reporting. In fact the global index was itself a failure time variate defined as the time to the earliest of the listed outcomes (with death from causes other than the diseases listed above it substituted for all-cause mortality). For each outcome the observed times (S) were days from randomization until the first occurrence of the specific outcome ($\delta = 1$), or until death from other diseases, loss to follow-up, or to date last known to be alive ($\delta = 0$).

Contrary to the hypothesis, there was a non-significant elevation (stratified logrank $p = 0.13$) in CHD incidence in the group randomized to CEE + MPA during the intervention phase, with an estimated hazard ratio (HR) of 1.18 with 95% CI of (0.95, 1.45). The corresponding CHD HR (95% CI) for CEE-alone was 0.94 (0.78, 1.14) with a stratified logrank $p = 0.53$. An elevated breast cancer risk with CEE + MPA (HR=1.24; 95% CI of 1.01–1.53, p=0.04) was consistent with earlier observational studies, but the possibility of a reduced breast cancer risk with CEE-alone (HR=0.79, 95% CI of 0.61 to 1.02, p =0.07), which became significant (p =0.02) with longer follow-up, was unexpected. Both CEE + MPA and CEE-alone yielded elevated stroke risk during the intervention phase, along with a reduced risk of hip fractures. Colorectal cancer risk may also be reduced with CEE + MPA, but any such reduction was restricted to early-stage cancers, and no colorectal cancer mortality difference emerged with longer-term follow-up. All-cause mortality was not significantly affected by either preparation, while the global index was in the adverse direction for CEE + MPA, and approximately balanced for CEE-alone.

Figure 2.3 provides corresponding information from disease events occurring during the post-intervention phase of the trials. These analyses also relied on the Cox model (2.5), with baseline stratification as in the intervention phase, with time from randomization as the basic time variable, and with entry into the "risk set" occurring at the end of the intervention period. The hazard ratios for most of the listed outcomes gravitated toward the null following the cessation of treatment, with some longer-term elevation in breast cancer risk with CEE + MPA as an exception. The interpretation of these post-intervention HRs is complicated by any selection that took place during the intervention phase. See Manson et al. (2013) for corresponding intervention evaluations over the combined intervention and post-intervention periods, evaluations that compare randomized groups and therefore have greater reliability and a simpler interpretation.

Naturally with a large-scale clinical trials of this type there are many relevant analyses beyond those ITT comparisons. For example, some HRs are decidedly variable over follow-up time within a particular study phase. For example, the CHD HR with CEE + MPA was large during the first 1–2 years from randomization, less so thereafter, while the corresponding breast cancer HR was somewhat less than one during the first two years from randomization, probably due to the treatment masking some tumor diagnoses on mammography, and increased rapidly and approximately linearly to about 2.2 by the end of the intervention period. Other relevant analyses attempt to estimate HRs among women who were adherent to their assigned hormone pills (whether active or placebo), though such analyses cannot be carried out with the purity of ITT analyses. Still other analyses attempt to explain treatment effects in terms of blood biomarkers measured at baseline and at one or more times during follow-up. The Cox model (2.5) can provide the framework for a wide range of analyses of these types, with much flexibility afforded by the semiparametric aspect of the model and by the time-varying stratification and regression variable features.

It is a mark of the value attributed to randomized controlled trial data that the WHI trials and a preceding secondary CHD prevention trial of CEE + MPA led to a sea change in the use of postmenopausal hormones in the United States and

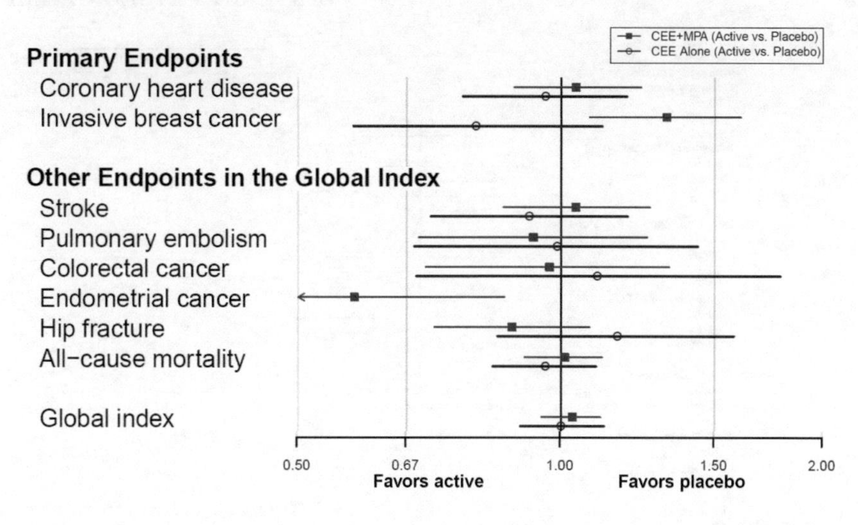

Figure 2.3 *Intention-to-treat hazard ratio parameter estimates and (asymptotic) 95% confidence intervals for various clinical outcomes, during the post-intervention phase of the Women's Health Initiative CEE + MPA and CEE-Alone postmenopausal hormone therapy randomized, placebo controlled trial. Adapted from a pre-publication version of Manson et al. (2013).*

around the world. The major change in CEE + MPA use has been hypothesized to have brought about a reduction by about 15,000–20,000 in the number of women in the United States alone who develop breast cancer each year since 2003, and to a cumulative reduction in medical care costs in excess of $32 billion.

Another prominent component of data analysis from this type of study involves treatment comparisons in study subsets. For example, only about 33% of women in the CEE + MPA trial, and 31% of women in the CEE-alone trial were in the age range 50–59 where decisions concerning the use of hormone therapy, especially after the sea change mentioned above, are typically made. Figure 2.4 shows HRs corresponding to Figure 2.2 according to baseline age in categories 50–59, 60–69 and 70–79. Most CIs are quite wide with modest numbers of disease events for some outcomes, particularly in the 50–59 age group. This type of subset analysis is accompanied by important multiple testing considerations. Nonetheless, it is evident that more precise information is needed among younger women to adequately inform hormone therapy decisions, concerning use of these preparations, that are very effective for control of vasomotor symptoms in spite of longer-term health concerns. The joint analysis of multiple failure time outcomes is one place to look for additional insight into the health effects of these prominent hormone therapy preparations, as will be considered in Chapters 5 and 6. The reader is referred to Manson et al. (2013) for information on numbers and crude rates for these various clinical outcomes, and for additional hormone therapy trial detail.

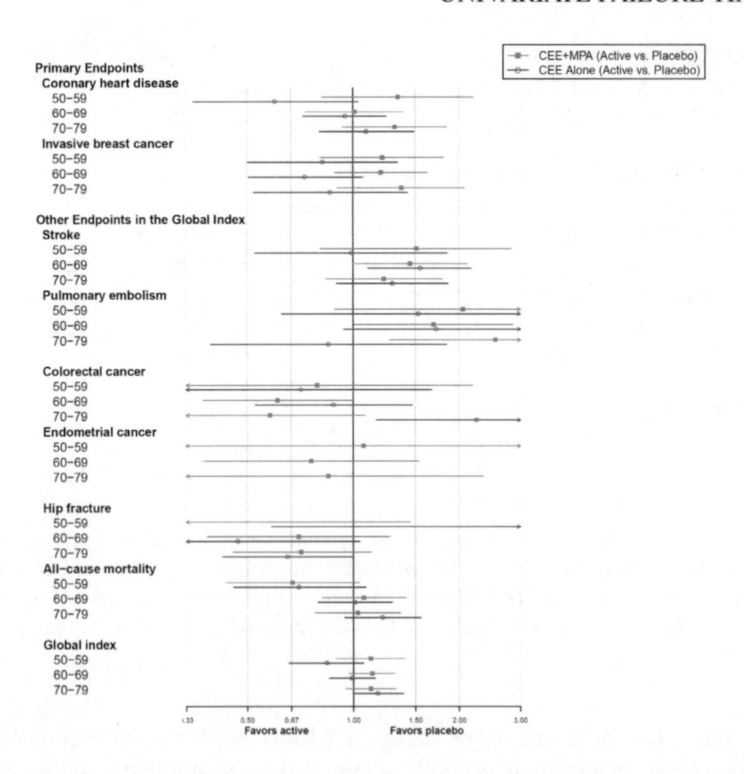

Figure 2.4 *Intention-to-treat hazard ratio parameter estimates and (asymptotic) 95% confidence intervals for various clinical outcomes by age group at randomization, for various clinical outcomes during the intervention phase of the Women's Health Initiative CEE + MPA and CEE-Alone randomized, placebo controlled trial. From Manson et al. (2013).*

2.9 Asymptotic Distribution Theory

The nonparametric and semiparametric aspects of the statistical models considered in this chapter preclude the application of standard parametric likelihood procedures to develop asymptotic theory for testing and estimation. The needed developments can, however, be based on empirical process distribution theory, or more specialized martingale convergence theory. A brief account of these approaches will be described here in a manner that will apply to some of the multivariate failure time testing and estimation procedures that will be described in subsequent chapters.

The estimates considered so far can be viewed as functions of processes that count failures over the cohort follow-up period. Let $N_k(t)$ denote the number of failures observed for the kth study subject over $[0,t]$, with $N_k(0) = 0$, including the possibility that $N_k(t) > 1$ for multivariate failure time counts, $k = 1, \ldots, n$. The counting process N_k is defined as a step function having right-continuous sample paths, so that the count $N_k(t)$ includes any failures at $T = t$. One can also define corresponding "at-risk" processes Y_k having left-continuous sample paths, so that $Y_k(t) = 1$ if the

kth individual is without prior censoring and still at risk for an observed failure at $T = t$, and $Y_k(t) = 0$ otherwise. Similarly, the covariate process Z_k may be defined to have left-continuous sample paths, so that $Z_k(t)$ can be "predicted" by the preceding values $Z_k(u), u < t$, precluding the inclusion of any jump in the covariate at $T = t$ in the specification of $Z_k(t), k = 1, \ldots, n$.

A standard approach to distribution theory development assumes $\{N_k, Y_k, Z_k\}$ to be independent and identically distributed (IID) for the n individuals in the study sample. Empirical process asymptotic results then apply to the types of transformations of these basic variables that appear in the specification of estimators for targeted parameters. These methods apply to the estimators considered in this chapter, as well as to many of the estimation procedures for multivariate failure time data to be described in subsequent chapters, even if the coordinate time axes for the multivariate failure times are unrelated.

When multivariate failure times arise through continued follow-up of individuals for second and subsequent failures on a single failure time axis, martingale methods can often be applied to derive asymptotic distributional results for estimators of interest. These methods can even somewhat relax the identically distributed assumption that attends the empirical process methods, and additionally can yield analytic variance estimators for tests and estimators of interest.

Here we give a brief, informal account of both approaches for the Cox model, by extracting key concepts and approaches from the seminal paper by Andersen and Gill (1982). Denote by $\mathscr{H}_t$ the collective failure, censoring and covariate information in the study cohort prior to time t. The Cox model (2.5), extended to allow a discrete failure probabilities at some t values, and extended to allow continued follow-up beyond a first failure to second and subsequent failures for individual study subjects, can be written

$$\begin{aligned} E\{N_k(dt); \mathscr{H}_t\} &= Y_k(t)\Lambda_k\{dt; Z_k(t), N_k(t^-)\} \\ &= Y_k(t)\Lambda_0(dt)\exp\{x_k(t)\beta\}, \end{aligned} \tag{2.15}$$

where independence of $\{N_k, Y_k, Z_k\}$ among the study subjects has been assumed along with independent censorship, and the modeled covariate x_k, with left-continuous sample paths, is defined such that $x_k(t)$ is a p-vector of functions derived from $Z_k(t)$ and $N_k(t^-)$, and possibly product terms between such functions and t.

Each counting process N_k can be decomposed into signal and noise process components such that

$$N_k(t) = \Lambda_k(t) + M_k(t),$$

where $\Lambda_k(dt) = Y_k(t)\Lambda_0(dt)\exp\{x_k(t)\beta\}$, and $M_k(dt) = N_k(dt) - \Lambda_k(dt)$ has expectation zero. In fact, the "noise" process M_k has the structure of a mean zero martingale for each k, meaning that $E\{M_k(t)\} = 0$ and $E\{M_k(t); \mathscr{H}_s\} = M_k(s)$ for every t and $s < t$. The (predictable) covariation process $\langle M_k, M_\ell \rangle$ for martingales M_k and M_ℓ is defined by

$$\langle M_k, M_\ell \rangle(t) = E\{M_k(t)M_\ell(t); \mathscr{H}_t\}.$$

The above independence assumption among $\{N_k, Y_k, Z_k\}, k = 1, \ldots, n$ leads to

$\langle M_k, M_\ell \rangle(t) = 0$ for all t and $k \neq \ell$, whence the martingales $M_k, k = 1, \ldots, n$ are said to be orthogonal. Also denote $\langle M_k \rangle(t) = \langle M_k, M_k \rangle(t)$.

With this background the estimating function (2.8) for β, based on data through follow-up time t, can be expressed as

$$U(\beta,t) = \sum_{k=1}^{n} \int_0^t \{x_k(u)' - \mathscr{E}(\beta,u)\}N_k(du) = \sum_{k=1}^{n} \int_0^t \{x_k(u)') - \mathscr{E}(\beta,u)\}M_k(du), \tag{2.16}$$

where $\mathscr{E}(\beta,u) = \sum_{j=1}^{n} Y_j(u)x_j(u)' \exp\{x_j(u)\beta\} / \sum_{j=1}^{n} Y_j(u) \exp\{x_j(u)\beta\}$.

Expression (2.16) is in the form of a stochastic integral of a predictable process with respect to a (square integrable) martingale, due to the left continuity (with right-hand limits) of x_k and Y_k, for each $k = 1, \ldots, n$ and one can apply a central limit theorem due to Rebolledo to show that $n^{-1/2}U(\beta,t)$ converges in probability, at the "true" β value, to a mean zero Gaussian process for $t \in (0, \tau]$ for any τ such that there is positive probability for an observed failure beyond τ for each $k = 1, \ldots, n$. Sufficient conditions for this convergence are that the covariation process for $n^{-1/2}U(\beta, \cdot)$, given by

$$\begin{aligned}\langle n^{-1/2}U(\beta,t) \rangle(t) =& n^{-1} \sum_{k=1}^{n} \int_0^t \{x_k(u) - \mathscr{E}(\beta,u)\}^{\otimes 2} \\ & [1 - \Lambda_0(\Delta u) \exp\{x_k(u)\beta\}] Y_k(u) \Lambda_0(du) \exp\{x_k(u)\beta\},\end{aligned}$$

where $a^{\otimes 2}$ denotes $a'a$ for a row vector a, converges in probability to a fixed function $V(\beta,t)$ as $n \to \infty$, and that the covariation process for related processes

$$n^{-1/2}U_\varepsilon(\beta,t) = n^{-1/2} \sum_{k=1}^{n} \int_0^t [\{x_k(u) - \mathscr{E}(\beta,u)\}' \mathbf{1}\{\|x_k(u) - \mathscr{E}(\beta,u)\|\} > \varepsilon] M_k(du)$$

converge in probability to zero, where $\|A\|$ denotes the maximum element of matrix A, and $\mathbf{1}(\cdot)$ is an indicator variable, for any $\varepsilon > 0$. The first condition is fulfilled under the stability of $n^{-1} \sum_{k=1}^{n} Y_k(t) \exp\{x_k(t)\beta\}$ and its first and second partial derivatives with respect to β, over $0 < t \leq \tau$ as $n \to \infty$, while the second is a Lindeberg condition that requires the influence of each study subject's data on the estimation of β to diminish to zero as the sample size becomes large. The Rebolledo theorem also gives $V(\beta, \cdot)$ as the covariation process for $n^{-1/2}U(\beta, \cdot)$.

The development just described applies under the extended Cox model (2.15), at the "true" value β. As a special case at $\beta = 0$ it provides asymptotic theory for the logrank test (2.11), and with minor modifications its weighted extension (2.12) with predictable weights.

Martingale convergence results can also be used to establish the consistency of $\hat{\beta}$ solving (2.16) for this true β, which we now denote by β_0. For β in an open neighborhood of β_0, the logarithm of the likelihood in (2.7) relative to that at β_0, for data through follow-up time t, with $0 < t \leq \tau$, can be written

$$n^{-1}\log\{L(\beta,t)/L(\beta_0,t)\} =$$
$$n^{-1}\sum_{k=1}^{n}\int_0^t \left(x_k(u)(\beta-\beta_0) - \log\left[\frac{n^{-1}\sum_{j=1}^n Y_j(t)\exp\{x_k(t)\beta\}}{n^{-1}\sum_{j=1}^n Y_j(t)\exp\{x_k(t)\beta_0\}}\right]\right)\Lambda_k(du)$$
$$+n^{-1}\sum_{k=1}^{n}\int_0^t \left(x_k(u)(\beta-\beta_0) - \log\left[n^{-1}\frac{\sum_{j=1}^n Y_j(t)\exp\{x_k(t)\beta\}}{\sum_{j=1}^n Y_j(t)\exp\{x_k(t)\beta_0\}}\right]\right)M_k(du) \tag{2.17}$$

The second term in (2.17) is a martingale with covariation process that converges to zero under stability conditional on $n^{-1}\sum_{k=1}^n Y_k(t)\exp\{x_k(t)\beta\}$ and its first and second derivatives with respect to β, over $0 < t \leq \tau$ and over an open neighborhood for β about β_0. An inequality due to Lenglart shows that the supremum over $0 < t \leq \tau$ of this second term converges in probability to zero at each β value in this open ball, so that the asymptotic behavior of (2.17) is governed by the first term. Under the stability conditions already mentioned and modest regularity conditions, this term converges to a function of β having unique maximum at β_0 with probability approaching one as $n \to \infty$, giving the desired consistency result.

Aside from a term that converges in probability to zero as $n \to \infty$ one can write, since $U(\hat{\beta},\tau) = 0$, that

$$0 = n^{-1/2}U(\beta_0,\tau) = \{n^{-1/2}(\hat{\beta}-\beta_0)\}\{n^{-1}I(\beta^*,\tau)\}$$

where $I(\beta,\tau) = n^{-1}\dfrac{\partial U(\beta,t)}{\partial \beta'} = n^{-1}\sum_{k=1}^n\int_0^t v_k(\beta,u)N_k(dt)$,

where $v_k(\beta,u) = \dfrac{\sum_{j=1}^n Y_j(u)x_j(u)'x_j(u)\exp\{x_j(u)\beta\}}{\sum_{j=1}^n Y_j(u)\exp\{x_j(u)\beta\}} - \mathscr{E}(\beta,u)^{\otimes 2}$,

and where each element of β_* is between the corresponding elements of $\hat{\beta}$ and β_0. The consistency of $\hat{\beta}$ for β is the key step in showing $I(\beta^*,\tau)$ to be a consistent estimator of $I(\beta_0,\tau)$ for every such β^* and in showing

$$\hat{V}(\hat{\beta},\tau) = n^{-1}\sum_{k=1}^n\int_0^t \{x_k(u)-\mathscr{E}(\hat{\beta},u)\}^{\otimes 2}[1-\hat{\Lambda}_0(\Delta u)\exp\{x_k(u)\hat{\beta}\}]$$
$$Y_k(u)\hat{\Lambda}_0(du)\exp\{x_k(u)\hat{\beta}\} \tag{2.18}$$

to be a consistent estimator of $V(\beta_0,\tau)$, where

$$\hat{\Lambda}_0(t) = \int_0^t \hat{\Lambda}_0(du) = \sum_{k=1}^n\int_0^t\left[\sum_{j=1}^n Y_j(u)\exp\{x_j(u)\beta'\}\right]^{-1} N_k(du). \tag{2.19}$$

It follows that $n^{1/2}(\hat{\beta}-\beta_0)$ converges in distribution to a mean zero normal distribution as $n \to \infty$, with variance consistently estimated by $I(\hat{\beta},\tau)^{-1}\hat{V}(\hat{\beta},\tau)I(\hat{\beta},\tau)^{-1}$

assuming that $I(\beta_0, \tau)$ converges to a positive definite matrix. With absolutely continuous failure times, one can set $\hat{\Lambda}_0(\Delta u) = 0$ in (2.19) and replace $\hat{V}(\hat{\beta}, \tau)$ by $I(\hat{\beta}, \tau)$, giving the variance estimator $I(\hat{\beta}, \tau)^{-1}$ for $n^{1/2}(\hat{\beta} - \beta_0)$ that is calculated in most software packages for the Cox model.

Martingale convergence results apply also to the baseline hazard process estimator $\hat{\Lambda}_0$ and yield an asymptotic mean zero Gaussian process for $\{n^{1/2}(\hat{\beta} - \beta_0), n^{1/2}(\hat{\Lambda}_0 - \Lambda_0)\}$ as $n \to \infty$. At $\beta_0 = 0$ the asymptotic distribution of $n^{1/2}(\hat{\Lambda}_0 - \Lambda_0)$ applies to the Nelson-Aalen estimator, and to the corresponding Kaplan–Meier estimator $n^{1/2}(\hat{F} - F)$ where $\hat{F}(t) = \prod_0^t \{1 - \hat{\Lambda}_0(du)\}$, and can be used to show the consistency of the Greenwood formula for estimating the variance process for $\hat{F}$ over $0 < t \leq \tau$.

The need to stop the follow-up at a finite $\tau < \infty$ in the support of the observed follow-up times is somewhat limiting in the developments sketched above. However, asymptotic results over the entire positive real line require additional assumptions and more complex developments. From a practical perspective there does not seem to be a risk in applying asymptotic formulae to all available data, without restricting the follow-up period, as is done with available Cox model software.

If one makes an identically distributed, as well as an independent, assumption for $\{N_k, Y_k, Z_k\}, k = 1, \ldots, n$, then the stability conditions alluded to above are satisfied for $0 < t \leq \tau$ and β in an open neighborhood of β_0. The asymptotic results listed above then hold under the conditions that the expectation of the supremum of $Y(t)|x(t)|^2 \exp\{x(t)\beta\}$ is less than infinity, for all $0 < t \leq \tau$ and β in an open neighborhood of β_0, to ensure that the Lindeberg condition holds, and the condition that $I(\beta_0, \tau)$ converges in probability to a positive definite matrix. See Andersen and Gill (1982) for additional detail.

2.10 Additional Univariate Failure Time Models and Methods

While the Cox model (2.5) is by far the most widely used regression model for the analysis of univariate absolutely continuous failure time data, a variety of other hazard rate regression models have been proposed, and may yield parsimonious models and valuable parameter interpretations in some settings. For example, the hazard rate model

$$\lambda\{t; Z(t)\} = \lambda_0\{te^{-x(t)\beta}\}e^{-x(t)\beta} \tag{2.20}$$

specifies a linear relationship $U = \log T = x(t)\beta + \varepsilon$, if $x(t) \equiv x$ with "error" variate ε having a fixed distribution. As a semiparametric class of models, this "accelerated failure time (AFT) model" is somewhat difficult to work with, as estimating functions for β are discontinuous. Nevertheless, these estimation challenges have been substantially addressed (e.g., Jin, Lin, Wei, & Ying, 2003), and this class of models may merit consideration for use in addition to the Cox model, toward ensuring that principal findings are not unduly model-dependent.

Other authors, rather than having $\log T$ on the left side of a regression model, consider linear models for an unspecified monotone transformation of T. These types of "transformation" models can incorporate considerable modeling flexibility, though parameter interpretation may be an issue. See, for example, Zeng and Lin (2007) for a substantial class of semiparametric regression models and their maximum likelihood estimation.

A rather different class of linear hazard rate models

$$\lambda\{t;Z(t)\} = \lambda_0(t) + x(t)\beta(t),$$

with regression parameters that may be time-dependent was introduced by Aalen (1980). The parameters in this model are restricted by $\lambda\{t;Z(t)\} \geq 0$, all (t,Z), but the additive form of the model makes it convenient for some purposes, such as for covariate measurement error correction; or for mediation analysis where one examines the ability of time-varying covariate measurements to provide an explanation for an observed relationship between hazard rates and a study treatment or exposure variable.

2.11 A Cox-Logistic Model for Continuous, Discrete or Mixed Failure Time Data

As previously noted, the Cox model (2.5) can be extended to include mass points at some values of t by writing

$$\Lambda\{dt;Z(t)\} = \Lambda_0(dt)\exp\{x(t)\beta\}$$

and applying the asymptotic formulae given above, including the sandwich-type estimator for the variance of $\hat{\beta}$. Some caution may be needed however, since $\Lambda\{dt;Z(t)\}$ is necessarily equal to or less than one at any mass point, possibly restricting the range of corresponding β-values. With small failure probabilities at any follow-up time t this constraint can likely be managed by careful specification of the regression variable. If there are large mass points, however, it may be preferable to instead apply a Cox-Logistic (CL) model given by

$$\frac{\Lambda\{dt,Z(t)}{1-\Lambda\{\Delta t,Z(t)\}} = \frac{\Lambda_0(dt)}{1-\Lambda_0(\Delta t)}\exp\{x(t)\beta\}, \tag{2.21}$$

where the failure time variate may have either a mass point or a continuity point at any $t > 0$, and the regression parameter β has an odds ratio interpretation. Note that (2.21) reduces to the Cox model (2.5) if T is everywhere absolutely continuous. More generally the semiparametric likelihood for (Λ_0,β) in (2.21), where $\Lambda_0(t) = \int_0^t \Lambda_0(ds)$, based on data as described in §2.3, can be written

$$L = \prod_{i=0}^{I}\left(\prod_{k\in D(t_i)}\Lambda\{dt_i;Z_k(t_i)\}\prod_{k\in R(t_i)-D(t_i)}\prod_{t_i}^{t_{i+1}\wedge S_k}[1-\Lambda\{du;Z_k(u)\}]\right) \tag{2.22}$$

where the product integral on the right ranges from $t_i < u \leq t_{i+1}\wedge S_k$, with $t_0 = 0$ and $t_{I+1} = \infty$, while $D(t_0)$ is empty. The maximum likelihood (ML) estimator places positive mass at each of $t_1,\ldots,t_I$, since otherwise $L = 0$, and the placement of any mass within the risk region away from these uncensored failure times can only diminish L on the basis of the product integral factors. Therefore the ML estimator places all mass within the risk region of the data at $t_1, \ldots, t_I$.

Set $\lambda_k(t_i) = \Lambda_k\{dt_i; Z(t_i)\}$, for all (k,i), and $\alpha_i = \log[\Lambda_0(dt_i)/\{1-\Lambda_0(dt_i)\}]$, $i = 1, \ldots, I$. The ML estimators of (Λ_0, β) then maximize

$$\log L = \sum_{i=1}^{I} \left(\sum_{k \in D(t_i)} \{\alpha_i + x_k(t_i)\beta\} + \sum_{k \in R(t_i)} \log\{1 - \lambda_k(t_i)\} \right),$$

and satisfy

$$\partial \log L/\partial \alpha_i = d_i - \sum_{k \in R(t_i)} \lambda_k(t_i) = 0, i = 1, \ldots, I \text{ and}$$

$$\partial \log L/\partial \beta = \sum_{i=1}^{I} \{ \sum_{k \in D(t_i)} x_k(t_i)' - \sum_{k \in R(t_i)} x_k(t_i)' \lambda_k(t_i)\} = 0, \text{ while} \tag{2.23}$$

while the elements of the corresponding Hessian are

$$-\partial^2 \log L/\partial \alpha_i \partial \alpha_m = \mathbf{I}(i = m) \sum_{k \in R(t_i)} \lambda_k(t_i)\{1 - \lambda_k(t_i)\},$$

$$-\partial^2 \log L/\partial \alpha_i \partial \beta = \sum_{k \in R(t_i)} x_k(t_i)' \lambda_k(t_i)\{1 - \lambda_k(t_i)\}, \text{ and}$$

$$-\partial^2 \log L/\partial \beta \partial \beta' = \sum_{i=1}^{I} (\sum_{k \in R(t_i)} x_k(t_i)' x_k(t_i) \lambda_k(t_i)\{1 - \lambda_k(t_i)\}).$$

The ML estimator of $\eta = (\alpha_1, \ldots, \alpha_I, \beta')'$, and hence of (Λ_0, β), can be obtained by iteratively updating a trial value η_0 to

$$\eta_0 + (-\partial^2 \log L/\partial \eta_0 \partial \eta_0')^{-1} \partial \log L/\partial \eta_0$$

until convergence is achieved, perhaps using starting values of $\alpha_i = \{d_i/(r_i - d_i)\}, i = 1, \ldots, I$ and $\beta = 0$. At convergence to $\hat{\eta}$ the inverse of $-\partial^2 \log L/\partial \hat{\eta} \partial \hat{\eta}'$ provides a candidate variance estimator for $\hat{\eta}$, and hence for $(\hat{\Lambda}_0, \hat{\beta})$, where $\hat{\Lambda}_0(t) = \sum_{t_i \leq t} \exp(\hat{\alpha}_i)/\{1 - \exp(\hat{\alpha}_i)\}$ for all $t \in R$.

These ML estimators, under the Cox-Logistic model, do not require any specialized likelihood procedures, or specialized maximum likelihood definitions and they allow for tied failure times, though the odds ratio parameter β in (2.21) differs somewhat from the hazard ratio parameter in (2.5), more so if there are large mass points.

In the absolutely continuous special case, these ML estimates differ slightly from the maximum partial likelihood estimates satisfying (2.8), and involve an iterative calculation for $(\alpha_1, \ldots, \alpha_I)$ as well as β. The absolutely continuous special case of (2.21) can also be embedded in a discrete-continuous model of the form (2.5). If this model form, say $\lambda_k(t_i) = \exp\{\gamma_i + x_k(t_i)\beta\}$, all (k,i), is substituted into the estimating functions (2.23) one obtains $\exp(\hat{\gamma}_i) = d_i / \sum_{k \in R} x_k(t_i) \exp\{x_k(t_i)\beta\}, i = 1, \ldots, I$ and estimating function for β that is precisely (2.8).

The corresponding Hessian-based variance estimator for β, following this substitution, agrees with the sandwich form variance estimator for $\hat{\beta}$ shown in §2.9.

The counting process approach to deriving asymptotic distribution theory for (β, Λ_0), under a mixed discrete and continuous version of (2.5) as outlined in §2.9, undoubtedly can be adapted to ML estimation of (β, Λ_0) under the Cox-Logistic model (2.21), though such adaptation has yet to appear in the literature.

BIBLIOGRAPHIC NOTES

Much more detailed accounts of many of the univariate failure time topics considered in this chapter can be found, for example, in Kalbfleisch and Prentice (2002), Andersen et al. (1993) and Fleming and Harrington (1991) among other books and review articles. Cox (1972), including its discussion component, provides insight into the stimulus and innovation arising from this seminal paper. Kalbfleisch and Prentice (1973), Breslow (1974), Cox (1975) and Johansen (1983) provide efforts to establish a likelihood basis for (2.7), while vigorous efforts to develop corresponding distribution theory for $(\hat{\beta}, \hat{\Lambda}_0)$ culminated in the elegant paper of Andersen and Gill (1982), which provided developments using both martingale convergence theory and empirical process convergence theory as outlined in §2.9. Begun, Hall, Huang, and Wellner (1983) show the maximum partial likelihood estimate solving (2.8) to be semiparametric efficient, with time-independent covariates and absolutely continuous failure times. Asymptotic distribution theory for the Kaplan–Meier estimator (2.3) was given in Breslow and Crowley (1974), and later in a simplified form using martingale methods (e.g., Andersen et al., 1993). See Kalbfleisch and Prentice (2002, Chapter 7) for an account of the history and application of the AFT model. A discrete and continuous hazard rate model of the form (2.5) was considered by Prentice and Kalbfleisch (2003). They showed that the solution to (2.8) consistently estimates β in this enlarged model, but that the correction noted above was needed to $I(\hat{\beta})^{-1}$ from (2.9) for variance estimation to allow for discrete components. Cox (1972) described the Cox-Logistic model (2.21) for discrete data, though its extension to a model for mixed discrete and continuous failure time data, as in (2.21) appears to be novel. The asymptotic distribution theory presented in §2.9 is adapted from a more complete version in Kalbfleisch and Prentice (2002). Marginal structural models were proposed by Robins et al. (2000). Detailed estimates of the US medical care cost saving resulting from the reduced use of CEE + MPA following the initial publication of the WHI hormone therapy trial results (Rossouw et al., 2002) is given in Roth et al. (2014).

EXERCISES AND COMPLEMENTS

Exercise 2.1

Plot the Kaplan–Meier estimates (2.3) for the CSP + MTX and MTX groups using the aplastic anemia A-GVHD data of Table 1.1. Calculate corresponding 95% confidence intervals $F(t)$ at $t = 180$ days using (2.4). Plot log $\{-\log \hat{F}(t)\}$ versus t for the two treatment groups. Are these separated by about the same distance across t, as would be expected under proportionality of hazard ratios between the two randomization groups? Apply the weighted logrank test (2.13) with $h(t) \equiv 1$ to formally compare A-GVHD rates between the two treatment groups. Repeat the comparison with $h(t) = \hat{F}(t)$, where $\hat{F}(t)$ is the Kaplan–Meier estimator for the A-GVHD data for the two treatment groups combined. Do the two tests yield similar (asymptotic) significance levels for this comparison?

Exercise 2.2

Calculate the partial likelihood function $L(\beta)$ in (2.7) for the aplastic anemia data of Table 1.1 with binary covariate $x_1(t) \equiv x_1$ that takes value zero for the groups of patients randomized to CSP + MTX and value one for those randomized to MTX alone. Plot log $L(\beta_1)$ versus β_1 over a fine grid of β_1 values. Is log $L(\beta_1)$ approximately quadratic and centered at the maximum partial likelihood estimator $\hat{\beta}_1$ with curvature $-I(\hat{\beta}_1)$? Calculate an asymptotic 95% confidence interval for β_1, and for the treatment hazard ratio e^{β_1}. Add $x_2 = x_1 \log t$ to the regression model and test $\beta_2 = 0$. Does this test yield evidence of departure from proportionality over follow-up time in the hazard ratio for A-GVHD?

Exercise 2.3

Augment the Cox model of Exercise 2.2 by defining $x_1(t) = x_1$ as before, but with $x_2(t) = x_2$ as an indicator variable for laminar air flow room (LAF) isolation $(x_2 = 1)$ or not $(x_2 = 0)$, and with $x_3(t) = x_3$ equal to the patient age in years at randomization. Does A-GVHD incidence appear to depend on LAF isolation or age? Was the estimated MTX versus CSP + MTX hazard ratio affected by the inclusion of these other variables? Repeat these analyses dropping x_2 from the regression model while stratifying baseline A-GVHD incidence on LAF isolation and on whether patient age at randomization was less than 20 years. How did this stratification affect the other regression parameter estimates?

Exercise 2.4

Show that inserting $\hat{\lambda}_i(\beta), i = 1, \ldots, I$ into (2.6) gives (2.7) up to a multiplicative factor that does not involve β. Suppose that the observation period for the kth study subject may begin at time $t_k^0 > 0$. Show that expressions (2.6)–(2.10) apply to (β, Λ_0) estimation under (2.5) with $R(t)$ redefined to include only study subjects under active follow-up at time t.

Exercise 2.5

Suppose that rather than using the profile likelihood (2.7), that has maximized over $\lambda_i, i = 1, \ldots, I$, that one proceeds with maximum likelihood estimation of the parameter $\eta = (\beta, \lambda_1, \ldots, \lambda_I)$ from the "parametric" likelihood (2.6). Show that the resulting maximum likelihood estimator of β is the same $\hat{\beta}$ that maximizes (2.7). Also using partition matrices show that the upper left p $\times$ p sub-matrix of $I(\hat{\eta})^{-1} = -\partial^2 \log L / \lambda \hat{\eta} \partial \hat{\eta}'$ is precisely the inverse of (2.9). Would the asymptotic inference on β be unaffected if one carried out profiling over Λ_0 numerically rather than analytically as in (2.7)?

Exercise 2.6

Consider the failure type–specific hazard rate models (2.12). Using an approximate likelihood of the form (2.6), show that the type-specific hazard ratio parameters $\beta_1, \ldots, \beta_q$ can be estimated by maximizing a profile likelihood that is the product of factors of the form (2.7) for each $j = 1, \ldots, q$ with the jth factor derived by censoring the follow-up period for an individual when failure of a type other than j occurs. Show that the type j baseline hazard function can be estimated by an expression like (2.10) with the failure times restricted to type j failures and with $R(t)$ redefined to include this additional censorship (Prentice et al., 1978).

Exercise 2.7

Show, under (2.5), that (2.8) provides an unbiased estimating function for β if $R(t)$ is composed only of cases occurring at time t_i and their matched controls, under nested case control sampling. Assuming that matched controls are drawn randomly from cohort members at risk for failure at each t_i, and independently for each case, show that the inverse of (2.9) provides a variance estimator for $\hat{\beta}$ under nested case–control sampling (Thomas, 1977; Prentice & Breslow, 1978).

Exercise 2.8

Show, under (2.5), that (2.8) provides an unbiased estimating function for β with $R(t_i)$ comprised of cases occurring at time t_i and subcohort members at risk for failure, under case–cohort sampling with subcohort a random sample of the entire cohort. Can you derive a variance estimator for this case–cohort regression parameter estimator (Prentice, 1986; Self & Prentice, 1988)?

Exercise 2.9

Suppose that $x(t) \equiv x$ in (2.5), and that x is measured with error, so that one observes $w = x + \varepsilon$ where x and ε are independent and normally distributed with ε having a mean of zero. Show that the induced hazard rate model for T given w is approximately of the same form (2.5) with $E(x|w)$ in place of x if the outcome is rare (i.e.,

$F(t;x)$ is close to one for all individuals and for all t in the study follow-up period). How could $E(x|w)$ be estimated if replicate w values having independent errors were available on a random subset of the study cohort? Devise a suitable variance estimator for the regression calibration estimator that replaces x in (2.5) by an estimator of $E(x|w)$ based on replicate data, and applies (2.8) (Prentice, 1982; Wang, Hsu, Feng, & Prentice, 1997; Carroll, Ruppert, Crainiceanu, & Stefanski, 2006)

Exercise 2.10

Show by direct calculation that the second equality in (2.16) holds. Also derive the expression for $\langle n^{1/2}U(\beta,\cdot)\rangle(t)$ given a few lines later.

Exercise 2.11

Apply Rebolledo's central limit theorem to derive the asymptotic distribution of $(\hat{\beta},\hat{\Lambda}_0)$ solving (2.23) under the Cox-logistic model (2.21). What conditions are needed to ensure a mean zero asymptotic Gaussian distribution for $\partial \log L/\partial \eta$ at the true β and Λ_0 values?

Chapter 3

Nonparametric Estimation of the Bivariate Survivor Function

3.1 Introduction

This chapter considers the long-standing statistical problem of nonparametric estimation of the bivariate survivor function F, given by $F(t_1,t_2) = P(T_1 > t_1, T_2 > t_2)$, for failure time variates $T_1 > 0$ and $T_2 > 0$ subject to independent right censorship, and the estimation of associated hazard rates. The application of these estimators to assess the nature and strength of association between the failure time variates will also be considered.

We have seen in Chapter 2 that the univariate survivor function can be estimated nonparametrically by plugging the empirical estimator of the hazard function into a product integral representation, which expresses the survivor function as a transformation on the hazard function, giving the familiar KM estimator. A similar approach applies to nonparametric estimation of the bivariate survivor function.

Bivariate failure time data allow empirical estimation of the marginal hazard rates for T_1 and T_2, as well as empirical estimation of the double failure hazard function Λ_{11} defined by

$$\Lambda_{11}(t_1,t_2) = \int_0^{t_1}\int_0^{t_2} \Lambda_{11}(ds_1,ds_2), \tag{3.1}$$

where $\Lambda_{11}(ds_1,ds_2) = P\{T_1 \in [s_1,s_1+ds_1), T_2 \in [s_2,s_2+ds_2); T_1 \geq s_1, T_2 \geq s_2\} = F(ds_1,ds_2)/F(s_1^-,s_2^-)$ as in (1.3). These empirical estimators are the principal building blocks for estimation of F, as will be elaborated in §3.2, and are also the principal building blocks for Cox-type regression extensions, as will be described in Chapter 4.

The bivariate survivor function estimator that arises from plugging empirical marginal single and double failure hazard estimators into a corresponding representation for F, however, has a distracting feature; namely, the estimator typically incorporates negative mass (probability) assignments. Such assignments occur because of a possibly poor correspondence between the single failure empirical and the double failure empirical hazard rate estimators. One response to this issue has been to consider alternate representations that express F in terms of its empirical single failure hazard rates and a modified double failure hazard rate estimator that adapts somewhat to the marginal hazard rate estimators. Popular estimators due to Dabrowska (1988) and Prentice and Cai (1992) fall in this category, but these do not fully resolve the negative mass issue (§3.2). It is natural to consider a nonparametric maximum likelihood approach to enforce probability function positivity requirements. However, a maximum likelihood approach that allows a separate parameter at each point on the grid formed by the uncensored T_1 and T_2 failure times is typically overparameterized, and does not yield a unique estimator of F unless additional constraints are imposed. Similarly, a mean parameter estimation approach is overparameterized if a free parameter is included in the nonparametric model at each uncensored grid point in the risk region of the data, and this approach also does not yield a unique estimator of F. These approaches will be briefly described in §3.3.

One use of a nonparametric estimator of F is characterization of the dependency between T_1 and T_2. Nonparametric estimation of cross ratio and concordance rate functions for this purpose is described in §3.4. Section 3.5 mentions some additional approaches to the estimation of F, and provides a general perspective on bivariate hazard rate and survivor function estimation.

3.2 Plug-In Nonparametric Estimators of F

3.2.1 The Volterra estimator

Suppose that (T_1,T_2) is subject to independent right censoring by variate (C_1,C_2). For example (C_1,C_2) may arise from a censoring "survivor" function G, where $G(t_1,t_2) = P(C_1 > t_1, C_2 > t_2)$ for all $t_1 \geq 0$ and $t_2 \geq 0$, with (T_1,T_2) independent of (C_1,C_2), a so-called random censorship model. The usual convention is that failures precede censorings in the event of tied times.

(T_1, T_2) subject to independent right censoring by (C_1, C_2), so observe
$S_i = T_i \wedge C_i$ and $\delta_i = I[S_i = T_i], i = 1, 2$, for a sample of size n

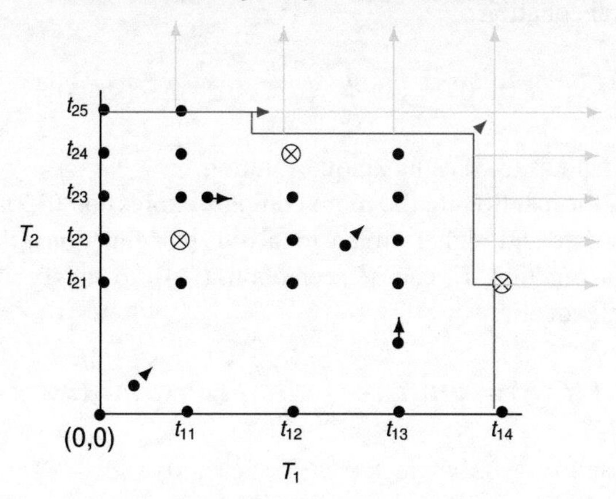

Risk region: $\{(t_1, t_2); S_1 \geq t_1,$ and $S_2 \geq t_2$ for one or more (S_1, S_2) in sample$\}$
$t_{11}, \ldots, t_{1I}$ – ordered uncensored T_1 failure times $(t_{10} = 0)$
$t_{21}, \ldots, t_{2J}$ – ordered uncensored T_2 failure times $(t_{20} = 0)$

Figure 3.1 *Bivariate failure time data structure (with) $\otimes$ indicating double failure, $\uparrow$ indicating failure on T_1 and censoring on T_2, $\rightarrow$ indicating failure on T_2, and censoring on T_1 and $\nearrow$ indicating censored value for both T_1 and T_2. A $\bullet$ denotes a grid point in the risk region of the data.*

Consider an independent random sample of size n from a study cohort, where one observes

$$S_{1k} = T_{1k} \wedge C_{1k}, \delta_{1k} = I[T_{1k} = S_{1k}], S_{2k} = T_{2k} \wedge C_{2k}, \delta_{2k} = I[T_{2k} = S_{2k}]$$

for $k = 1, \ldots, n$. For convenience these data will be referred to as arising from "individual" k, for $k = 1, \ldots, n$. Denote by $t_{11} < t_{12} < \cdots < t_{1I}$ and by $t_{21} < t_{22} < \cdots < t_{2J}$ the respective ordered uncensored T_1 and T_2 values in the sample, and set $t_{10} = t_{20} = 0$, as illustrated in Figure 3.1. The marginal (single failure) hazard rate functions can be denoted by $\Lambda_{10}(\cdot, 0)$ and $\Lambda_{01}(0, \cdot)$ where, for example,

$$\Lambda_{10}(t_1, 0) = \int_0^{t_1} \Lambda_{10}(ds_1, 0) \text{ and } \Lambda_{10}(ds_1, 0) = P\{T_1 \in [s_1, s_1 + ds_1); T_1 \geq s_1\}. \quad (3.2)$$

Product integral transformations give corresponding marginal survivor functions $F(\cdot, 0)$ and $F(0, \cdot)$ via

$$F(t_1, 0) = \prod_0^{t_1} \{1 - \Lambda_{10}(ds_1, 0)\} \text{ and } F(0, t_2) = \prod_0^{t_2} \{1 - \Lambda_{01}(0, ds_2)\}.$$

These marginal distributions have an equivalent expression in the form of Péano series. For example, one can write

$$F(t_1, 0) = 1 + \sum_{j=1}^{\infty} \int_0^{t_1} \int_{s_1}^{t_1} \int_{s_2}^{t_1} \cdots \int_{s_{j-1}}^{t_1} \prod_{m=1}^{j} \{-\Lambda_{10}(ds_m, 0)\}. \quad (3.3)$$

This Péano series representation derives from the fact that $F(\cdot,0)$ satisfies a homogeneous integral equation

$$F(t_1,0) = 1 + \int_0^{t_1} F(s_1^-,0)\{-\Lambda_{10}(ds_1,0)\}$$

for all $t_1 \geq 0$, that has (3.3) as its unique solution.

The reason for mentioning the more complex expression (3.3) here is that it generalizes to bivariate and higher dimensional survivor functions. Specifically, the bivariate survivor function, F, can be seen, as in (1.4), to satisfy the inhomogeneous Volterra integral equation

$$F(t_1,t_2) = \psi(t_1,t_2) + \int_0^{t_1}\int_0^{t_2} F(s_1^-,s_2^-)\Lambda_{11}(ds_1,ds_2), \tag{3.4}$$

for all $t_1 \geq 0$ and $t_2 \geq 0$, where $\psi(t_1,t_2) = F(t_1,0) + F(0,t_2) - 1$, which also has unique solution in Péano series form given by

$$F(t_1,t_2) = \psi(t_1,t_2) + \sum_{j=1}^{\infty} \int_0^{t_1}\int_{s_{11}}^{t_1}\cdots\int_{s_{1,j-1}}^{t_1}\int_0^{t_2}\int_{s_{21}}^{t_2}\cdots\int_{s_{2,j-1}}^{t_2} \psi(s_{11}^-,s_{21}^-)\prod_{m=1}^{j}\Lambda_{11}(ds_{1m},ds_{2m}) \tag{3.5}$$

for all $t_1 \geq 0$ and $t_2 \geq 0$. This expression shows that F is uniquely determined by its marginal single failure hazard rate and its double failure hazard rate functions. F can be estimated nonparametrically by inserting empirical estimators for each such hazard rate function. The resulting "Volterra" estimator has been attributed to Peter Bickel (Dabrowska, 1988).

In spite of the complex form of (3.5) this estimator is simply calculated recursively. To see this, denote by $d_{ij}^{11}, d_{ij}^{10}, d_{ij}^{01}$ and d_{ij}^{00} the 2×2 table counts for the number of double failures at (t_{1i},t_{2j}), the number of "individuals" having $T_1 = t_{1i}$ with T_2 known to be greater than t_{2j}, the number of individuals having $T_2 = t_{2j}$ with T_1 known to be greater than t_{1i}, and the number of individuals known to have T_1 greater than t_{1i} and T_2 greater than t_{2j} in the sample, respectively. Explicitly

$$\begin{aligned}
d_{ij}^{11} &= \#\{k; S_{1k} = t_{1i}, \delta_{1k} = 1, \text{ and } S_{2k} = t_{2j}, \delta_{2k} = 1\},\\
d_{ij}^{10} &= \#\{k; S_{1k} = t_{1i}, \delta_{1k} = 1, \text{ and } S_{2k} > t_{2j} \text{ if } \delta_{2k} = 1, \text{ or } S_{2k} \geq t_{2j} \text{ if } \delta_{2k} = 0\}\\
d_{ij}^{01} &= \#\{k; S_{1k} > t_{1i} \text{ if } \delta_{1k} = 1, \text{ or } S_{1k} \geq t_{1i} \text{ if } \delta_{1k} = 0; \text{ and } S_{2k} = t_{2j}, \delta_{2k} = 1\},\\
d_{ij}^{00} &= \#\{k; S_{1k} > t_{1i} \text{ if } \delta_{1k} = 1, \text{ or } S_{1k} \geq t_{1i} \text{ if } \delta_{1k} = 0; \text{ and } S_{2k} > t_{2j} \text{ if } \delta_{2k} = 1,\\
&\qquad \text{or } S_{2k} \geq t_{2j} \text{ if } \delta_{2k} = 0\}.
\end{aligned}$$

Also denote by $r_{ij} = \#\{k; S_{1k} \geq t_{1i}, S_{2k} \geq t_{2j}\} = d_{ij}^{11} + d_{ij}^{10} + d_{ij}^{01} + d_{ij}^{00}$ the size of the risk set at uncensored data grid point (t_{1i},t_{2j}) for all $i \geq 0$, $j \geq 0$. The step function empirical marginal hazard function estimators $\hat{\Lambda}_{10}(\cdot,0)$ and $\hat{\Lambda}_{01}(0,\cdot)$ are determined by $\hat{\Lambda}_{10}(\Delta t_{1i},0) = d_{i0}^{10}/r_{i0}$ for $i = 1,\ldots,I$ and $\hat{\Lambda}_{01}(0,\Delta t_{2j}) = d_{0j}^{01}/r_{0j}$, for $j = 1,\ldots,J$, and the step function empirical double failure hazard rate function $\hat{\Lambda}_{11}$ is determined by $\hat{\Lambda}_{11}(\Delta t_{1i}, \Delta t_{2j}) = d_{ij}^{11}/r_{ij}$ for all $(t_{1i}, t_{2j}) \in R$. The Volterra nonparametric estimator $\hat{F}$ arises by inserting these empirical estimators into (3.5). As such it is readily calculated, starting with the KM marginal survivor function estimators

$$\hat{F}(t_1, 0) = \prod_{\{t_{1i} \leq t_1\}} \{1 - d_{i0}^{10}/r_{i0}\} \text{ and } \hat{F}(0, t_2) = \prod_{\{t_{2j} \leq t_2\}} \{1 - d_{0j}^{01}/r_{0j}\},$$

using the recursive form

$$\hat{F}(t_{1i}, t_{2j}) = \hat{F}(t_{1i}, t_{2j}^-) + \hat{F}(t_{1i}^-, t_{2j}) - \hat{F}(t_{1i}^-, t_{2j}^-)\{1 - \hat{\Lambda}_{11}(\Delta t_{1i}, \Delta t_{2j})\}, \tag{3.6}$$

which derives from the fact that $\hat{F}(\Delta t_{1i}, \Delta t_{2j}) = \hat{F}(t_{1i}^-, t_{2j}^-)\hat{\Lambda}_{11}(\Delta t_{1i}, \Delta t_{2j})$, at all grid points away from the coordinate axes in the risk region of the data.

While the Volterra estimator has the desirable asymptotic properties that one might expect from its empirical single failure and double failure hazard rate components, it also has the distracting feature of typically incorporating negative probability assignments. This occurs because of a possibly poor agreement between the marginal single failure hazard rates and the double failure hazard rates. Figure 3.1 shows the four types of observations according to whether δ_{1k} and δ_{2k} take values zero or one. The KM marginal survivor functions assign positive mass along all uncensored data grid lines in each direction, but the empirical double failure hazard rate function assigns positive point mass within the risk region of the data only at grid points where $d_{ij}^{11} > 0$. As a result, for example, the probability assignment along a grid line where there are no doubly censored observations is entirely pushed to the half-line beyond the risk region of the data by $\hat{F}$, causing the mass assignments along half-lines where there are doubly censored observations to compensate through possible negative probability assignments beyond the risk region. Gill, van der Laan, and Wellner (1995) noted that nonparametric plug-in estimators due to Dabrowska (1988) and Prentice and Cai (1992) have the property of nonparametric efficiency if T_1, T_2, C_1, C_2 were completely independent, whereas this did not appear to be the case for the Volterra estimator, and those authors speculated that the Volterra estimator may be "much inferior" to these other estimators. These other estimators are perhaps the most widely used of available nonparametric estimators of F.

3.2.2 The Dabrowska and Prentice–Cai estimators

These estimators use the KM marginal survivor function estimators, but do so in conjunction with a double failure estimator that acknowledges the KM estimators to some extent. Both estimators focus on representations for the ratio of F to the product of its corresponding marginal survivor functions.

Denote this ratio by Q, so that

$$Q(t_1, t_2) = \begin{cases} F(t_1, t_2)/\{F(t_1, 0)F(0, t_2)\} & \text{if } F(t_1, 0)F(0, t_2) > 0 \\ 0 \text{ otherwise.} & \end{cases}$$

The Dabrowska (1988) representation expresses this ratio by the two-dimensional product integral

$$Q(t_1,t_2) = \begin{cases} \prod_{s_1 \le t_1} \prod_{s_2 \le t_2} [1 + \frac{\Lambda_{11}(ds_1,ds_2) - \Lambda_{10}(ds_1,s_2^-)\Lambda_{01}(s_1^-,ds_2)}{\{1-\Lambda_{10}(\Delta s_1,s_2^-)\}\{1-\Lambda_{01}(s^-)1,\Delta s_2)\}}] & \\ \quad \text{if } \{1-\Lambda_{10}(\Delta s_1,s_2^-)\}\{1-\Lambda_{01}(s_1^-,\Delta s_2)] > 0. & \\ 0 \quad \text{otherwise} & \end{cases} \tag{3.7}$$

The Dabrowska estimator arises by inserting empirical hazard rates into (3.7).

Note that the integral in (3.7) involves a comparison between the double failure hazard rate $\Lambda_{11}(ds_1,ds_2)$ and the product of single failure hazard rates $\Lambda_{10}(ds_1,s_2^-)\Lambda_{01}(s_1^-,ds_2)$ that would obtain under local independence between T_1 and T_2 at (s_1,s_2). These single failure hazard rates can be estimated empirically by $\hat{\Lambda}_{10}(\Delta t_{1i},t_{2j}^-) = (d_{ij}^{11} + d_{ij}^{10})/r_{ij}$ and $\hat{\Lambda}_{01}(t_{1i}^-,\Delta t_{2j}) = (d_{ij}^{11} + d_{ij}^{01})/r_{ij}$ at uncensored data grid point $(t_{1i},t_{2j}) \in R$ in defining the Dabrowska estimator. As a result the Dabrowska estimator differs from the Volterra estimator. Specifically the Volterra representation (3.5) fully determines the single failure hazard rates away from the coordinate axes via

$$\Lambda_{10}(ds_1,s_2^-) = F(ds_1,s_2^-)/F(s_1^-,s_2^-) \text{ and } \Lambda_{01}(s_1^-,ds_2) = F(s_1^-,ds_2)/F(s_1^-,s_2^-)$$

at all $s_1 > 0$ and $s_2 > 0$, but the estimators of these hazard rates induced from empirical estimators for marginal single failure and double failure hazard rates generally do not agree with the single failure empirical rates used by the Dabrowska estimator. Note that if either $\hat{\Lambda}_{10}(\Delta t_{1i},t_{2j}^-) = 0$ or $\hat{\Lambda}_{01}(t_{1i}^-,\Delta t_{2j}) = 0$ then the product integral factor in (3.7) takes the local independence value of one at all such grid points away from the boundary of the risk region. Hence, the Dabrowska estimator defines mass assignments via a modified double failure hazard rate function that makes a local independence assignment at grid point (t_{1i},t_{2j}) when there are no empirical data along one or both of $T_1 = t_{1i}$ and $T_2 = t_{2j}$ at or beyond (t_{1i},t_{2j}). This helps to explain the nonparametric efficiency of the Dabrowska estimator under the complete independence of the failure and censoring variates. In doing so, however, the Dabrowska estimator typically assigns substantial negative mass within the risk region of the data, even as sample size n becomes large.

The Dabrowska estimator is a step function taking value

$$\hat{F}(t_{1i},t_{2j}) = \prod_{\ell \le i}\{1 - d_{\ell 0}^{10}/r_{\ell 0}\} \prod_{m \le j}\{1 - d_{0m}^{01}/r_{0m}\} \prod_{\ell \le i}\prod_{m \le j} \left\{ \frac{d_{\ell m}^{00} r_{\ell m}}{(d_{\ell m}^{10} + d_{\ell m}^{00})(d_{\ell m}^{01} + d_{\ell m}^{00})} \right\} \tag{3.8}$$

at grid point $(t_{1i},t_{2j}) \in R$ where $d_{ij}^{00} > 0$. It can be calculated recursively starting with KM marginal survivor function estimators, with

$$\hat{F}(t_{1i},t_{2j}) = \begin{cases} \frac{\hat{F}(t_{1i},t_{2j}^-)\hat{F}(t_{1i}^-,t_{2j})}{\hat{F}(t_{1i}^-,t_{2j}^-)} \left\{ \frac{d_{ij}^{00} r_{ij}}{(d_{ij}^{10}+d_{ij}^{00})(d_{ij}^{01}+d_{ij}^{00})} \right\} & \text{if } d_{ij}^{00} > 0 \\ 0 \text{ otherwise} & \end{cases} \tag{3.9}$$

at grid points $(t_{1i},t_{2j}) \in R$ away from the coordinate axes. The Prentice–Cai (1992) representation derives from the fact that Q satisfies the homogeneous Volterra integral equation

$$Q(t_1,t_2) = 1 + \int_0^{t_1}\int_0^{t_2} Q(s_1^-,s_2^-)B(ds_1,ds_2), \tag{3.10}$$

where

$$\begin{aligned}B(ds_1,ds_2) =& \{\Lambda_{11}(ds_1,ds_2) - \Lambda_{10}(ds_1,s_2^-)\Lambda_{01}(0,ds_2) - \Lambda_{10}(ds_1,0)\Lambda_{01}(s_1^-,ds_2)\\ &+ \Lambda_{10}(ds_1,0)\Lambda_{01}(0,ds_2)\}/[\{1-\Lambda_{10}(ds_1,0)\}\{1-\Lambda_{01}(0,ds_2)\}]\end{aligned}$$

which has Péano series solution

$$Q(t_1,t_2) = 1 + \sum_{j=1}^{\infty}\int_0^{t_1}\int_{s_{11}}^{t_1}\cdots\int_{s_{1,j-1}}^{t_1}\int_0^{t_2}\int_{s_{21}}^{t_2}\cdots\int_{s_{2,j-1}}^{t_2}\prod_{m=1}^{j} B(ds_{1m},ds_{2m}). \tag{3.11}$$

The Prentice–Cai estimator starts with KM marginal survivor function estimators and is readily calculated recursively by setting $\hat{Q}(t_{1i},0) = 1, i = 1,\ldots,I$ and $\hat{Q}(0,t_{2j}) = 1, j = 1,\ldots,J$ and then calculating

$$\hat{F}(t_{1i},t_{2j}) = \begin{cases}\hat{F}(t_{1i},0)\hat{F}(0,t_{2j})\hat{Q}(t_{1i},t_{2j}) & \text{if } \hat{F}(t_{1i},0)\hat{F}(0,t_{2j}) > 0,\\ 0 & \text{otherwise}\end{cases}$$

where $\hat{Q}(t_{1i},t_{2j}) = \hat{Q}(t_{1i},t_{2j}^-) + \hat{Q}(t_{1i}^-,t_{2j}) - \hat{Q}(t_{1i}^-,t_{2j}^-)\{1-\hat{B}(\Delta t_{1i},\Delta t_{2j})\}$, with

$$\begin{aligned}\hat{B}(\Delta t_{1i},\Delta t_{2j}) =& \{\hat{\Lambda}_{11}(\Delta t_{1i},\Delta t_{2j}) - \hat{\Lambda}_{10}(\Delta t_{1i},t_{2j}^-)\hat{\Lambda}_{01}(0,\Delta t_{2j})\\ &- \hat{\Lambda}_{10}(\Delta t_{1i},0)\hat{\Lambda}_{01}(t_{1i}^-,\Delta t_{2j}) + \hat{\Lambda}_{10}(\Delta t_{1i},0)\hat{\Lambda}_{01}(0,\Delta t_{2j})\}/\\ &[\{1-\hat{\Lambda}_{10}(\Delta t_{1i},0)\}\{1-\hat{\Lambda}_{01}(0,\Delta t_{2j})\}],\end{aligned}$$

at all grid points $i > 0$ and $j > 0$ with $(t_{1i},t_{2j}) \in R$ where $\hat{F}(t_{1i},0)\hat{F}(0,t_{2j}) > 0$. This estimator also uses empirical estimators of single failure hazards away from the coordinate axes, but includes these in a different manner than does the Dabrowska estimator. It is of interest to examine whether these plug-in estimator variations materially affect their performance as estimators of F.

3.2.3 *Simulation evaluation*

Table 3.1 gives simulation summary statistics for the three nonparametric estimators described above with failure times generated under a Clayton–Oakes model (1.7) with unit exponential marginal survivor functions, given by $F(t_1,0) = e^{-t_1}$ and $F(0,t_2) = e^{-t_2}$, at values $\theta = 0$ (independence between T_1 and T_2) and $\theta = 2$ (constant cross ratio of 3), and various sample sizes n. The censoring variates C_1 and C_2 were taken to have exponential distributions, with C_1 and C_2 independent of each other and of (T_1,T_2). The common censoring hazard rate, c, was chosen to give a specified fraction of T_1 and T_2 values that were uncensored: either 1/6, 1/3, or 1. All three estimators are evidently quite accurate at the T_1 and T_2 (marginal) percentiles

Table 3.1 *Simulation summary statistics for the Volterra, Dabrowska, and Prentice–Cai estimators* ($\hat{F}_V, \hat{F}_D, \hat{F}_{PC}$) *under Clayton–Oakes model* (1.7) *at parameter values* $\theta = 0$ *(independence) and* $\theta = 2$ *(cross-ratio of 3), and certain sample sizes n and censoring rates.*

$\{F(t_1,0),F(0,t_2)\}$	F	$\hat{F}$	Sample mean (sample standard deviation)*			
Clayton–Oakes Parameter			$\theta=0$			
Sample Size n			500	1000	250	250
% Uncensored: T_1, T_2 and (T_1, T_2)			16.7 16.7 2.8	16.7 16.7 2.8	33.3 33.3 11.1	100 100 100
(0.85,0.85)	0.723	$\hat{F}_V$	0.722 (0.025)	0.722 (0.018)	0.722 (0.031)	0.722 (0.028)
		$\hat{F}_D$	0.722 (0.025)	0.722 (0.018)	0.722 (0.031)	0.722 (0.028)
		$\hat{F}_{PC}$	0.722 (0.025)	0.722 (0.018)	0.722 (0.031)	0.722 (0.028)
(0.85,0.70)	0.595	$\hat{F}_V$	0.594 (0.038)	0.595 (0.026)	0.594 (0.037)	0.595 (0.031)
		$\hat{F}_D$	0.594 (0.037)	0.595 (0.026)	0.594 (0.037)	0.595 (0.031)
		$\hat{F}_{PC}$	0.593 (0.037)	0.595 (0.026)	0.594 (0.037)	0.595 (0.031)
(0.85,0.55)	0.468	$\hat{F}_V$	0.467 (0.064)	0.468 (0.043)	0.468 (0.045)	0.468 (0.031)
		$\hat{F}_D$	0.466 (0.066)	0.468 (0.041)	0.468 (0.044)	0.468 (0.031)
		$\hat{F}_{PC}$	0.462 (0.063)	0.466 (0.041)	0.468 (0.044)	0.468 (0.031)
(0.70,0.70)	0.490	$\hat{F}_V$	0.489 (0.050)	0.490 (0.033)	0.489 (0.041)	0.489 (0.032)
		$\hat{F}_D$	0.488 (0.047)	0.491 (0.031)	0.490 (0.040)	0.489 (0.032)
		$\hat{F}_{PC}$	0.489 (0.046)	0.491 (0.031)	0.490 (0.040)	0.489 (0.032)
(0.70,0.55)	0.385	$\hat{F}_V$	0.381 (0.075)	0.386 (0.053)	0.386 (0.049)	0.385 (0.030)
		$\hat{F}_D$	0.380 (0.086)	0.387 (0.054)	0.386 (0.046)	0.385 (0.030)
		$\hat{F}_{PC}$	0.379 (0.066)	0.385 (0.046)	0.386 (0.045)	0.386 (0.030)
(0.55,0.55)	0.303	$\hat{F}_V$	0.298 (0.095)	0.299 (0.076)	0.303 (0.057)	0.303 (0.028)
		$\hat{F}_D$	0.303 (0.117)	0.306 (0.084)	0.303 (0.048)	0.303 (0.028)
		$\hat{F}_{PC}$	0.316 (0.072)	0.313 (0.058)	0.305 (0.047)	0.303 (0.028)

$\{F(t_1,0),F(0,t_2)\}$	F	$\hat{F}$	Sample mean (sample standard deviation)			
Clayton–Oakes Parameter			$\theta=2$			
Sample Size n			500	1000	250	250
% Uncensored: T_1, T_2 and (T_1, T_2)			16.7 16.7 5.3	16.7 16.7 5.3	33.3 33.3 16.3	100 100 100
(0.85,0.85)	0.752	$\hat{F}_V$	0.752 (0.025)	0.752 (0.018)	0.752 (0.030)	0.752 (0.027)
		$\hat{F}_D$	0.752 (0.025)	0.752 (0.018)	0.752 (0.030)	0.752 (0.027)
		$\hat{F}_{PC}$	0.752 (0.025)	0.752 (0.017)	0.752 (0.031)	0.752 (0.027)
(0.85,0.70)	0.642	$\hat{F}_V$	0.642 (0.037)	0.643 (0.026)	0.641 (0.036)	0.642 (0.030)
		$\hat{F}_D$	0.642 (0.036)	0.643 (0.025)	0.641 (0.036)	0.643 (0.030)
		$\hat{F}_{PC}$	0.641 (0.036)	0.643 (0.025)	0.641 (0.035)	0.643 (0.030)
(0.85,0.55)	0.521	$\hat{F}_V$	0.520 (0.064)	0.522 (0.043)	0.522 (0.044)	0.521 (0.031)
		$\hat{F}_D$	0.520 (0.063)	0.522 (0.041)	0.522 (0.043)	0.521 (0.031)
		$\hat{F}_{PC}$	0.517 (0.060)	0.521 (0.041)	0.521 (0.043)	0.521 (0.031)
(0.70,0.70)	0.570	$\hat{F}_V$	0.571 (0.050)	0.569 (0.033)	0.569 (0.039)	0.569 (0.031)
		$\hat{F}_D$	0.571 (0.046)	0.569 (0.030)	0.569 (0.037)	0.569 (0.031)
		$\hat{F}_{PC}$	0.570 (0.044)	0.569 (0.030)	0.569 (0.037)	0.569 (0.031)
(0.70,0.55)	0.480	$\hat{F}_V$	0.479 (0.086)	0.480 (0.055)	0.481 (0.044)	0.480 (0.031)
		$\hat{F}_D$	0.480 (0.084)	0.481 (0.054)	0.481 (0.043)	0.480 (0.031)
		$\hat{F}_{PC}$	0.477 (0.071)	0.479 (0.045)	0.481 (0.043)	0.480 (0.031)
(0.55,0.55)	0.422	$\hat{F}_V$	0.412 (0.111)	0.414 (0.087)	0.424 (0.048)	0.422 (0.031)
		$\hat{F}_D$	0.422 (0.118)	0.423 (0.094)	0.424 (0.048)	0.422 (0.031)
		$\hat{F}_{PC}$	0.423 (0.076)	0.423 (0.060)	0.424 (0.046)	0.422 (0.031)

*Sample mean and sample standard deviation based on 1000 simulated samples at each sampling configuration. Samples contributed to summary statistics at all (t_1,t_2) values that were in the risk region of the data. The three estimators reduce to the ordinary empirical estimator in the absence of censoring.

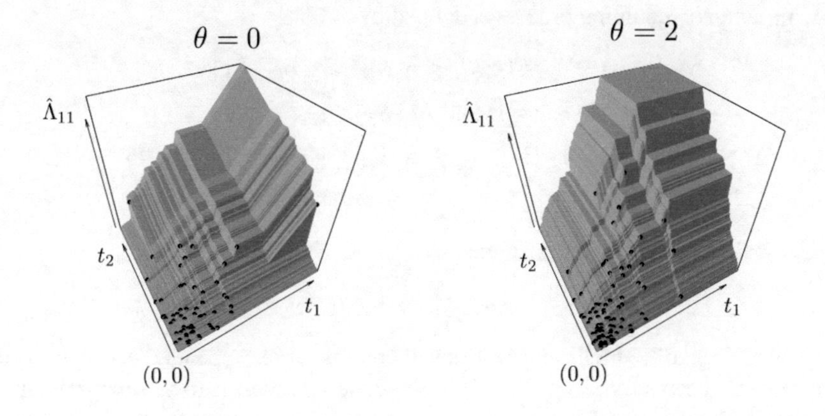

Figure 3.2 *Empirical double failure hazard function estimators $\hat{\Lambda}_{11}$ with failure time generated under the Clayton–Oakes model (1.7) with unit exponential marginal and cross ratio $C(t_1,t_2) \equiv 1+\theta$, at sample size $n = 500$ and mutually independent censoring times with each failure time having a 2/3 probability of censoring. The dots denote double failure times.*

shown, as was also the case under these same configurations, but with smaller sample size. Note also that the moderate sample size efficiencies evidently do not differ materially among the three estimators. In fact, it is not likely possible to much improve on the efficiencies of these estimators nonparametrically in spite of the previously mentioned negative mass assignments. Also, it seems that the Volterra estimator is likely to be quite competitive as a nonparametric estimator of F, especially if the expected number of double failures in the sample is not too small (e.g., 13.89 at $\theta = 0$ in the first configuration of Table 3.1). With this reassurance we will build on empirical marginal single and double hazard functions that yield the Volterra estimator in regression extensions described in later chapters.

Figure 3.2 displays the double failure hazard rate estimator for random samples generated as above at both $\theta = 0$ and $\theta = 2$, with $n = 500$ and a 2/3rds probability of censoring for both T_1 and T_2. Note the greater concentration of probability and of double failures around the $t_1 = t_2$ diagonal at $\theta = 2$ compared to $\theta = 0$.

3.2.4 *Asymptotic distributional results*

Empirical process methods apply to each of the estimators described in §3.2.2 to show strong consistency and weak convergence to a Gaussian process and to show bootstrap applicability.

Briefly, consider a failure time region $[0,\tau_1] \times [0,\tau_2]$ with $F(\tau_1,\tau_2)G(\tau_1,\tau_2) > 0$. For a sufficiently large sample size n the risk region of the data includes (τ_1,τ_2) with probability arbitrarily close to one. Hence we assume $[0,\tau_1] \times [0,\tau_2] \subset R$. Denote by

N_{10}, N_{01} and N_{11} counting processes defined by

$$N_{10}(t_1,t_2) = n^{-1}\#\{k; S_{1k} \le t_1, S_{2k} > t_2, \delta_{1k} = 1\}$$
$$N_{01}(t_1,t_2) = n^{-1}\#\{k; S_{1k} > t_1, S_{2k} \le t_2, \delta_{2k} = 1\}$$
$$N_{11}(t_1,t_2) = n^{-1}\#\{k; S_{1k} \le t_1, S_{2k} \le t_2, \delta_{1k} = 1, \delta_{2k} = 1\}$$

and by Y the "at-risk" process defined by

$$Y(t_1,t_2) = n^{-1}\#\{k; S_{1k} \ge t_1, S_{2k} \ge t_2\}.$$

The Glivenko–Cantelli and Donsker theorems (see Appendix A) apply to the empirical processes $(N_{10}, N_{01}, N_{11}, Y)$ to show these processes to be supremum norm consistent for, and weakly convergent in a Gaussian manner to, their target over $[0,\tau_1] \times [0,\tau_2]$ as $n \to \infty$.

Also define hazard processes $\Lambda_{10}, \Lambda_{01}$ and Λ_{11} according to

$$\hat{\Lambda}_{10}(t_1,t_2) = \int_0^{t_1} Y(u_1,t_2)^{-1} N_{10}(du_1,t_2),$$
$$\hat{\Lambda}_{01}(t_1,t_2) = \int_0^{t_2} Y(t_1,u_2)^{-1} N_{01}(t_1,du_2),$$
$$\hat{\Lambda}_{11}(t_1,t_2) = \int_0^{t_1}\int_0^{t_2} Y(u_1,u_2)^{-1} N_{11}(du_1,du_2).$$

The continuity and (weakly continuous) compact differentiability of these hazard process transformations (Gill & Johansen, 1990) then show $(\hat{\Lambda}_{10}, \hat{\Lambda}_{01}, \hat{\Lambda}_{11})$ to be strongly consistent for and weakly convergent to its corresponding target $(\Lambda_{10}, \Lambda_{01}, \Lambda_{11})$ over $[0,\tau_1] \times [0,\tau_2]$. As evidenced by the representations (3.5), (3.7) and (3.11), the three plug-in nonparametric estimators of F each derive from transformation on the hazard function estimators $(\hat{\Lambda}_{10}, \hat{\Lambda}_{01}, \hat{\Lambda}_{11})$ over $[0,\tau_1] \times [0,\tau_2]$. In fact, each such representation is a continuous and (weakly continuously) compact differentiable transformation on the hazard functions $(\Lambda_{10}, \Lambda_{01}, \Lambda_{11})$, so that the properties of strong consistency; that is,

$$\sup_{(t_1,t_2)\in[0,\tau_1]\times[0,\tau_2]} |\hat{F}(t_1,t_2) - F(t_1,t_2)| \xrightarrow{P} 0,$$

weak convergence of $n^{1/2}(\hat{F} - F)$ to a mean zero Gaussian process, and bootstrap applicability for variance estimation (among other purposes) follow from corresponding properties for the hazard function estimators. See Gill et al. (1995) for a thorough account of these developments for each of the three estimators, including the use of empirical process convergence results to establish bootstrap applicability.

3.3 Maximum Likelihood and Estimating Equation Approaches

There is a long history of attempts to estimate F via maximum likelihood. The nonparametric likelihood

$$L = \prod_{k=1}^{n} [F(dS_{1k}, dS_{2k})^{\delta_{1k}\delta_{2k}} \{-F(dS_{1k}, S_{2k})\}^{\delta_{1k}(1-\delta_{2k})}$$
$$\{-F(S_{1k}, dS_{2k})\}^{(1-\delta_{1k})\delta_{2k}} F(S_{1k}, S_{2k})^{(1-\delta_{1k})(1-\delta_{2k})}] \quad (3.12)$$

can be maximized by placing mass (probability) at uncensored failure time grid points (t_{1i}, t_{2j}) within the risk region $R = \{(t_1, t_2); S_{1k} \geq t_1, S_{2k} \geq t_2 \text{ for some } k\}$ and along grid half-lines beyond the risk region in each direction.

However, L as a nonparametric likelihood with parameters that include $\{F(t_{1i}, t_{2j}), \text{ at all } (t_{1i}, t_{2j}) \in R\}$ is overparameterized and, without further restriction, generally does not yield a unique maximizer.

The overparameterization occurs because of the inability to determine a meaningful double failure hazard rate estimator at grid points $(t_{1i}, t_{2j}) \in R$ where $d_{ij}^{10} = d_{ij}^{01} = d_{ij}^{11} = 0$. The response to this overparameterization has primarily been to impose constraints so that F has a reduced set of parameters that can be uniquely estimated. One semiparametric approach involves copula models that express F in terms of its marginal survivor functions and a fixed dimensional parameter that governs dependence between T_1 and T_2. This formulation embraces certain regression generalizations, as discussed below in Chapter 4, but it typically embraces only a limited class of dependencies between the two failure time variates. Another approach involves the imposition of smoothness constraints, or data reduction, so that a unique maximizer for a smaller set of parameters emerges with high probability as sample size increases (e.g., Tsai, Leurgans, & Crowley, 1986). Van der Laan's (1996) repaired maximum likelihood procedure stands out among such estimators, as being nonparametric efficient if a certain data reduction bandwidth goes to zero at a sufficiently slow rate as sample size increases. However, this estimator has some practical limitations, and has not proven to have moderate sample size properties that are better than those for simpler plug-in estimators. Additionally, this type of estimator does not reduce to the standard empirical bivariate survivor function estimator in the absence of censoring.

Similarly, a mean parameter estimation approach is overparameterized if a free parameter is included at each uncensored data grid point in the risk region of the data. Hence, this approach also does not yield a unique nonparametric estimator.

A topic closely tied to the nonparametric estimation of F concerns whether or not the bivariate failure time data are useful, beyond the respective univariate failure time data, for nonparametric estimation of the marginal survivor functions $F(\cdot, 0)$ and $F(0, \cdot)$. For example, in the absence of censoring the empirical joint survivor function, with its empirical (Kaplan–Meier) marginal survivor function estimators is the accepted nonparametric estimator. Estimators that impose smoothing constraints on the bivariate survivor function may be able to slightly enhance the efficiency of marginal survivor function estimators, but in doing so may run the risk of introducing bias into these survivor function estimators. Hence, it is natural to focus on two-stage estimators that first estimate marginal distribution parameters using only the pertinent marginal censored data, followed by estimation of joint distribution parameters at specified marginal distribution parameter estimates.

3.4 Nonparametric Assessment of Dependency

3.4.1 Cross ratio and concordance function estimators

Now consider the application of nonparametric survivor function estimators of the type described in §3.2 for assessing the nature and magnitude of any dependence between the failure time variates T_1 and T_2.

The presence of right censoring implies that it will typically only be possible to assess dependency over a finite sample space for (T_1, T_2). Accordingly, consider the estimation of pairwise dependency over $[0, \tau_1] \times [0, \tau_2]$ where (τ_1, τ_2) is in the support of the observation times (S_1, S_2). Local dependence at (t_1, t_2) in this region can be defined in terms of the cross ratio $\alpha(t_1, t_2)$, or equivalently its reciprocal

$$\begin{aligned}\alpha^{-1}(t_1,t_2) &= \Lambda_{10}(dt_1,t_2^-)\Lambda_{01}(t_1^-,dt_2)/\Lambda_{11}(dt_1,dt_2)\\ &= F(dt_1,t_2^-)F(t_1^-,dt_2)/\{F(dt_1,dt_2)F(t_1^-,t_2^-)\},\end{aligned}$$

which can be integrated with respect to the failure time probability element, $F(dt_1,dt_2)/\int_0^{\tau_1}\int_0^{\tau_2} F(ds_1,ds_2)$, over this space to give an average cross ratio measure $C(\tau_1, \tau_2)$ over $[0, \tau_1] \times [0, \tau_2]$, where

$$\begin{aligned}C(\tau_1,\tau_2) &= \int_0^{\tau_1}\int_0^{\tau_2} F(dt_1,dt_2)\Big/\int_0^{\tau_1}\int_0^{\tau_2} \alpha^{-1}(t_1,t_2)F(dt_1,dt_2)\\ &= \int_0^{\tau_1}\int_0^{\tau_2} F(t_1^-,t_2^-)\Lambda_{11}(dt_1,dt_2)\Big/\\ &\quad \int_0^{\tau_1}\int_0^{\tau_2} F(t_1^-,t_2^-)\Lambda_{10}(dt_1,t_2^-)\Lambda_{01}(t_1^-,dt_2). \qquad (3.13)\end{aligned}$$

Empirical estimates $\hat{C}(\tau_1, \tau_2)$ of the average cross ratio measure $C(\tau_1, \tau_2)$ are readily obtained by inserting estimators that derive from a suitable survivor function estimator $\hat{F}$, such as the Volterra, Dabrowska or Prentice–Cai estimators. Note that the weighting function $F(ds_1, ds_2)$ in (3.13) derives from the failure time distribution, and does not involve the censoring rates, so that average cross ratio estimates arising from studies having different censoring patterns can be compared.

As a process over $[0, \tau_1] \times [0, \tau_2]$, the average cross ratio estimator $\hat{C}$, defined by $\hat{C}(t_1, t_2)$ for $(t_1, t_2) \in [0, \tau_1] \times [0, \tau_2]$, has the form of a function of a stochastic integral that inherits such properties as a strong consistency, weak convergence to a Gaussian process, and applicability of bootstrap sampling procedures, from those for the generating survivor function estimator $\hat{F}$.

Another nonparametric dependency measure is Kendall's tau, which in the absence of censoring assesses concordance between the paired (T_1, T_2) values via $E\{\text{sign}(T_1^{(1)} - T_1^{(2)})(T_2^{(1)} - T_2^{(2)})\}$ where $(T_1^{(1)}, T_2^{(1)})$ and$(T_1^{(2)}, T_2^{(2)})$ are independent variates having survivor function F. Oakes (1989) proposed the corresponding local dependence measure at (t_1, t_2) as

$$\text{tau}(t_1,t_2) = E\{\text{sign }(T_1^{(1)} - T_1^{(2)})(T_2^{(1)} - T_2^{(2)})|T_1^{(1)} \wedge T_1^{(2)} = t_1, T_2^{(1)} \wedge T_2^{(2)} = t_2\},$$

which can be estimated with right censored data. In fact, the cross ratio and local concordance dependency measures have the simple monotonic relationship

$$\text{tau}(t_1,t_2) = \{\alpha(t_1,t_2) - 1\}/\{\alpha(t_1,t_2) + 1\} \tag{3.14}$$

so that values of $\alpha(t_1,t_2)$ of one (local independence), zero (maximal negative dependence) and ∞ (maximal positive independence) correspond to tau (t_1,t_2) values of $0, -1$ and 1, respectively. A summary concordance measure $\mathscr{T}(\tau_1,\tau_2)$ can be obtained by averaging tau(t_1,t_2) according to the probability element,

$$2F(t_1^-,t_2^-)F(dt_1,dt_2) + 2F(t_1^-,dt_2)F(dt_1,t_2^-),$$

of the componentwise minima $T_1^{(1)} \wedge T_1^{(2)}$ and $T_2^{(1)} \wedge T_2^{(2)}$ giving

$$\mathscr{T}(\tau_1,\tau_2) = \frac{\int_0^{\tau_1}\int_0^{\tau_2} F(t_1^-,t_2^-)F(dt_1,dt_2) - \int_0^{\tau_1}\int_0^{\tau_2} F(t_1^-,dt_2)F(dt_1,t_2^-)}{\int_0^{\tau_1}\int_0^{\tau_2} F(t_1^-,t_2^-)F(dt_1,dt_2) + \int_0^{\tau_1}\int_0^{\tau_2} F(t_1^-,dt_2)F(dt_1,t_2^-)} \tag{3.15}$$

which also takes values in $[-1,1]$. The concordance estimator $\hat{\mathscr{T}}(\tau_1,\tau_2)$ is obtained by everywhere inserting $\hat{F}$ for F in (3.15). As a process $\hat{\mathscr{T}}$ inherits strong consistency, weak convergence to a Gaussian process and bootstrap applicability from these same properties for $\hat{F}$. Of course, dependency estimators over other subsets of the risk region of the data are readily specified from $\hat{C}$ or $\hat{\mathscr{T}}$. For example, an average cross ratio estimator over a rectangular region $(t_1,\tau_1] \times (t_2,\tau_2]$ is given by $\hat{C}(\tau_1,\tau_2) - \hat{C}(\tau_1,t_2) - \hat{C}(t_1,\tau_2) + \hat{C}(t_1,t_2)$.

3.4.2 *Australian twin study illustration*

These data were described in §1.7.2. Here we regard the ages at appendectomy or censoring for the 1218 MZ and the 735 DZ twins as random samples from respective twin pair cohorts for illustration purposes. The joint survivor function F for the paired ages at appendectomy occurrence can be characterized by its marginal single and double failure hazard rates. Table 3.2 shows average cross ratio and average concordance estimates using the cumulative data through certain specified ages, based on the Dabrowska survivor function estimator, under an arbitrary designation of first and second membership within each pair. It is evident that cross ratios and concordances are larger at younger ages, and they appear to be somewhat larger for MZ than for DZ twins. For example for MZ twins an asymptotic 95% confidence interval for the average cross ratio, $C(10,10)$ up to age 10 is $\exp\{\log(7.69 \pm 1.96(0.36)\} = (3.85, 16.67)$ indicating quite a strong dependency. The corresponding confidence interval for DZ twins is $(1.75, 10.0)$. Over the region $(20,60] \times (20,60]$ the average cross ratio estimate is 1.32 with 95% CI of $(0.80, 2.22)$ for MZ twins and 1.30 with 95% CI of $(0.61, 2.78)$ for DZ twins, indicating rather limited association between ages at appendectomy for either MZ or DZ twins after age 20. As elaborated in Table 3.2 footnotes, bootstrap procedures were used for confidence interval calculation.

One can use the asymptotic distributions for $\hat{C}$ or $\hat{\mathscr{T}}$ to test equality of average cross ratios between MZ and DZ twins. For example, a comparison at age 30 based

Table 3.2 *Average cross ratio and concordance estimators of ages at appendectomy occurrence, through selected ages for the members of monozygotic (MZ) and dizygotic (DZ) twin pairs in the Australian twin Study (Duffy et al., 1990).*

		Age of Second Twin[a]		
Age of First Twin[a]		10	30	50
		Average Cross Ratio Estimate ($\hat{C}$)		
10	MZ	7.69 (0.36)[b]	4.17 (0.22)	3.70 (0.24)
	DZ	4.17 (0.44)	1.59 (0.47)	1.85 (0.54)
30	MZ	3.13 (0.26)	3.03 (0.10)	2.78 (0.10)
	DZ	2.94 (0.27)	1.92 (0.16)	1.64 (0.17)
50	MZ	2.56 (0.27)	2.56 (0.11)	2.38 (0.10)
	DZ	2.70 (0.26)	1.72 (0.17)	1.69 (0.15)
		Average Concordance Estimate ($\hat{\mathscr{T}}$)		
10	MZ	0.78 (0.083)[c]	0.62 (0.067)	0.59 (0.075)
	DZ	0.61 (0.150)	0.26 (0.205)	0.30 (0.203)
30	MZ	0.53 (0.095)	0.51 (0.031)	0.48 (0.036)
	DZ	0.50 (0.101)	0.32 (0.071)	0.28 (0.071)
50	MZ	0.47 (0.107)	0.46 (0.039)	0.43 (0.038)
	DZ	0.47 (0.107)	0.29 (0.071)	0.28 (0.063)

Source: (Fan, Prentice, & Hsu, 2000)
[a]The designations first and second are arbitrary within a pair.
[b]In parentheses are bootstrap estimates of the standard deviation of $\log\hat{C}(t_1,t_2)$, based on 200 bootstrap samples.
[c]In parentheses are bootstrap estimates of the standard deviation of $\hat{\mathscr{T}}(t_1,t_2)$, based on 200 bootstrap samples.

on $\log\hat{C}(30,30)$ would compare $\{\log(3.03)-\log(1.92)\}/\{(0.10)^2+(0.16)^2\}^{1/2}=$ 2.41 to a standard normal distribution, providing evidence for stronger dependency between MZ twins than DZ twins in ages of appendectomy through age 30. A corresponding test of equality of average concordance rates $\mathscr{T}(30,30)$ through age 30 for MZ and DZ twins takes value 2.45, in good agreement with the test based on $\hat{C}(30,30)$. These analyses may suggest a genetic component to the appendectomy risk given the complete sharing of genetic material for MZ twins versus partial sharing for DZ twins, though the possibility of greater "environmental" factor sharing by MZ versus DZ twins may also need to be considered, as may the details of ascertainment and follow-up of the study cohort, in making a substantive interpretation of these data.

This illustration points to the need for more flexible methods to accommodate various statistical features and generalizations. For example, it is natural to restrict marginal hazard rates to be identical for twin pair members, possibly enhancing the efficiency of the dependency assessments shown in Table 3.2. Also the data set included year of births for each twin pair, as well as additional pair, and pair member, characteristics and exposures. These and other features will be included in regression generalizations in later chapters, culminating in Chapter 6 where semiparametric models for marginal single and double failure hazard rates will be considered, with nonparametric components that coincide for failures, such as those for members of a twin pair here, that are defined to be of the same "type."

3.4.3 *Simulation evaluation*

Table 3.3 gives simulation summary statistics for the average cross ratio estimator $\hat{C}$ and average concordance estimator $\hat{\mathscr{T}}$ with data generated as for Table 3.1. Table 3.2 shows simulation results at $\theta = 2$ using the Prentice–Cai estimator $\hat{F}_{PC}$, with sample means and sample standard deviations at the same (t_1,t_2) values as in Table 3.1. Note that $\hat{C}$ tends to slightly overestimate C and $\hat{\mathscr{T}}$ tends to somewhat underestimate $\mathscr{T}$ at these configurations. Also the cross ratio and concordance rate estimators are not very precisely estimated, especially in the heavier censoring scenarios, as is to be expected since the estimator precision at (t_1,t_2) depends directly on the number of double failures in $[0,t_1) \times [0,t_2)$. The precision also depends on the reliability of $\hat{F}(t_1,t_2)$, leading to some instability as (t_1,t_2) move into the tails for the failure distribution. These simulations suggest that rather precise estimators of marginal single and double failure hazard functions are needed for a nonparametric assessment of dependency between a pair of censored failure time variates. The same features seen in Table 3.3 were evident if the Volterra or Dabrowska estimators substituted for thc Prentice–Cai estimator.

3.5 Additional Estimators and Estimation Perspectives

3.5.1 *Additional bivariate survivor function estimators*

As noted above, semiparametric estimators may also be considered for estimation of the survivor function F. For example, with absolutely continuous failure times (T_1,T_2) one could use likelihood maximization to apply the Clayton–Oakes model (1.7) with nonparametric marginals. The related constancy of the corresponding cross ratio function may be too restrictive for many applications, but this model can be extended (Nan, Lin, Lisabeth, & Harlow, 2006) to allow the cross ratio to vary over a fixed grid defined by the elements of partitions of the T_1 and T_2 axes. Specifically, if $a_{11},a_{12},\ldots$ denote the cut points for a partition of the T_1 axis, while $a_{21},a_{22},\ldots$ denote T_2 axis cut points, while $a_{10} = a_{20} = 0$, then a constant cross ratio $1+\gamma_{\ell m}$ at all continuity points in $\Omega_{\ell m} = (a_{1,\ell-1},a_{1\ell}] \times (a_{2,m-1},a_{2m}]$ is implied by the survivor function model

$$F(t_1,t_2) = \{F(t_1,a_{2,m-1})^{-\gamma_{\ell m}} + F(a_{1,\ell-1},t_2)^{-\gamma_{\ell m}} - F(a_{1,\ell-1},a_{2,m-1})^{-\gamma_{\ell m}}\}^{-1/\gamma_{\ell m}} \vee 0. \tag{3.16}$$

for all (ℓ,m).

This class of models can presumably provide a good fit to many data sets. Log-likelihood derivatives can be calculated recursively for joint estimation of marginal hazard rates in intervals defined by uncensored observations for the two time variables, and corresponding asymptotic theory for marginal hazard rate and cross ratio parameters is available and can be expected to provide good approximations to the distribution of parameter estimates if the number of double failures within each $\Omega_{\ell m}$

Table 3.3 *Simulation summary statistics for the average cross ratio estimation* ($\hat{C}$) *and average concordance estimator* ($\hat{\mathscr{T}}$) *under the sampling configurations of Table 3.1 with* $\theta = 2$*, using the Prentice–Cai estimator* $\hat{F}_{PC}$.

Clayton–Oakes Parameter			$\theta = 2$			
Sample size (n)			500	1000	250	250
Percent Uncensored: T_1, T_2 and (T_1, T_2)			16.7 16.7 2.8	16.7 16.7 2.8	33.3 33.3 11.1	100 100 100
		$C(t_1,t_2)$	$\hat{C}$ sample mean (sample standard deviation)			
$\{F(t_1,0), F(0,t_2)\}$	(0.85,0.85)	3	3.039 (0.984)	3.033 (0.671)	3.146 (1.071)	3.136 (0.884)
	(0.85,0.70)	3	3.091 (1.016)	3.027 (0.671)	3.128 (0.919)	3.098 (0.681)
	(0.85,0.55)	3	3.104 (1.310)	3.050 (0.848)	3.129 (0.959)	3.089 (0.594)
	(0.70,0.70)	3	3.132 (1.003)	3.015 (0.624)	3.089 (0.713)	3.057 (0.491)
	(0.70,0.55)	3	3.112 (1.300)	3.042 (0.787)	3.092 (0.720)	3.051 (0.426)
	(0.55,0.55)	3	3.217 (1.458)	3.095 (0.985)	3.100 (0.683)	3.030 (0.369)
		$\mathscr{T}(t_1,t_2)$	$\hat{\mathscr{T}}$ sample mean (sample standard deviation)*			
	(0.85,0.85)	0.5	0.475 (0.127)	0.491 (0.081)	0.484 (0.139)	0.493 (0.113)
	(0.85,0.70)	0.5	0.481 (0.125)	0.490 (0.079)	0.492 (0.109)	0.498 (0.083)
	(0.85,0.55)	0.5	0.472 (0.138)	0.488 (0.089)	0.492 (0.104)	0.500 (0.072)
	(0.70,0.70)	0.5	0.488 (0.112)	0.491 (0.072)	0.496 (0.082)	0.500 (0.060)
	(0.70,0.55)	0.5	0.475 (0.129)	0.489 (0.083)	0.496 (0.080)	0.500 (0.053)
	(0.55,0.55)	0.5	0.480 (0.134)	0.488 (0.095)	0.498 (0.075)	0.499 (0.046)

*Based on 1000 simulated samples at each sampling configuration. Samples contributed to summary statistics at all (t_1, t_2) values that were in the risk region of the data.

rectangle is not too small. The related calculations, however, are somewhat tedious and results may depend on choice of failure time axis partitions. Consequently this class of estimators does not appear to have received much use in applications.

Note that the Dabrowska estimator avoids negative mass if there is censoring on only one of the two failure time variates. Prentice (2014) considered a nonparametric estimator of F that applied the Dabrowska estimator to all data except doubly censored observations that are interior to the risk region of the data in a first stage, followed by the inclusion of the omitted doubly censored data using a self-consistency argument. Some benefit from this maneuver for estimating the failure distribution function $\underline{F}$, where

$$\underline{F}(t_1,t_2) = F(t_1,t_2) - F(t_1,0) - F(0,t_2) + 1$$

were suggested by simulation studies, but the possibility of negative mass assignments remained.

3.5.2 *Estimation perspectives*

While this chapter focuses on bivariate survivor function estimation, it seems that a focus on marginal single and double failure hazard rates may be preferable, with the Volterra nonparametric survivor function estimator from (3.5) and (3.6) as a consequence. This perspective is supported by the natural empirical estimators that obtain for the of set marginal hazard function estimators, and by the apparent competitive moderate and large sample properties of the Volterra estimator compared to other nonparametric survivor function estimators.

Additionally one can see that bivariate failure time data under independent right censorship directly support the estimation of these marginal single and double hazard rates, nothing more, nothing less. In fact the minimal requirement for the censoring to be "independent" is that the condition of no T_1 censoring in $[0,t_1)$ can be added without changing the marginal hazard rate $\Lambda_{10}(dt_1,0)$, the condition of no T_2 censoring in $[0,t_2)$ can be added without changing the marginal hazard rate $\Lambda_{01}(0,t_2)$, and the condition of no T_1 censoring in $[0,t_1)$ and no T_2 censoring in $[0,t_2)$ can be added without altering the double hazard rate $\Lambda_{11}(dt_1,dt_2)$, for all $t_1 \geq 0$ and $t_2 \geq 0$.

Along the same lines, one can consider that the principal value of bivariate failure time data, as compared to separate univariate failure time data sets, is in the ability to examine the double failure occurrence patterns. Such double failures may be of clinical interest as patients develop each of two important outcomes, or of public health interest as cohort study participants develop each of two study diseases. The rates of occurrence of such dual events may provide information and insights into intervention and disease mechanisms beyond marginal hazard rate analyses. Furthermore the marginal single and double failure hazard rate estimators come together to allow nonparametric estimation of related pairwise dependency functions as important byproducts. Perhaps most importantly, the nonparametric marginal single and double failure hazard rates of this chapter generalize readily to semiparametric models for these hazard rates given covariates, including covariates that are evolving in time. This approach is central to subsequent chapters.

Independent censoring relative to Λ_{11} requires censoring rates for the later of the two outcomes to be unaffected by the occurrence of the former. The plausibility of this assumption needs to be carefully considered for pairs of non-fatal outcomes, or for pairs comprised of a non-fatal followed by a fatal outcome. The assumption would be implausible if T_1 and T_2 were each composite outcomes having both fatal and non-fatal components, with fatal components that are not nested for the two variates. These issues will be discussed further in §4.9.2.

BIBLIOGRAPHIC NOTES

There is a long history of studies of nonparametric maximum likelihood approaches to bivariate survivor function estimation (Campbell, 1981; Hanley & Parnes, 1983; Tsai et al., 1986; van der Laan, 1996; Akritas & Van Keilegom, 2003; Prentice, 2014). Plug-in nonparametric estimators of this survivor function have been studied in Dabrowska (1988), Prentice and Cai (1992), and Gill et al. (1995). Gill and Johansen (1990) provide a detailed account of product integration, and describe the use of empirical process theory and stochastic integration to develop distribution theory for the Dabrowska estimator. Gill et al. (1995) extend this approach in a thorough manner to include each of the Volterra, Dabrowska and Prentice–Cai estimators. See Kalbfleisch and Prentice (2002, Chapter 10) for additional simulation comparisons, including other plug-in estimators (e.g., Campbell & Földes, 1982), whose moderate sample size efficiency is unfavorable compared to the three plug-in estimators highlighted here. Prentice (2014) applied self-consistency to develop an approach to the bivariate survivor function estimation, building on the work of (Efron, 1967) and (Tsai & Crowley, 1985). This approach relieved but did not eliminate the negative mass assignment issue. Van der Laan showed the potential of nonparametric maximum likelihood approaches to address this bivariate survivor function estimator problem in a nonparametric efficient manner. Nan et al. (2006) considered the use of constant cross ratio models over a grid for the analysis of bivariate failure time data as did Bandeen-Roche and Ning (2008). Fan, Hsu, and Prentice (2000) and Fan, Prentice, and Hsu (2000) consider estimators of dependency over a finite failure time region, including the average cross ratio and concordance measures described in §3.4.

EXERCISES AND COMPLEMENTS

Exercise 3.1

Develop the Volterra integral equation (3.4) from first principals for a discrete, continuous or mixed discrete and continuous failure time variate (T_1, T_2).

Exercise 3.2

By repeatedly replacing $F(s_1^-, s_2^-)$ on the right side of (3.4) using this same integral equation, and reversing the order of integration, see the Péano series representation

(3.5) emerge. Also show the equivalence of (3.3) and the usual product integral expression for the univariate survivor function.

Exercise 3.3

Consider discrete failure times (T_1, T_2). Show by massive cancellations that $Q(t_1, t_2)$ in (3.7) reduces to $F(t_1, t_2)/\{F(t_1, 0)F(0, t_2)\}$. See Dabrowska (1988) for the development of (3.7) with mixed discrete and continuous failure times.

Exercise 3.4

Show that inserting empirical estimators for all hazard rates in (3.9) into (1.6) gives the Dabrowska estimator (3.8). Show that the recursive calculation (3.9) then follows.

Exercise 3.5

Show that the concordance estimator (3.15) follows from (3.14) and the distribution shown for the componentwise minima.

Exercise 3.6

Show that each of the Volterra, Dabrowska and Prentice–Cai estimators reduces to the usual empirical estimator in the absence of censoring.

Exercise 3.7

Compute and display the empirical marginal single and double failure hazard rate estimators for the three small data sets ($n = 50$) shown below, obtained by generating observations randomly from the Clayton–Oakes model (1.7) with respective θ values of 3, 0 and -0.5 ($\theta + 1$ is the constant cross ratio). Unit exponential marginal failure distributions, and independent exponentially distributed censoring times that were independent of each other with a 1/3 probability of censoring, apply to each data set. Comment on, and contrast, the pattern of double failures, and the pattern of double hazard rate contours, for the three data sets.

Table 3.4 *Data simulated under Clayton–Oakes model (1.7) at various θ values and $n = 50$, with each observed time having a 1/3 probability of being censored.*

$\theta = 3$				$\theta = 0$				$\theta = -0.5$			
$S1$	$\delta 1$	$S2$	$\delta 2$	$S1$	$\delta 1$	$S2$	$\delta 2$	$S1$	$\delta 1$	$S2$	$\delta 2$
0.647	1	0.363	1	0.410	1	0.084	0	0.078	0	0.744	1
0.370	1	0.091	1	0.623	1	0.236	1	0.405	1	2.150	1
0.099	1	0.036	1	0.062	1	0.157	1	0.313	0	0.429	1
0.522	1	0.425	1	0.220	1	1.076	0	0.381	1	1.017	1
0.100	1	0.726	1	0.643	1	1.086	1	1.003	1	1.305	0
0.043	1	0.461	0	0.358	1	0.972	0	2.112	1	0.339	1
1.777	0	1.509	0	0.933	1	0.500	1	0.072	1	0.214	1
0.298	0	2.479	1	0.139	1	0.927	1	0.131	1	0.670	0
0.032	1	0.055	1	0.703	0	0.306	1	0.773	1	0.051	0
0.261	1	0.051	1	0.792	1	0.672	1	0.158	1	2.342	0
0.507	1	0.192	1	0.504	1	0.527	1	1.116	0	0.284	1
0.426	1	0.244	1	0.498	0	0.432	1	0.003	1	0.469	1
0.826	1	1.331	1	0.363	0	2.126	1	0.032	1	0.905	1
0.143	1	0.369	1	1.134	1	0.121	1	0.485	1	1.391	1
1.622	1	1.499	1	1.193	0	0.503	1	0.611	1	1.132	0
2.400	0	0.713	0	1.006	1	0.009	1	0.665	1	0.635	1
0.050	1	0.363	1	0.316	1	1.158	0	0.102	0	0.194	1
0.357	1	0.088	1	0.805	1	0.045	0	2.151	0	0.118	1
1.560	1	1.392	0	0.270	0	0.039	1	1.309	0	0.756	0
0.774	1	0.905	1	1.763	1	0.779	1	0.553	0	1.100	1
0.337	1	0.432	1	0.301	1	0.374	1	0.037	1	2.251	0
0.294	1	0.144	1	0.602	0	0.259	1	0.475	1	1.173	1
1.090	1	0.381	1	0.164	1	1.679	0	1.902	0	0.165	1
0.074	1	0.168	1	0.100	1	0.067	1	0.611	1	0.801	0
0.338	1	0.917	1	0.741	0	0.152	1	0.075	1	3.647	1
0.536	0	3.755	0	0.119	0	0.664	1	1.672	0	0.412	0
0.295	1	0.130	1	0.147	0	0.752	0	0.339	0	0.495	1
1.432	1	0.028	0	0.541	0	0.323	1	0.498	1	0.741	1
0.510	1	0.402	1	0.912	1	0.542	1	0.121	1	0.532	1
1.253	1	1.428	1	0.067	1	0.099	1	0.140	1	2.699	1
0.283	1	0.043	1	0.152	1	0.351	0	0.966	0	0.156	1
0.883	1	1.097	0	1.856	0	1.343	1	0.013	1	0.833	0
0.365	0	3.164	1	0.034	1	0.102	1	0.498	1	0.713	1
0.102	1	0.290	1	0.674	1	0.246	0	0.123	1	0.374	0
0.088	1	0.769	1	0.706	1	0.213	1	0.099	0	0.265	1
0.037	1	0.142	0	1.436	1	1.462	0	1.750	1	0.217	1
0.536	1	0.388	0	0.047	1	1.925	1	0.253	1	0.165	1
0.766	1	0.164	0	0.054	1	0.102	1	0.213	1	0.181	1
0.136	1	0.952	0	0.648	0	0.581	1	0.136	0	0.457	1
0.685	1	0.386	1	0.193	1	0.368	1	0.095	0	0.090	1
0.690	0	0.871	1	2.272	1	1.869	1	0.119	0	1.177	0
0.863	1	1.299	1	1.483	1	0.168	1	0.877	1	1.042	1
1.988	1	1.640	1	0.841	0	0.268	1	0.034	0	0.245	0
0.287	0	0.224	1	0.253	0	2.875	0	0.11	1	0.784	1
0.681	0	0.811	1	0.921	1	0.246	1	0.113	0	0.905	0
1.408	0	1.713	1	0.003	1	1.430	1	1.020	0	0.136	1
0.192	0	0.527	1	3.294	1	0.312	1	0.042	1	1.720	1
3.208	1	0.055	0	0.072	1	0.383	1	1.827	1	0.240	1
0.194	1	0.353	0	0.118	1	1.613	0	0.289	0	1.091	0
1.932	1	1.637	0	0.975	0	3.030	1	0.441	0	0.192	1

Chapter 4

Regression Analysis of Bivariate Failure Time Data

4.1 Introduction

Many applications of bivariate failure time data involve the evaluation of treatments, or assessments of study subject characteristics or exposures, in relation to the failure rates for two failure time variates $T_1 > 0$ and $T_2 > 0$. The time axes for these two variates may be the same or entirely unrelated. Some simplifications occur when the two time axes are the same, as will be discussed in Chapter 7.

As noted in Chapter 2, failure time regression data analysis methods are well developed for univariate failure time data, including analyses that examine hazard rates in relation to a preceding covariate history that may be evolving in time. With bivariate failure times we would like to extend these methods to the analysis of hazard rates in relation to a bivariate covariate $z(t_1,t_2)$ that takes value $\{z_1(t_1,t_2), z_2(t_1,t_2),\ldots\}$ at follow-up time (t_1,t_2). Let Z denote the (bivariate) covariate history up to time (t_1,t_2), so that $Z(t_1,t_2) = \{z(s_1,s_2); s_1 = t_1$ if $t_1 = 0, s_1 < t_1$ if $t_1 > 0$, and $s_2 = t_2$ if $t_2 = 0, s_2 < t_2$ if $t_2 > 0\}$. The sample paths for Z will be assumed to be continuous from the left, so that $Z(t_1,t_2)$ does not include jumps in the covariate process at (t_1,t_2). In this Chapter methods will be considered for relating hazard rates for T_1 and T_2 separately and jointly to their preceding covariate history.

Of particular interest will be methods for estimating marginal hazard rates $\Lambda_{10}\{dt_1,0;Z(t_1,0)\}$ for $t_1 \geq 0$ and $\Lambda_{01}\{0,dt_2;Z(0,t_2)\}$ for $t_2 \geq 0$ and double failure hazard rates $\Lambda_{11}\{dt_1,dt_2;Z(t_1,t_2)\}$ for $t_1 \geq 0$ and $t_2 \geq 0$ in relation to their preceding covariate histories. Analyses of this type will permit an assessment of covariate effects on marginal single and double failure hazard rates; and may also permit an assessment of the nature of dependency between T_1 and T_2 given Z, throughout the study follow-up period. It is useful to consider first the independent censoring conditions needed for estimating these hazard rate processes, and their relationship to the likelihood function for failure time distribution parameters.

4.2 Independent Censoring and Likelihood-Based Inference

Consider observations $S_{1k} = T_{1k} \wedge C_{1k}$, $\delta_{1k} = I[T_{1k} = S_{1k}]$, $S_{2k} = T_{2k} \wedge C_{2k}$, $\delta_{2k} = I[T_{2k} = S_{2k}]$ and $Z(S_{1k}, S_{2k})$, $k = 1,\ldots,n$, for a randomly selected cohort from a study population. As above, denote by Λ_{10} given Z and Λ_{01} given Z the marginal single outcome hazard processes given Z, and by Λ_{11} given Z the dual outcome hazard process given Z, so that

$$\begin{aligned}
\Lambda_{10}\{t_1,0;Z(t_1,0)\} &= \int_0^{t_1} \Lambda_{10}\{ds_1,0;Z(s_1,0)\} \text{ with} \\
\Lambda_{10}\{ds_1,0;Z(s_1,0)\} &= P\{T_1 \in [s_1,s_1+ds_1); T_1 \geq s_1; Z(s_1,0)\}, \\
\Lambda_{01}\{0,t_2;Z(0,t_2)\} &= \int_0^{t_2} \Lambda_{01}\{0,ds_2;Z(0,s_2)\} \text{ with} \\
\Lambda_{01}\{0,ds_2;Z(0,s_2)\} &= P\{T_2 \in [s_2,s_2+ds_2); T_2 \geq s_2, Z(0,s_2)\}, \text{ and} \\
\Lambda_{11}\{t_1,t_2;Z(t_1,t_2)\} &= \int_0^{t_1}\int_0^{t_2} \Lambda_{11}\{ds_1,ds_2;Z(s_1,s_2)\} \text{ with} \\
\Lambda_{11}\{ds_1,ds_2;Z(s_1,s_2)\} &= P\{(T_1,T_2) \in [s_1,s_1+ds_1) \times [s_2,s_2+ds_2); \\
&\qquad T_1 \geq s_1, T_2 \geq s_2, Z(s_1,s_2)\}. \quad (4.1)
\end{aligned}$$

Independent censoring requires that absence of T_1 censoring in $[0,s_1)$, of T_2 censoring in $[0,s_2)$, and of T_1 or T_2 censoring in $[0,s_1)\times[0,s_2)$ can be added, respectively, to the conditioning events in the above expressions without changing these hazard rates. These conditions ensure that marginal single and dual outcome hazard rates can be estimated by individuals at risk in the study cohort at $(t_1,0),(0,t_2)$ and (t_1,t_2) respectively for all (t_1,t_2) in the study follow-up period. Estimation of dual outcome hazard rates can add to information about the influence of treatments or exposures, encoded in Z, on the outcomes under consideration, beyond the standard single outcome hazard rate analyses described in Chapter 2.

In §4.6 we consider semiparametric Cox-type regression models for each of the hazard rates in (4.1), and a plug-in estimating equation approach is described for parameter estimation. In contrast, nearly all of the multivariate failure time literature uses a likelihood-based approach for regression modeling and estimation. A likelihood approach can begin with a specification of a joint probability model for the failure time and covariate processes, to which censoring is brought in under a "coarsening-at-random" assumption (e.g., van der Laan & Robins, 2003). This approach is attractive conceptually and offers the potential of efficient estimation of failure distribution parameters. However it can be quite challenging to develop the requisite probability models in the correct context; for example, dual outcome hazard rates Λ_{11} given Z are typically constrained in a complex manner by corresponding single outcome hazard rates and vice versa. To explore this interface further suppose that the covariate process is time-independent, so that $Z(t_1,t_2)\equiv z(0,0)$ or, if stochastic covariates are included they are external to the failure process in the sense that sample paths for Z are unaffected by the failure times (T_1,T_2). One can then entertain a joint survivor function F given Z, defined by

$$F\{t_1,t_2;Z(t_1,t_2)\}=\text{pr}\{T_1\geq t_1,T_2\geq t_2,Z(t_1,t_2)\}.$$

This joint survivor function can be expressed in terms of single and dual outcome hazard rates according to

$$F\{t_1,0;Z(t_1,0)\}=\prod_0^{t_1}[1-\Lambda_{10}\{ds_1,0,Z(s_1,0)\}],\text{ and}$$

$$F\{0,t_2;Z(0,t_2)\}=\prod_0^{t_2}[1-\Lambda_{01}\{0,ds_2,Z(0,s_2)\}]$$

on the coordinate axes, and

$$\begin{aligned}F\{t_1,t_2;Z(t_1,t_2)\}&=F\{t_1,0;Z(t_1,0)\}+F\{0,t_2;Z(0,t_2)\}-1\\&\quad+\int_0^{t_1}\int_0^{t_2}F\{s_1^-,s_2^-;Z(s_1,s_2)\}\Lambda_{11}\{ds_1,ds_2;Z(s_1,s_2)\}\end{aligned}$$

away from these axes. The latter expression is an inhomogeneous Volterra integral equation at any specified covariate history Z, with Péano series solution

$$F\{t_1,t_2;Z(t_1,t_2)\} = \Psi\{t_1,t_2;Z(t_1,0),Z(0,t_2)\} + \sum_{j=1}^{\infty} \int_0^{t_1}\int_{s_{11}}^{t_1}\cdots\int_{s_{1,j-1}}^{t_1}\int_0^{t_2}\int_{s_{21}}^{t_2}\cdots\int_{s_{2,j-1}}^{t_2} \Psi\{s_{11}^-,s_{21}^-;Z(s_{11},s_{21})\}\prod_{m=1}^{j}\Lambda_{11}\{ds_{1m},ds_{2m};Z(s_{1m},s_{2m})\}, \tag{4.2}$$

where $\Psi\{t_1,t_2;Z(t_1,0),Z(0,t_2)\} = F(t_1,0;Z(t_1,0)\} + F\{0,t_2;Z(0,t_2)\} - 1$, which generalizes (3.5). It follows that the joint survivor function F given Z is identifiable over the follow-up period of the study under the independent censoring conditions described above. In fact, the likelihood for F given Z can be written

$$L = \prod_{k=1}^{n}\Big(F\{dS_{1k},dS_{2k};Z_k(S_{1k},S_{2k})\}^{\delta_{1k}\delta_{2k}}[-F\{dS_{1k},S_{2k};Z_k(S_{1k},S_{2k})\}]^{\delta_{1k}(1-\delta_{2k})} [-F\{S_{1k},dS_{2k};Z_k(S_{1k},S_{2k})\}]^{(1-\delta_{1k})\delta_{2k}}F\{S_{1k},S_{2k};Z_k(S_{1k},S_{2k})\}^{(1-\delta_{1k})(1-\delta_{2k})}\Big). \tag{4.3}$$

The discerning reader might ask at this point "Since (4.3) is conveniently expressed in terms of the function F given Z, why not simply specify a convenient model for $F\{t_1,t_2;Z(t_1,t_2)\}$, rather than specifying single and dual outcome hazard functions given Z, and estimate model parameters by maximizing (4.3)?" This is essentially the copula approach to bivariate failure time regression.

4.3 Copula Models and Estimation Methods

4.3.1 Formulation

Still with fixed or external covariates, any of the univariate hazard rate regression models discussed in Chapter 2 could be used to define marginal hazard rate models $\Lambda_{10}\{dt_1,0;Z(t_1,0)\}$ and $\Lambda_{01}\{0,dt_2;Z(0,t_2)\}$, from which standardized variates

$$V_1 = \int_0^{T_1}\Lambda_{10}\{dt_1,0;Z(t_1,0)\} \text{ and } V_2 = \int_0^{T_2}\Lambda_{01}\{0,dt_2;Z(0,t_2)\}$$

can be defined. With absolutely continuous failure times, V_1 and V_2 will have unit exponential distributions. The copula approach to absolutely continuous bivariate failure time modeling then specifies a joint survivor function, $F_0(\cdot,\cdot;\theta)$ for (V_1,V_2) with parameter θ that governs the dependence between V_1 and V_2 given Z. Under this specification one can write

$$F\{t_1,t_2;Z(t_1,t_2)\} = F_0\left[\int_0^{t_1}\Lambda_{10}\{du_1,0;Z(u_1,0)\},\int_0^{t_2}\Lambda_{01}\{0,du_2;Z(0,u_2)\};\theta\right], \tag{4.4}$$

and can apply (4.3) for maximum likelihood estimation of marginal hazard rate parameters and the dependency parameter θ. The formulation is not conducive to allowing dependence between T_1 and T_2 given Z to depend on an evolving covariate, but the parameter θ can be allowed to depend on a baseline covariate vector $z = z(0,0)$.

There is a wealth of literature on possible choices of copula functions, with corresponding discussion of the nature of the dependencies between T_1 and T_2 that are implied by specific copula model specifications (e.g., Nelsen, 2007). Prominent examples include the Clayton–Oakes copula

$$F_0(v_1, v_2; \theta) = (e^{v_1\theta} + e^{v_2\theta} - 1)^{-1/\theta} \vee 0 \tag{4.5}$$

for $\theta \in [-1, \infty)$, and the normal transformation copula

$$F_0(v_1, v_2; \theta) = \phi\{\phi^{-1}(1 - e^{-v_1}), \phi^{-1}(1 - e^{-v_2}); \theta\} \tag{4.6}$$

for $\theta \in [-1, 1]$, where $\phi(\cdot)$ is the univariate standard normal density and $\phi\{\cdot, \cdot; \theta\}$ is the standard bivariate normal survivor function with correlation θ between the two standard normal variates. These are special cases of the class of Archimedean copulas. Both models approach the lower Fréchet and upper Fréchet boundaries as θ approaches the lower and upper extremes of its parameter space respectively, and both are absolutely continuous at all points away from these boundaries.

4.3.2 *Likelihood-based estimation*

The application of a copula model (4.4) to absolutely continuous, independently censored failure time regression data through maximization of (4.3) is conceptually simple since

$$\begin{aligned} F\{t_1, t_2; Z(t_1, t_2)\} &= F_0\{v_1, v_2; \theta(z)\}, \\ -F\{dt_1, t_2; Z(t_1, t_2)\} &= -F_0\{dv_1, v_2; \theta(z)\} dt_1/dv_1, \\ -F\{t_1, dt_2; Z(t_1, t_2)\} &= -F_0\{v_1, dv_2; \theta(z)\} dt_2/dv_2, \text{ and} \\ F\{dt_1, dt_2; Z(t_1, t_2)\} &= F_0\{dv_1, dv_2; \theta(z)\}(dt_1/dv_1)(dt_2/dv_2), \end{aligned}$$

where

$$\begin{aligned} v_1 &= \int_0^{t_1} \Lambda_{10}\{du_1, 0; Z(u_1, 0)\}, dt_1/dv_1 = 1/\Lambda_{10}\{dt_1, 0; Z(t_1, 0)\}, \\ v_2 &= \int_0^{t_2} \Lambda_{01}\{0, du_2; Z(0, u_2)\}, \text{ and } dt_2/dv_2 = 1/\Lambda_{01}\{0, dt_2; Z(0, t_2)\}. \end{aligned}$$

Maximum likelihood estimation with parametric models for marginal hazard rate and copula parameters then involves summing, over the sample, derivatives of the logarithms of these quantities with respect to parameters in $\Lambda_{10}\{\cdot, 0; Z(\cdot, 0)\}$ and $\Lambda_{01}\{0, \cdot; Z(0, \cdot)\}$, and θ. The maximum likelihood estimating function involves the derivative functions $F_0\{dv_1, v_2; \theta(z)\}, F_0\{v_1, dv_2; \theta(z)\}$ and $F_0\{dv_1, dv_2; \theta(z)\}$ in a rather intimate fashion, for all model parameters, suggesting a possible sensitivity of marginal hazard rate parameter estimates to the choice of F_0. This sensitivity can be avoided by a two-stage estimation procedure wherein parameters in the marginal hazard rate models are estimated first based on the respective marginal failure time data, then θ is estimated by maximizing (4.3) with all marginal hazard rate parameters fixed at the first stage estimates (e.g., Shih & Louis, 1995).

Much of the development work on bivariate failure time regression methods based on copula models has assumed the Clayton–Oakes copula (4.5), usually with $\theta \geq 0$ thereby precluding negative dependency between T_1 and T_2 given Z. This emphasis seems appropriate based on the useful interpretation of the copula parameter θ in terms of the cross ratio, which under the Clayton–Oakes model does not depend on the follow-up times, either in terms of the original variates (T_1, T_2) or the transformed variates (V_1, V_2). However, it may be awkward to specify fully parametric models for marginal hazard rates, and inadequate modeling may lead to biased estimators of marginal hazard rate regression parameters. Hence, regression estimation procedures in this context have typically used semiparametric procedures for marginal hazard rates, most notably Cox models. Pipper and Martinussen (2003), building on the approach used in Glidden and Self (1999), express the Clayton–Oakes model in a frailty model form (see §4.4) and derive likelihood-based estimating equations for marginal regression parameters and for the single cross ratio parameter that is assumed to not depend on covariates. Their development allowed clusters of more than two failure time variates under a rather restrictive higher dimensional version of the Clayton–Oakes model. Asymptotic distributional results required a specialized development because of the semiparametric modeling of marginal hazard rates. In simulation studies these authors showed that meaningful efficiency gain in marginal hazard ratio parameters relative to analyses based on marginal T_1 or T_2 data only, could be achieved under the assumed Clayton–Oakes model, if dependencies between T_1 and T_2 given Z were strong. However, this form of data analysis needs to be accompanied by the requirement that the cross ratio function is a constant independent of follow-up time for the failure time variates, and is also independent of regression variables, since otherwise bias may attend marginal hazard ratio parameter estimates.

Glidden (2000) considered this same statistical model, and focused on estimation of the cross ratio. Marginal hazard rates were estimated using standard Cox model estimating equations with a working independence model (given Z) between failure times. Asymptotic distributional results were obtained, and the cross ratio estimator behaved well in simulation studies. Simulations in Pipper and Martinussen (2003) show similar performance of Glidden's cross ratio parameter estimator with theirs.

4.3.3 *Unbiased estimating equations*

Prentice and Hsu (1997) consider a mean and covariance parameter estimating equation approach for marginal hazard ratio and corresponding dependency parameters. Specifically Cox model estimating equations, expressed in terms of marginal martingales as in (2.16), were considered for two or more failure time variates. The elements of these equations were weighted according to the inverse of the estimated covariance matrix for the set of marginal martingales for each study subject, with a corresponding set of unbiased estimating equations for marginal martingale covariance parameters. The pairwise covariance models were assumed to the take a form derived from a copula model for each pair of failure time variates. For example a Clayton–Oakes model could be assumed, with cross ratio of the form $1+\theta e^{x(0,0)\gamma}$, where $x(0,0) = \{x_1(0,0), x_2(0,0), \ldots\}$ is defined from $z(0,0)$ with possibly distinct θ and γ parameters for each pair of failure time variates. Asymptotic distribution theory was provided for estimates of marginal hazard ratio parameters, that may benefit in efficiency from the inverse covariance weighting, and for the dependency (e.g., cross ratio) parameters, which may be derived from estimating equations having an identity working weight matrix. Estimator performance was satisfactory in simulation studies.

The main limitation of this estimating equation approach is the need to specify a copula model to generate the model for marginal martingale covariances, and the related inability to allow dependencies between failure time variates given Z to depend on covariates that evolve over time. Simulation studies under pairwise Clayton–Oakes models indicated that the estimated cross ratio parameters approximately target an average cross ratio value over the study follow-up period, under departure from a cross ratio model that is time-independent.

Note that this estimating equation approach allows marginal hazard ratio regression parameters to have some components in common across failure times, and is readily adapted to settings in which baseline marginal hazard ratio functions are common among certain failure time variates. All of the methods described in this section also adapt readily to stratification of the baseline marginal hazard rates on covariate values, as in (2.11).

To summarize, the copula approach to bivariate failure time regression has some attractive features in terms of ease of application and parameter interpretation when the copula is well chosen. There are also some limitations: Most substantially, a copula model with a single or a low-dimensional parameter typically embraces only a modest class of dependencies between T_1 and T_2, given Z. For example, (4.5) gives a cross ratio of the form $1+\theta(z)$, where $z = z(0,0)$, at all continuity points (t_1,t_2). While this simple form is attractive for the interpretation of θ, it follows that the cross ratio function not only doesn't allow for an evolving covariate, but importantly does not depend on either time component throughout the failure time space. This may be acceptable with short follow-up periods and small failure rates, but some provision for temporal variations in the cross ratio can be expected to be needed in applications, as was evident for example, in the illustration of §3.4.2.

Related to this, Nan et al. (2006) generalize the Clayton–Oakes model to allow the cross ratio $1+\theta(z)$ to vary over the elements of a grid formed by fixed partitions of the time axes, in conjunction with Cox model marginals. This model, carefully applied, can presumably provide a good fit to many data sets, and can also allow the cross ratio to depend on covariate data $Z(a_1,a_2)$ where (a_1,a_2) is the lower left corner of rectangles in the failure time grid. However, the method requires the specification of time axis partitions that may be somewhat arbitrary, and may also require a moderately large number of double failures in each element of the failure time grid for good estimator behavior (Bandeen-Roche & Ning, 2008). Before considering even more general semiparametric models for single and dual outcome hazard rates it is instructive to consider the common approach to generating dependency models in statistics by means of random effects, which in the context of multivariate failure time data are usually referred to as frailties.

4.4 Frailty Models and Estimation Methods

A frailty modeling approach to bivariate failure time data analysis would assume that T_1 and T_2 are independent, given Z and a hypothetical shared frailty variate W, which is usually assumed to affect the hazard rates, given Z and W, in a multiplicative fashion. For example, Cox-type model marginal hazard rate models

$$\Lambda_{10}\{dt_1,0;Z(t_1,0),W\} = \Lambda_{10}(dt_1,0)W\exp\{x(t_1,0)\beta_{10}\}, \text{ and}$$
$$\Lambda_{01}\{0,dt_2;Z(0,t_2),W\} = \Lambda_{01}(0,dt_2)W\exp\{x(0,t_2)\beta_{01}\} \tag{4.7}$$

may be considered. The frailty variate W is hypothetical and not observed, and models for the joint survivor function F given Z, and for its related marginal single and dual outcome hazard rate functions, need to be induced by integrating over a specified distribution for W, a distribution that is usually taken to have mean one to allow parameter identifiability. A popular choice of frailty model is a gamma distribution that has been rescaled to have mean one and variance $\theta \geq 0$. Andersen et al. (1993, Chapter 9) give a detailed account of the induced hazard rates under a gamma frailty distribution, and note that an additional assumption that censoring rates are non-informative concerning W needs to be made. The induced marginal hazard rates under a gamma frailty distribution, as with most other mixing distributions involves the parameters in the frailty distribution. Hence, in this class of models the frailty parameters are not simply reflecting dependencies between T_1 and T_2 given Z, but also influence the marginal hazard rates. For this reason a frailty modeling approach may not be the best approach if primary interest resides in marginal hazard rate regression parameters. Hougaard (1986) proposed the use of an infinite mean positive stable frailty distribution to avoid implications of the frailty model parameter for marginal rates of proportional hazards form. Also, under a gamma frailty distribution a θ-dependent transformation on T_1 and T_2 leads to a copula model form (4.5) with $\theta \geq 0$ for the transformed variates in (4.7), providing another way of avoiding this problem in the special case of (4.5).

As a means of inducing marginal single and dual outcome hazard rate regression models frailty models with few parameters, like copula models, tend to embrace a rather limited class of dependencies, and are not conducive to allowing such dependencies to depend on evolving covariates. In addition the models induced for marginal single and dual outcome hazard rates are typically complex and related parameters may lack a ready interpretation.

Fundamentally, these issues arise because frailty models derive their parameter interpretation from models (4.7) that condition on the hypothesized frailty variate. As such they are suited to such purposes as the assessment of failure rate regression effects within "clusters" of correlated failure times, and to the estimation of frailty factors for specific clusters. These may be important analytic foci in some contexts as is illustrated by applications in the books by Hougaard (2000) and Duchateau and Janssen (2010). Also, the limited class of dependencies mapped out by a frailty distribution having a small number of parameters could potentially be offset by allowing the frailty factor in (4.7) to depend in some way on (t_1,t_2).

Rather than further reviewing these aspects of the frailty modeling approach, in §4.6 we consider models and methods for directly estimating marginal single and dual outcome hazard rate parameters, with bivariate failure time regression data. These are population-averaged inference targets. Univariate failure time regression data analyses are likely to apply hazard rate regression models, as discussed in Chapter 2. In many applications it would seem undesirable to change the target of marginal distribution inference, simply because data on one or more companion failure time variates and related covariates are also available for use in data analysis, arguing against a frailty modeling approach for these inferential targets.

4.5 Australian Twin Study Illustration

In §3.4.2 we saw that average cross ratios for age at appendectomy were larger at younger compared to older ages, for both monozygotic and dizygotic twins, in the Australia Twin Study illustration. Glidden (2000) applied a constant cross ratio model to these data, with marginal hazard ratio parameters estimated using Cox models as applied to the respective univariate failure time data. Cross ratio estimates (standard errors) of 2.80 (0.27) for MZ twins and 1.83 (0.25) for DZ twins were obtained. The unweighted estimating equation approach of Prentice and Hsu (1997) yielded similar values of 2.69 (0.25) and 1.82 (0.25) for MZ and DZ twins respectively. These cross ratio estimates presumably have an interpretation as average cross ratios over the study follow-up period, with averaging that is somewhat dependent on censoring, but they fail to reveal the noteworthy age dependencies for the cross ratio function, which may be important to the interpretation of study results.

4.6 Regression on Single and Dual Outcome Hazard Rates

4.6.1 *Semiparametric regression model possibilities*

In Sections 4.3 and 4.4 bivariate failure time regression models were considered, with dependency between T_1 and T_2 given Z modeled parametrically. One might alternatively hope to apply semiparametric regression models to describe such dependency, in conjunction with semiparametric regression models for marginal single failure hazard rates. Additionally, it would be desirable for the dependency models to accommodate external covariates that are evolving in relation to the time axes. Upon specifying such models, one could consider a likelihood-based estimation procedure that maximizes (4.3) over its semiparametric parameters.

While this likelihood maximization approach is simple conceptually, its application is not at all straightforward. For example, one could consider a semiparametric regression model for $\Lambda_{11}\{dt_1,dt_2;Z(t_1,t_2)\}$, along with semiparametric regression models for marginal hazard rates $\Lambda_{10}\{dt_1,0;Z(t_1,0)\}$ and $\Lambda_{01}\{0,dt_2;Z(0,t_2)\}$. However, even though F given Z can be uniquely expressed in terms of these quantities alone, as shown in §4.2, probability function positivity requirements place substantial constraints on the modeling of Λ_{11} given Λ_{10} and Λ_{01} (and given pertinent covariate histories), and vice versa, greatly complicating model specification for a likelihood-based approach. Alternatively, one could consider modeling covariance rates

$$\Omega_{11}\{dt_1,dt_2;Z(t_1,t_2)\} = \frac{[\Lambda_{11}\{dt_1,dt_2;Z(t_1,t_2)\} - \Lambda_{10}\{dt_1,t_2^-;Z(t_1,t_2)\}\Lambda_{01}\{t_1^-,dt_2;Z(t_1,t_2)]}{[1-\Lambda_{10}\{\Delta t_1,t_2^-;Z(t_1,t_2)\}][1-\Lambda_{01}\{t_1^-,\Delta t_2;Z(t_1,t_2)\}]}$$

in addition to marginal hazard rates, as $F\{\cdot,\cdot;Z(\cdot,\cdot)\}$ has an explicit expression as a function of these quantities. However, these covariance rates are also substantially restricted by the marginal single failure hazard rate specifications, and by related negative mass avoidance requirements, again complicating a likelihood maximization approach.

Semiparametric regression modeling of the cross ratio process $\alpha\{t_1,t_2;Z(t_1,t_2)\} = \Lambda_{11}\{dt_1,dt_2;Z(t_1,t_2)\}/[\Lambda_{10}\{dt_1,t_2^-;Z(t_1,t_2)\}\Lambda_{01}\{t_1^-,dt_2;Z(t_1,t_2)\}]$ is evidently free from such constraints with absolutely continuous failure times, but the absence of an explicit expression for $F\{t_1,t_2;Z(t_1,t_2)\}$ in terms of marginal hazard rates and cross ratios substantially complicates likelihood maximization using this modeling idea, and no such methodology has appeared in the literature.

In summary, there is currently no available likelihood maximization–based approach to bivariate failure time regression with flexible semiparametric models for marginal single failure hazard rates and corresponding dependency functions.

4.6.2 *Cox models for marginal single and dual outcome hazard rates*

Fundamentally, regression analysis of independently censored bivariate failure time data allows estimation of marginal single and double failure hazard rates, given corresponding, possibly evolving, covariate values. Hence, an alternative approach, building on the plug-in estimation approach described in Chapter 3, simply applies empirical-type estimators to regression models for marginal single and dual outcome hazard rates, and brings these together to estimate $F\{\cdot,\cdot;Z(\cdot,\cdot)\}$ and related quantities.

For absolutely continuous, discrete or mixed failure time variates (T_1,T_2), consider marginal single outcome hazard rate models

$$\Lambda_{10}\{dt_1,0;Z(t_1,0)\} = \Lambda_{10}(dt_1,0)\exp\{x(t_1,0)\beta_{10}\} \text{ for } t_1 \geq 0, \tag{4.8}$$

and

$$\Lambda_{01}\{0,dt_2;Z(0,t_2)\} = \Lambda_{01}(0,dt_2)\exp\{x(0,t_2)\beta_{01}\} \text{ for } t_2 \geq 0, \tag{4.9}$$

and also consider a Cox-type dual outcome hazard rate model

$$\Lambda_{11}\{dt_1,dt_2;Z(t_1,t_2)\} = \Lambda_{11}(dt_1,dt_2)\exp\{x(t_1,t_2)\beta_{11}\} \text{ for } t_1 \geq 0 \text{ and } t_2 \geq 0. \tag{4.10}$$

There are connections between (4.10) and the single outcome hazard models

(4.8) and (4.9), but the time-dependent modeling options for the regression vector $x(t_1,t_2) = \{x_1(t_1,t_2), x_2(t_1,t_2)\ldots\}$ formed from $\{(t_1,t_2)$ and $Z(t_1,t_2)\}$ provides the potential for a good fit of (4.10) to available data, as is the case also for the single outcome hazard rates through the specification of $x(t_1,0) = \{x_1(t_1,0), x_2(t_1,0),\ldots\}$ and $x(0,t_2) = \{x_1(0,t_2), x_2(0,t_2),\ldots\}$. Baseline stratification in (4.8)–(4.10) can add further valuable flexibility. If (4.8)–(4.10) each provide a good fit to available data, so will the corresponding estimator of F given Z and related quantities.

The parameters in (4.8)–(4.10) can be readily estimated in a manner analogous to (2.8) and (2.10) even when Z includes internal time-varying covariates. Specifically, subject to the adequacy of their respective models, β_{10} can be estimated as the solution, $\hat{\beta}_{10}$, to

$$\sum_{i=1}^{I}\left\{\sum_{k\in D(\Delta t_{1i},0)} x_k(t_{1i},0) - d_{i0}^{10}\frac{\sum_{k\in R(t_{1i},0)} x_k(t_{1i},0)e^{x_k(t_{1i},0)\beta_{10}}}{\sum_{k\in R(t_{1i},0)} e^{x_k(t_{1i},0)\beta_{10}}}\right\} = 0, \tag{4.11}$$

with $\hat{\Lambda}_{10}(t_1,0) = \sum_{t_{1i}\le t_1}\{d_{i0}^{10}/\sum_{k\in R(t_{1i},0)} e^{x_k(t_{1i},0)\hat{\beta}_{10}}\}$, for all $(t_1,0)\in R$;

β_{01} can be estimated as the solution, $\hat{\beta}_{01}$, to

$$\sum_{j=1}^{J}\left\{\sum_{k\in D(0,\Delta t_{2j})} x_k(0,t_{2j}) - d_{0j}^{01}\frac{\sum_{k\in R(0,t_{2j})} x_k(0,t_{2j})e^{x_k(0,t_{2j})\beta_{01}}}{\sum_{k\in R(0,t_{2j})} e^{x_k(0,t_{2j})\beta_{01}}} = 0\right\}, \tag{4.12}$$

with $\hat{\Lambda}_{01}(0,t_2) = \sum_{t_{2j}\le t_2}\{d_{0j}^{01}/\sum_{k\in R(0,t_{2j})} e^{x_k(0,t_{2j})\hat{\beta}_{01}}\}$ for all $(0,t_2)\in R$; and β_{11} can be estimated as the solution, $\hat{\beta}_{11}$, to

$$\sum_{i=1}^{I}\sum_{j=1}^{J}\left\{\sum_{k\in D(\Delta t_{1i},\Delta t_{2j})} x_k(t_{1i},t_{2j}) - d_{ij}^{11}\frac{\sum_{k\in R(t_{1i},t_{2j})} x_k(t_{1i},t_{2j})e^{x_k(t_{1i},t_{2j})\beta_{11}}}{\sum_{k\in R(t_{1i},t_{2j})} e^{x_k(t_{1i},t_{2j})\beta_{11}}}\right\} = 0, \tag{4.13}$$

with $\hat{\Lambda}_{11}(t_1,t_2) = \sum_{t_{1i}\le t_1}\sum_{t_{2j}\le t_2}\{d_{ij}^{11}/\sum_{k\in R(t_{1i},t_{2j})} e^{x_k(t_{1i},t_{2j})\hat{\beta}_{11}}\}$ for all $(t_1,t_2)\in R$, where, for example, $D(\Delta t_{1i},0)$ is the set of d_{i0}^{10} individuals failing at $T_1 = t_{1i}$, and $D(\Delta t_{1i},\Delta t_{2j})$ is the set of d_{ij}^{11} individuals having double failure at (t_{1i},t_{2j}).

With fixed or external time-dependent covariates the single and dual outcome hazard rate estimators can be brought together to estimate the survivor function semiparametrically, under (4.8)–(4.10), in a manner that extends the plug-in Volterra estimator of Chapter 3. At any uncensored data grid point $(t_{1i},t_{2j})\in R$ away from the coordinate axes one has

$$\hat{F}\{\Delta t_{1i},\Delta t_{2j};Z(t_{1i},t_{2j})\} = \hat{F}\{t_{1i}^-,t_{2j}^-;Z(t_{1i},t_{2j})\}\hat{\Lambda}_{11}\{\Delta t_{1i},\Delta t_{2j};Z(t_{1i},t_{2j})\}$$

from which

$$\hat{F}\{t_{1i},t_{2j};Z(t_{1i},t_{2j})\} = \hat{F}\{t_{1i},t_{2j}^-;Z(t_{1i},t_{2j}\} + \hat{F}\{t_{1i}^-,t_{2j};Z(t_{1i},t_{2j})\}$$
$$- \hat{F}\{t_{1i}^-,t_{2j}^-;Z(t_{1i},t_{2j})\}[1-\hat{\Lambda}_{11}\{\Delta t_{1i},\Delta t_{2j};Z(t_{1i},t_{2j})\}],$$

with $\hat{\Lambda}_{11}\{\Delta t_{1i},\Delta t_{2j};Z(t_{1i},t_{2j})\} = \hat{\Lambda}_{11}(\Delta t_{1i},\Delta t_{2j})\exp\{x(t_{1i},t_{2j})\hat{\beta}_{11}\}$, giving a simple recursive procedure, starting with

$$\hat{F}\{t_{1i},0;Z(t_{1i},0)\} = \prod_{\ell=1}^{i}[1-\hat{\Lambda}_{10}(\Delta t_{1\ell},0)e^{x(t_{1\ell},0)\hat{\beta}_{10}}] \text{ and}$$

$$\hat{F}\{0,t_{2j};Z(0,t_{2j})\} = \prod_{m=1}^{j}[1-\hat{\Lambda}_{01}(0,\Delta t_{2m})e^{x(0,t_{2m})\hat{\beta}_{01}}],$$

for estimating F by the step function $\hat{F}\{t_1,t_2;Z(t_1,t_2)\}$ at any $(t_{1i},t_{2j}) \in R$ at any covariate history Z.

4.6.3 Dependency measures given covariates

From these estimates, one can estimate average cross ratios $C\{\tau_1,\tau_2;Z(\tau_1,\tau_2)\}$ given Z, over $[0,\tau_1]\times[0,\tau_2]$ with $(\tau_1,\tau_2)\in R$, analogous to (3.13) via

$$\hat{C}\{\tau_1,\tau_2;Z(\tau_1,\tau_2)\} = \int_0^{\tau_1}\int_0^{\tau_2} \hat{F}\{t_1^-,t_2^-;Z(t_1,t_2)\}\hat{\Lambda}_{11}\{dt_1,dt_2;Z(t_1,t_2)\} \Big/$$
$$\int_0^{\tau_1}\int_0^{\tau_2} \hat{F}\{t_1^-,t_2^-;Z(t_1,t_2)\}\hat{\Lambda}_{10}\{dt_1,t_2^-;Z(t_1,t_2)\}\hat{\Lambda}_{01}\{t_1^-,dt_2;Z(t_1,t_2)\}$$

and estimate concordances between T_1 and T_2 over $[0,\tau_1]\times[0,\tau_2]$, given Z, analogous to (3.15), by

$$\hat{\mathscr{T}}\{\tau_1,\tau_2;Z(\tau_1,\tau_2)\} = \Big[\int_0^{\tau_1}\int_0^{\tau_2} \hat{F}\{t_1^-,t_2^-;Z(t_1,t_2)\}\hat{F}\{dt_1,dt_2;Z(t_1,t_2)\}$$
$$- \int_0^{\tau_1}\int_0^{\tau_2} \hat{F}\{dt_1,t_2^-;Z(t_1,t_2)\}\hat{F}\{t_1^-,dt_2;Z(t_1,t_2)\}\Big] \Big/$$
$$\Big[\int_0^{\tau_1}\int_0^{\tau_2} \hat{F}\{t_1^-,t_2^-;Z(t_1,t_2)\}\hat{F}\{dt_1,dt_2;Z(t_1,t_2)\}$$
$$+ \int_0^{\tau_2}\int_0^{\tau_2} \hat{F}\{dt_1,t_2^-;Z(t_1,t_2)\}F\{t_1^-,dt_2;Z(t_1,t_2)\}\Big].$$

These estimates can be used, for example, to examine how the strength of dependency between T_1 and T_2 varies with Z, or to examine how the strength of dependency, given Z, varies over the follow-up period of a study.

If Z includes internal stochastic covariates then F given Z typically lacks a survivor function interpretation. Whether or not the estimators $\hat{C}$ given Z and $\hat{\mathscr{T}}$ given Z provide useful basis for assessing residual dependence between T_1 and T_2 after allowing for Z that includes internal covariates, is a question for future research.

4.6.4 Asymptotic distribution theory

Any of the hazard rate models (4.8)–(4.10) may be misspecified, and the dual outcome hazard rate regression model need not be mutually consistent with the single outcome hazard rate regression models. Nonetheless the solutions

$\{\hat{\beta}_{10}, \hat{\beta}_{01}, \hat{\beta}_{11}, \hat{\Lambda}_{10}(\cdot,0), \hat{\Lambda}_{01}(0,\cdot), \hat{\Lambda}_{11}(\cdot,\cdot)\}$ quite generally have a joint asymptotic Gaussian distribution over $(t_1,t_2) \in [0,\tau_1] \times [0,\tau_2]$ with (τ_1,τ_2) in the support of the observed times (S_1,S_2). In applications one can expect some asymptotic bias in these estimators relative to parameters in (4.8)–(4.10) because of regression model misspecification, but as noted above, if each such model is in reasonably good agreement with the data, then this agreement can also be expected to extend to estimators $\hat{F}$ given Z and to related processes derived from $\hat{F}$, such as average cross ratio and concordance estimators, given Z with fixed or external covariates.

The block diagonal Hessian matrix $\hat{I}(\beta) = \text{diag}\{\hat{I}_{10}(\beta_{10}), \hat{I}_{01}(\beta_{01}), \hat{I}_{11}(\beta_{11})\}$, where, for example,

$$\hat{I}_{10}(\beta_{10}) = \sum_{i=1}^{I} d_{i0}^{10} \left[\frac{\sum_{k\in D(t_{1i},0)} x_k(t_{1i},0)' x_k(t_{1i},0) e^{x_k(t_{1i},0)\beta_{10}}}{\sum_{\ell\in R(t_{1i},0)} e^{x_k(t_{1i},0)\beta_{10}}} - \left\{ \frac{\sum_{k\in R(t_{1i},0)} x_k(t_{1i},0)' e^{x_k(t_{1i},0)\beta_{10}}}{\sum_{k\in R(t_{1i},0)} e^{x_k(t_{1i},0)\beta_{10}}} \right\}^{\otimes 2} \right],$$

and

$$\hat{I}_{11}(\beta_{11}) = \sum_{i=1}^{I}\sum_{j=1}^{J} d_{ij}^{11} \left[\frac{\sum_{k\in R(t_{1i},t_{2j})} x_k(t_{1i},t_{2j})' x_k(t_{1i},t_{2j}) e^{x_k(t_{1i},t_{2j})\beta_{11}}}{\sum_{\ell\in R(t_{1i},t_{2j})} e^{x_k(t_{1i},t_{2j})\beta_{11}}} - \left\{ \frac{\sum_{k\in R(t_{1i},t_{2j})} x_k(t_{1i},t_{2j}) e^{x_k(t_{1i},t_{2j})\beta_{11}}}{\sum_{k\in R(t_{1i},t_{2j})} e^{x_k(t_{1i},t_{2j})\beta_{11}}} \right\}^{\otimes 2} \right],$$

that derives from differentiating the negative of left sides of (4.11)–(4.13) with respect to $\beta = (\beta_{10}', \beta_{01}', \beta_{11}')'$, can be used in a Newton procedure to compute $\hat{\beta} = (\hat{\beta}_{10}', \hat{\beta}_{01}', \hat{\beta}_{11}')'$.

Note, however, that $\hat{I}(\hat{\beta})^{-1}$ will typically not provide a consistent variance estimator for $\hat{\beta}$ because of the possibility of discrete elements in the distribution of (T_1,T_2) given Z, and because of a lack of complete ordering of the bivariate space, precluding the type of conditioning argument used in §2.3 for estimating the variance of $\hat{\beta}_{11}$. However, as detailed below, a sandwich-form variance estimator for $\hat{\beta}$ can be calculated.

For asymptotic distribution theory development, over a follow-up period $[0,\tau_1] \times [0,\tau_2]$, where (τ_1,τ_2) is in the support of (S_1,S_2) given Z, it is convenient to reconstrue (4.11)–(4.13) as

$$\sum_{k=1}^{n} \int_0^{\tau_1} \{x_k(t_1,0) - E_{10}(t_1,0;\beta_{10})\} M_{10k}(dt_1,0;\beta_{10}) = 0 \tag{4.14}$$

$$\sum_{k=1}^{n} \int_0^{\tau_2} \{x_k(0,t_2) - E_{01}(0,t_2;\beta_{01})\} M_{01k}(0,dt_2;\beta_{01}) = 0, \text{ and} \tag{4.15}$$

$$\sum_{k=1}^{n} \int_0^{\tau_1}\int_0^{\tau_2} \{x_k(t_1,t_2) - E_{11}(t_1,t_2;\beta_{11})\} M_{11k}(dt_1,dt_2;\beta_{11}) = 0 \tag{4.16}$$

where, for example,

$$E_{10}(t_1,0;\beta_{10}) = n^{-1}\sum_{\ell=1}^{n} Y_{1\ell}(t_1)x_\ell(t_1,0)\exp\{x_\ell(t_1,0)\beta_{10}\} \Big/ \left[n^{-1}\sum_{\ell=1}^{n} Y_{1\ell}(t_1)\exp\{x_\ell(t_1,0)\beta_{10}\}\right], \tag{4.17}$$

$$E_{11}(t_1,t_2;\beta_{11}) = n^{-1}\sum_{\ell=1}^{n} Y_{1\ell}(t_1)Y_{2\ell}(t_2)x_\ell(t_1,t_2)\exp\{x_\ell(t_1,t_2)\beta_{11}\} \Big/ \left[n^{-1}\sum_{\ell=1}^{n} Y_{1\ell}(t_1)Y_{2\ell}(t_2)\exp\{x_\ell(t_1,t_2)\beta_{11}\}\right], \tag{4.18}$$

$$M_{10k}(dt_1,0;\beta_{10}) = N_{1k}(dt_1) - Y_{1k}(t_1)\exp\{x_k(t_1,0)\beta_{10}\}\Lambda_{10}(dt_1,0),$$
$$M_{01k}(0,dt_2;\beta_{01}) = N_{2k}(dt_2) - Y_{2k}(t_2)\exp\{x_k(0,t_2)\beta_{01}\}\Lambda_{01}(0,dt_2),$$
$$M_{11k}(dt_1,dt_2;\beta_{11}) = N_{1k}(dt_1)N_{2k}(dt_2) - Y_{1k}(t_1)Y_{2k}(t_2)\exp\{x_k(t_1,t_2)\beta_{11}\}\Lambda_{11}(dt_1,dt_2),$$

and where N_{1k}, N_{2k}, Y_{1k} and Y_{2k} are the counting and at-risk processes for the kth individual. See Exercise (4.6) for elaboration of the arguments leading to (4.14)–(4.16).

It turns out that the centering processes E_{10}, E_{01} and E_{11} in (4.14)–(4.16) can be replaced under mild conditions by e_{10}, e_{01}, and e_{11} where, for example, e_{10} is the ratio of the expectation of the numerator to the expectation of the denominator in (4.17) and e_{11} is similarly the ratio of the numerator expectation to denominator expectation in (4.18), without affecting the asymptotic distribution of the left sides of (4.14)–(4.16). This property is shown for (4.14) and (4.15), in a more general context using empirical process methods, in Spiekerman and Lin (1998), and their methods extend readily to two dimensions for (4.16). Having made these replacements, and assuming that $\{N_{1k}, Y_{1k}, N_{2k}, Y_{2k}, Z(S_{1k}, S_{2k})\}$ are independent and identically distributed for $k = 1, \ldots, n$, one has that the left sides of (4.14)–(4.16) are summations over IID random variables to which, following standardization by $n^{-1/2}$ factors, the central limit theorem can be applied. It follows readily that the standardized left sides of (4.14)–(4.16) converge to a mean zero Gaussian process under (4.8)–(4.10), with variance

$$A(\beta) = E\begin{pmatrix} \int_0^{\tau_1}\{x(t_1,0) - e_{10}(t_1,0;\beta_{10})\}M_{10}(dt_1,0;\beta_{10}) \\ \int_0^{\tau_2}\{x(0,t_2) - e_{01}(0,t_2;\beta_{01})\}M_{01}(0,dt_2;\beta_{01}) \\ \int_0^{\tau_1}\int_0^{\tau_2}\{x(t_1,t_2) - e_{11}(t_1,t_2;\beta_{11})\}M_{11}(dt_1,dt_2;\beta_{11}) \end{pmatrix}^{\otimes 2}$$

where E denotes expectation.

The consistency of $\hat\beta_{10}, \hat\beta_{01}$, and $\hat\beta_{11}$ as estimators of β_{10}, β_{01} and β_{11} follows from the fact that the solutions to (4.11)–(4.13) each maximize a function that can be shown to be uniquely maximized at the true regression parameter with probability approaching one as the sample size becomes large. The arguments are very similar to those applied to (2.17), using the mean zero properties of M_{10}, M_{01} and M_{11} under (4.8)–(4.10), almost sure bounded total variation constraints on the modeled covariates, and the strong embedding theorem of Shorack and Wellner (1986) (see Appendix A).

A Taylor series expansion

$$n^{1/2}(\hat{\beta}-\beta)=\{I(\beta^*)/n\}^{-1}n^{-1/2}U(\beta)$$

where $U(\beta)$ refers to the left sides of (4.11)–(4.13) and the elements of β^* are on the line segment between the true β element and the corresponding element of $\hat{\beta}$, then yields an asymptotic distribution for $n^{1/2}(\hat{\beta}-\beta)$ that has mean zero and variance consistently estimated by

$$\{\hat{I}(\hat{\beta})/n\}^{-1}\hat{A}(\hat{\beta})\{\hat{I}(\hat{\beta})/n\}^{-1} \tag{4.19}$$

assuming that the semidefinite matrices $\hat{I}_{10}(\beta_{10}), \hat{I}(\beta_{01})$ and $\hat{I}(\beta_{11})$ each approach a positive definite matrix at the pertinent true β-value as $n \to \infty$. Also in this sandwich variance formula is the empirical estimator

$$\hat{A}(\hat{\beta})=\frac{1}{n}\sum_{k=1}^{n}\begin{pmatrix} \int_0^{\tau_1}\{x_k(t_1,0)-E_{10}(t_1,0;\hat{\beta}_{10})\}\hat{M}_{10k}(dt_1,0;\hat{\beta}_{10}) \\ \int_0^{\tau_2}\{x_k(0,t_2)-E_{01}(0,t_2;\hat{\beta}_{01})\}\hat{M}_{01k}(0,dt_2;\hat{\beta}_{01}) \\ \int_0^{\tau_1}\int_0^{\tau_2}\{x_k(t_1,t_2)-E_{11}(t_1,t_2;\hat{\beta}_{11})\}\hat{M}_{11k}(dt_1,dt_2;\hat{\beta}_{11}) \end{pmatrix}^{\otimes 2}$$

and the hat on M_{10k}, M_{01k} and M_{11k} refers to evaluation at baseline rates $\hat{\Lambda}_{10}$, $\hat{\Lambda}_{01}$ and $\hat{\Lambda}_{11}$ respectively. In fact, the asymptotic Gaussian convergence extends to joint mean zero Gaussian field convergence for $n^{1/2}(\hat{\Lambda}_{10}-\Lambda_{10})$, $n^{1/2}(\hat{\Lambda}_{01}-\Lambda_{01})$ and $n^{1/2}(\hat{\Lambda}_{11}-\Lambda_{11})$ under a small extension of the empirical process–based developments in Spiekerman and Lin (1998). Specifically, these standardized processes collectively converge in probability to a sum of IID mean zero random processes to which the central limit theorem applies. A corresponding sandwich covariance function estimator leads to pointwise confidence intervals for baseline hazard rates. These results extend to hazard processes at a general covariate history Z by suitable recentering of the modeled regression variables. Furthermore, these asymptotic Gaussian results for parameters in any one of (4.8)–(4.10) continue to apply under departure from the other two hazard rate models. Also, the IID contributions of each individual can be perturbed by multiplying by a standard normal variate that is independent among individuals, and is independent of all available data, leading to a resampling procedure for more general inference on the three hazard processes. This can be used, for example, for confidence band estimation for baseline hazard rates at any specified covariate history Z. These developments are described in considerable detail in Spiekerman and Lin (1998) and Lin et al. (2000), with extensions to include dual outcome hazard rates in Prentice and Zhao (2019).

4.6.5 Simulation evaluation of marginal hazard rate estimators

In this section we consider some moderate sample size properties of the semiparametric (Cox) model estimation of single and dual outcome hazard rates procedures described in Subsections 4.6.2–4.6.4. To do so, absolutely continuous failure times, given a fixed covariate vector $z = (z_1, z_2, \ldots)$, were generated under a Clayton–Oakes survivor function model

$$F(t_1,t_2;z) = \{F_0(t_1,0)^{-\theta \exp\{z(\beta_{10}-\gamma)\}} + F_0(0,t_2)^{-\theta \exp\{z(\beta_{01}-\gamma)\}} - 1\}^{-e^{z\gamma}/\theta} \quad (4.20)$$

for $\theta \geq 0$, where F_0 denotes the survivor function at $z = 0$. The resulting failure time variates have Cox model marginal hazard rates $\Lambda_{10}(dt_1,0;z) = \Lambda_{10}(dt_1,0)e^{z\beta_{10}}$ and $\Lambda_{01}(0,dt_2;z) = \Lambda_{01}(0,dt_2)e^{z\beta_{01}}$ and corresponding local cross ratios

$$\Lambda_{11}(dt_1,dt_2;z)/\{\Lambda_{10}(dt_1,t_2;z)\Lambda_{01}(t_1,dt_2;z)\} = 1 + \theta e^{-z\gamma}$$

that do not depend on (t_1,t_2).

The rather special case where $\beta_{10} = \beta_{01} = \gamma$ is of interest in that the induced dual outcome hazard rates are then

$$\Lambda_{11}(dt_1,dt_2;z) = \Lambda_{11}(dt_1,dt_2)e^{z\gamma}(e^{z\gamma}+\theta)/(1+\theta), \quad (4.21)$$

which is also of Cox model form with dual outcome hazard ratio $e^{z\gamma}(e^{z\gamma}+\theta)/(1+\theta)$ that is also independent of (t_1,t_2). Hence for a binary covariate z the dual outcome hazard rate function conforms to (4.10) with hazard ratio $e^{\beta_{11}} = e^{\gamma}(e^{\gamma}+\theta)/(1+\theta)$ under this model.

Data for various parameter values (β,θ) and various sample sizes n were generated under this special case of (4.20), with unit exponential marginal survivor functions at $z = 0$, with exponentially distributed censoring variates that were independent of each other and of the failure time variates, at each value of a binary variate z, that took values 0 and 1 with probability 0.5. Censoring was introduced by specifying exponential censoring distributions with rate parameters equal to 5 for each of C_1 and C_2, or no censoring.

Table 4.1 shows simulation summary statistics for $(\hat{\beta}_{10}, \hat{\beta}_{01}, \hat{\beta}_{11})$ at (θ,γ) values of $(2,0)$ and $(2,\log 2)$ and sample sizes of $n = 500$ or 1000 with substantial censoring or $n = 250$ with no censoring. These simulations provide little evidence of bias in regression parameter estimates even though there are only about 27 expected double failures at $(\theta,\gamma) = (2,0)$ with censoring at $n = 500$. Table 4.1 also provides regression simulation summary statistics for the sample mean of standard deviation estimates derived from the sandwich variance estimator (4.19), along with corresponding asymptotic 95% confidence coverage rates from the same simulations. The average of standard deviation estimates based on (4.19) was close to corresponding sample standard deviation estimates, and asymptotic 95% confidence integrals had close to nominal coverage rates under these sampling configurations.

Table 4.2 shows corresponding summary statistics for survivor function estimators $\hat{F}$ and for the average cross ratio and concordance estimators $\hat{C}$ and $\hat{\mathscr{T}}$ at selected percentiles of the marginal distributions for T_1 and T_2 at $(\theta,\gamma) = (2,\log 2)$, at both $z = 0$ and $z = 1$. The survivor function estimates do not show evidence of bias, as was also the case at smaller sample sizes (e.g., = 250) with substantial censoring, at either z-value. Average cross ratio estimates tend to be somewhat upward biased, and average concordance estimates somewhat downward biased under the configuration

Table 4.1 *Simulation summary statistics for marginal single outcome hazard ratio parameters β_{10} and β_{01} and for dual outcome hazard ratio parameter β_{11}, and for related estimators from sandwich-form variance estimators, under the Clayton–Oakes model (4.20) with $\beta_{10} = \beta_{01} = \gamma$ and a binary covariate z. This model implies marginal hazard ratio (for $z = 1$ versus $z = 0$) of e^{γ} for both T_1 and T_2, and double failure hazard ratio of $e^{\gamma}(e^{\gamma} + \theta)/(1+\theta)$.*

		($\theta = 2, \gamma = 0$)											
Sample size (n)		500				1000				250			
T_1 and T_2 failing %		16.7				16.7				100			
Double failure %		5.3				5.3				100			
	True	Sample[a] Mean	Sample[b] SD	Sand.[b] SD	95% CI[b] Cov.	Sample Mean	Sample SD	Sand. SD	95% CI Cov.	Sample Mean[a]	Sample SD	Sand. SD	95% CI Cov.
β_{10}	0	0.006	0.227	0.222	0.951	−0.002	0.160	0.156	0.947	0.000	0.126	0.127	0.950
β_{01}	0	−0.008	0.224	0.221	0.952	0.000	0.157	0.156	0.948	0.000	0.128	0.127	0.946
β_{11}	0	−0.007	0.440	0.420	0.949	−0.004	0.293	0.289	0.957	−0.002	0.169	0.167	0.947
		($\theta = 2, \gamma = \log 2$)											
Sample size (n)		500				1000				250			
T_1 and T_2 failing %		22.6				22.6				100			
Double failure %		8.2				8.2				100			
β_{10}	0.693	0.705	0.203	0.198	0.941	0.695	0.145	0.139	0.940	0.698	0.135	0.134	0.947
β_{01}	0.693	0.697	0.199	0.197	0.955	0.693	0.139	0.139	0.951	0.698	0.135	0.133	0.945
β_{11}	0.981	1.004	0.381	0.364	0.951	0.976	0.259	0.259	0.951	0.989	0.192	0.186	0.945

[a]Based on 1000 simulations at each sampling configuration.

[b] Abbreviations: Sample SD is sample standard deviation of the regression parameter estimates; Sand. SD is the corresponding average of standard deviation estimates derived from the sandwich form estimation of variance for $\hat{\beta}$, and 95% CI Cov. is the fraction of simulated samples from which the approximate 95% confidence interval, formed from $\hat{\beta}$ and its sandwich-form variance estimator, includes the true β.

Table 4.2 *Simulation summary statistics for survivor function* ($\hat{F}$), *cross ratio* ($\hat{C}$) *and concordance* ($\hat{\mathcal{T}}$) *estimators at selected marginal survivor function percentiles under Clayton–Oakes model* (4.20) *with* $\beta_{10} = \beta_{01} = \gamma = \log 2$ *and cross ratio parameter* $\theta = 2$, *at both* $z = 0$ *and* $z = 1$.

Sample size (n)		1000	250		1000	250		1000	250
T_1 and T_2 censoring rate (%)		77.4	0		77.4	0		77.4	0
	F	$\hat{F}$		C	$\hat{C}$		$\mathcal{T}$	$\hat{\mathcal{T}}$	
$\{F(t_1,0;z), F(0,t_2;z)\}$		Mean (SD)*	Mean (SD)		Mean (SD)	Mean (SD)		Mean (SD)	Mean (SD)
					$z = 0$				
(0.85, 0.85)	0.752	0.752 (0.021)	0.754 (0.028)	3	3.075 (0.794)	3.090 (0.696)	0.5	0.492 (0.096)	0.498 (0.085)
(0.85, 0.70)	0.642	0.643 (0.029)	0.644 (0.034)	3	3.128 (0.951)	3.066 (0.550)	0.5	0.493 (0.107)	0.500 (0.067)
(0.85, 0.55)	0.521	0.521 (0.047)	0.522 (0.038)	3	3.282 (1.489)	3.058 (0.502)	0.5	0.490 (0.138)	0.501 (0.061)
(0.70, 0.70)	0.570	0.571 (0.039)	0.571 (0.037)	3	3.157 (1.071)	3.046 (0.460)	0.5	0.493 (0.117)	0.501 (0.055)
(0.70, 0.55)	0.480	0.481 (0.064)	0.480 (0.039)	3	3.200 (1.443)	3.039 (0.448)	0.5	0.486 (0.143)	0.500 (0.054)
(0.55, 0.55)	0.422	0.423 (0.102)	0.423 (0.040)	3	3.149 (1.802)	3.041 (0.448)	0.5	0.470 (0.169)	0.500 (0.054)
					$z = 1$				
(0.85, 0.85)	0.739	0.739 (0.020)	0.739 (0.032)	2	2.019 (0.532)	2.116 (0.880)	0.333	0.318 (0.122)	0.312 (0.186)
(0.85, 0.70)	0.623	0.623 (0.025)	0.624 (0.037)	2	2.020 (0.470)	2.086 (0.643)	0.333	0.324 (0.102)	0.327 (0.139)
(0.85, 0.55)	0.501	0.502 (0.032)	0.503 (0.039)	2	2.034 (0.533)	2.085 (0.570)	0.333	0.325 (0.108)	0.333 (0.119)
(0.70, 0.70)	0.538	0.538 (0.029)	0.540 (0.039)	2	2.002 (0.422)	2.069 (0.484)	0.333	0.324 (0.091)	0.335 (0.103)
(0.70, 0.55)	0.445	0.444 (0.035)	0.446 (0.040)	2	2.011 (0.476)	2.051 (0.419)	0.333	0.324 (0.097)	0.336 (0.090)
(0.55, 0.55)	0.379	0.379 (0.043)	0.380 (0.040)	2	2.029 (0.541)	2.036 (0.352)	0.333	0.326 (0.104)	0.336 (0.076)

*Sample mean and standard deviation (SD) based on 1000 simulated samples at each sampling configuration.

with no censoring. These biases disappear as the sample size at any particular configuration becomes large. They reflect somewhat asymmetric sampling distributions for $\hat{C}$ and $\hat{\mathscr{T}}$ in samples of moderate numbers of dual failures, and biases may be able to be reduced by simple transformation (e.g., apply asymptotic normal distributional approximation to $\log \hat{C}$ rather than to $\hat{C}$). See Prentice and Zhao (2019) for closely related simulations.

4.7 Breast Cancer Followed by Death in the WHI Low-Fat Diet Intervention Trial

In §1.7.5 a brief description was given of the Women's Health Initiative Dietary Modification randomized trial that contrasted a low-fat dietary pattern intervention (40%) with a usual diet comparison group (60%) in respect to various clinical outcomes. At the end of an 8.5-year average intervention period the Cox model hazard ratio estimate and asymptotic 95% confidence interval were 0.92 (0.84,1.01) with logrank significance level of $p = 0.09$, for the invasive breast cancer primary outcome, with 671 and 1093 breast cancer cases respectively in the intervention and comparison groups (Prentice et al., 2006). Similarly, the estimated hazard ratio (95% CI) for total mortality was 0.98 (0.91, 1.06) based on 989 and 1519 deaths in the respective randomization groups. These analyses stratify baseline rates on age at randomization in 5-year categories and randomization status in the companion hormone therapy trials (CEE active, CEE placebo, CEE + MPA active, CEE + MPA placebo, not randomized).

What can be said about the dual outcome of breast cancer and death? This outcome occurs only when death (from any cause) follows breast cancer. Also the two outcomes share the same follow-up time axis and have a potential censoring time equal to time from a randomization to the earlier of the end date for the intervention period (3/31/05) or for a small fraction of women, time to earlier loss to follow-up. Additionally, follow-up for breast cancer is discontinued at the time of death, for women who died without a breast cancer diagnosis. An independent censoring assumption in this context requires that death ascertainment does not change following a breast cancer diagnosis, a reasonable assumption here since all death ascertainment procedures, including matching to the U.S. National Death Index, continued for participating women throughout and beyond the intervention period.

The special structure of this composite outcome implies that dual outcomes occur along this single time axis (follow-up time from randomization) and occur at death following breast cancer, with censored times at the earlier of the cutoff time for data analysis, loss to follow-up or death without breast cancer. In analyses that stratify baseline rates for the dual outcome as for the single outcomes, the composite outcome of incident breast cancer followed by death from any cause had an estimated dual outcome hazard ratio (95% CI) of 0.64 (0.44, 0.93), with 40 and 94 women experiencing the dual event in the intervention and comparison groups during the intervention period. Hence, this composite outcome analysis provides stronger evidence of intervention benefit (logrank $p = 0.02$) than was the case for either outcome separately, in spite of a much smaller number of dual outcome events compared to either outcome separately. A corresponding analysis with outcome of death attributed to breast cancer gave a similar hazard ratio estimate of 0.67, but with broader 95% CI of (0.43, 1.06), and $p = 0.08$, since there were only 27 and 61 deaths attributed to breast cancer in the respective randomization groups. These results are perhaps not too surprising for an intervention that is hypothesized to reduce the risk of multiple important diseases, including breast cancer where any favorable influence may be larger for more serious subtypes (e.g., estrogen receptor–positive, progesterone receptor–negative tumors) or for which disease or associated treatments may affect the risk of death beyond that attributed to breast cancer itself. See Chlebowski et al. (2017) for a closely related analysis that regards breast cancer followed by death from any cause as a "marked" point process, and for additional subgroup analyses, and analyses over longer-term follow-up.

The dual outcome hazard ratios of the type just illustrated do not have any simple connection to the corresponding single outcome hazard ratios. The interpretation of dual outcome hazard ratio is essentially the same as that for the single outcome hazard ratio. For example, in the present illustration the rate with which postmenopausal US women develop breast cancer and die within an average 8.5 year follow-up period is lower by an estimated factor of $1.00 - 0.64 = 36\%$ in the dietary intervention group versus the comparison group. Furthermore the magnitude of this dual outcome hazard ratio can be examined in relation to the time from randomization to breast cancer diagnosis and time from breast cancer diagnosis to death by defining $x(t_1, t_2) = \{z, zt_1, z(t_2 - t_1)\}$ where z denotes intervention ($z = 1$) or comparison group ($z = 0$) randomization status in (4.10). The solution $\hat{\beta}_{11} = (0.184, 0.008, -0.125)'$ to (4.13) has corresponding sandwich standard error estimates of $(0.714, 0.117, 0.123)'$. A test of zero value for the two interaction coefficients, using the sandwich covariance estimator for $\hat{\beta}$ has significance level $p = 0.09$, providing some modest evidence of dual outcome hazard ratio variation over the study follow-up period. If the zt_1 interaction component is dropped leaving $x(t_1, t_2) = \{z, z(t_2 - t_1)\}$, one obtains $\hat{\beta}_{11} = (0.226, -0.220)$ with corresponding standard deviation estimates of $(0.346, 0.101)$, giving nominally significant ($p = 0.03$) evidence for a dual outcome hazard ratio that decreases with increasing time from breast cancer diagnosis to death. This is consistent with a recent trial report (Chlebowski et al., 2018) indicating improved post-diagnosis survival in the intervention versus comparison group. Note that these latter analyses condition on post-randomization information and therefore do not constitute a comparison between randomized groups. In contrast the dual outcome hazard ratio analyses described here do not involve such conditioning and enjoy intention-to-treat status, suggesting a DO-ITT (dual outcome intention-to-treat) acronym for this type of data analysis (with apologies to Nike!).

Similarly, with non-fatal outcomes one can, for example, define a hazard ratio regression model as $\{zI(t_1 < t_2), zI(t_1 \geq t_2)\}$ to compare dual outcome hazard ratios according to which outcome occurs first, potentially providing insight into intervention mechanisms. This modeling special case will be illustrated in Chapter 6.

4.8 Counting Process Intensity Modeling

In settings such as the WHI low-fat diet intervention trial just discussed, where T_1 and T_2 are on the same time axis and have a common censoring time $C_1 = C_2 = C$, one can also consider regression analyses based on modeling the counting process intensity. Specifically T_1 and T_2 can be considered as differing failure types, and type-specific failure rate regression models can be specified. For example, one might specify semiparametric models of the form

$$\Lambda_k(dt;H_t) = Y_k(t)\Lambda_k(dt)\exp\{x_k(t)\beta_k\} \tag{4.22}$$

for a type k hazard rate, $k = 1,2$, at follow-up time t. Here, the conditioning event H_t includes all failure, censoring and covariate information prior to time t, including the failure counting process history. Hence the rate of failure of a particular type is modeled conditional on the counting process prior to time t for the companion failure type. As a result the modeled covariate $x_k(t) = \{x_{k1},(t),\ldots,x_{kp}(t)\}$ needs to allow for possible dependence on whether or not the companion failure type has occurred and, also, on the timing of such occurrence. For example, in the above WHI breast cancer illustration, the all-cause mortality rate needs to be modeled according to whether or not the study participant has experienced an earlier breast cancer diagnosis during trial follow-up. One could relax (4.22) to allow a separate baseline mortality rate function $\Lambda_{21}(dt)$ or $\Lambda_{22}(dt)$ according to whether a breast cancer diagnosis had not occurred, or had occurred, prior to time t, and the corresponding regression parameter can be relaxed to β_{21} or β_{22} accordingly. Estimators of model parameters in (4.22), or in these generalizations, and associated distribution theory arise naturally from the procedures summarized in §2.9, as will be elaborated in a more general context in Chapter 7. Note, however, that the interpretation of hazard ratio parameters in these models may be quite different from that for regression parameters in (4.8)–(4.10), which model single and dual outcome hazard rates given preceding covariate histories, but not counting process histories for the potentially correlated times. Related to this, inference on intensity model parameters, such as β_{22} in the approach to all-cause mortality rates among women with a post-randomization breast cancer diagnosis, may often be of medical or scientific interest, but may typically lack the basis in randomization enjoyed by the single and dual outcome hazard ratio parameters in (4.8)–(4.10) in the low-fat diet trial. On the other hand, analyses based on (4.8)–(4.10) may typically require a stronger independent censoring condition than do those based on (4.22), since censoring rates in intensity process modeling can depend on the prior counting process information in the intensity rate definition. For example, in the breast cancer illustration, independent censoring using (4.8)–(4.10) would require censoring processes for mortality to be unaltered when a woman experiences a breast cancer diagnosis. As noted above, this is a plausible assumption in view of outcome ascertainment procedures that include National Death Index matching for all participating women throughout the study follow-up period.

4.9 Marginal Hazard Rate Regression in Context

4.9.1 Likelihood maximization and empirical plug-in estimators

There are several points concerning the single and dual outcome hazard rate regression models of §4.6 that merit additional comment. These are essentially empirical plug-in methods that extend the nonparametric estimators of §3.2 to include hazard ratio regression components for both single and dual hazard rates. As such they embrace models that may not be fully compatible with any probability model for the overall data. This feature may make it difficult to construct suitable simulation models to evaluate estimator performance. For example, we used the rather specialized model (4.20) with $\beta_{10} = \beta_{01} = \gamma$ to study moderate sample properties of single and dual hazard ratio parameter estimates. If $\beta_{10} = \beta_{01} = \gamma$ is relaxed under (4.20) one retains a constant hazard ratio for single outcome hazard rates but the dual outcome hazard ratio then has a complex form. Simulations reported in Prentice and Zhao (2019) show that survival probabilities given the binary covariate, z, can be well estimated under this more relaxed model simply by defining $x(t_1,t_2) = \{z, z\log t_1, z\log t_2\}$, or by other simple time-dependent modeling of the dual outcome hazard ratio.

One might expect, from a theoretical perspective, a likelihood-based estimation procedure would have advantages, including the possibility of semiparametric efficiency, compared to the proposed empirical plug-in approach. However, a likelihood-based approach for the type of data considered in this chapter may require complex calculations, and optimality properties may be realized very slowly, as $n \to \infty$, as is known to be the situation in the absence of regression variables for van der Laan's (1996) repaired maximum likelihood estimator of the bivariate survivor function. This estimator may have nonparametric efficiency properties, but it does not appear to materially improve upon the simple plug-in estimators discussed in Chapter 3.

A key feature of the single and dual outcome hazard ratio modeling approach is the ease of calculation and interpretation of hazard ratio parameters. These methods allow the user to extend the familiar hazard ratio interpretation from single outcomes to combined single and dual outcomes. Misspecified models for one or more of these hazard rate functions of course can lead to biases in corresponding regression parameter estimates, but doesn't affect the asymptotic distribution for hazard rate parameter estimates for the remaining hazard rate functions. As with univariate Cox model parameter estimates one can imagine applications that begin with simple proportionality assumptions for dual as well as single outcome hazard ratios for simple summary analyses, with product terms between measured covariates and the follow-up time variables subsequently included for more refined hazard ratio analyses.

4.9.2 Independent censoring and death outcomes

Many applications of single and dual outcome hazard ratio methods will involve outcome pairs on the same time axis on each study individual, as in §4.7. In such contexts the single and dual hazard rates can be implicitly regarded as conditioning on the continued survival of the individual at all follow-up times. T_1 and T_2 may then each represent time from a specified time origin to certain non-fatal outcomes. Independent censoring for the dual outcome then requires the censoring rate at follow-up time (t_1, t_2) given $Z(t_1, t_2)$ for either outcome to be unaffected by the occurrence of the companion outcome, and assumption that needs to be carefully considered in each application setting, and relaxed as necessary. An impressive feature of the empirical process developments and sandwich variance estimator sketched above, in that additional aspects of the bivariate counting process can be added to the conditioning event in hazard rate specification, as may be necessary for an independent censoring assumption to be plausible, without invalidating the asymptotic distributional results. Note, however, that the interpretation of hazard rate parameters will be affected by such inclusion.

In addition to paired non-fatal outcomes, the dual outcome hazard rate estimation procedure can be applied to a paired non-fatal outcome (T_1) and an overall or cause-specific death outcome (T_2). By definition information for estimating T_1 or (T_1, T_2) hazard rates ceases to accumulate at the death of the individual, and dual outcome hazard rate estimators only assign mass on or above the $t_1 = t_2$ diagonal. Independent censoring in this context requires censoring rates for the death outcome, given Z, to be unaffected by the occurrence of the non-fatal outcome.

The scenario of the preceding paragraph can be extended slightly by allowing T_1 to include a fatal component that is also a T_2 outcome, as was the situation in the illustration of §4.7 since some breast cancers were only ascertained by death certificate, so that $T_1 = T_2$ for the dual outcome of breast cancer and death from any cause for these outcomes. These data are most naturally thought of as incorporating some measurement error in T_1 ascertainment that prevented a more accurate dual outcome, with $T_1 < T_2$, from being recorded. The practical implications of such a delay in breast cancer diagnosis is likely to be small in this trial context, which included its substantial efforts to ensure equal outcome ascertainment procedures in the two randomization groups.

4.9.3 *Marginal hazard rates for competing risk data*

The bivariate failure time data considered in this chapter differs from classical competing risk data comprised of univariate failure time data that is accompanied by a failure type, with death accompanied by cause of death category as motivating example. Competing risk failure time data can be considered as a "marked" point process that admits the estimation of type-specific hazard rates, as in (2.12). Competing risk data have sometimes been modeled using hypothetical latent failure times. For example T_1 may represent time to death attributed to cancer, while T_2 is time to death from all other causes. It has long been recognized (Tsiatis, 1975) that the joint distribution of such hypothetical times is wholly unidentifiable from such data. In the terminology of this chapter, there is no possibility of estimating either single or dual outcome hazard rates for (T_1, T_2) from classical competing risk data, without making strong additional assumptions on the latent failure time distribution. Any such assumption is untestable with these data, so other sources of information are needed for justification. For example, in some industrial application mechanistic considerations may be used to support an assumption of independence between T_1 and T_2 given covariates, but such an assumption would usually be suspect for differing disease processes acting on an individual, for example in a biomedical context.

In comparison the breast cancer incidence (T_1) and all-cause mortality (T_2) outcomes considered in §4.7 represent genuinely bivariate outcomes, since trial participants continued to be followed for death following a breast cancer diagnosis. The (identifiable) single outcome hazard rates in this context implicitly condition on the continued survival of the study participant, so that T_1 is time from randomization to breast cancer diagnosis, $\hat{\Lambda}_{10}\{t_1, 0; Z(t_1, 0)\}$ is the estimated cumulative breast cancer hazard at follow-up time t_1, and $\hat{F}\{t_1, 0; Z(t_1, 0)\}$ is the estimated breast cancer–free survival probability at time t_1 for an individual having (fixed or external) covariate history $Z(t_1, 0)$. These estimators have ready and useful interpretation with this type of data, as do marginal hazard estimators for T_2 and (upper wedge) dual outcome hazard estimators as illustrated in §4.7.

Data of the type just considered are sometimes referred to as semicompeting risk data. There is a related literature on the estimation of the marginal distribution for a hypothetical latent non-fatal outcome, say $\tilde{T}_1$, that is regarded as being censored in a dependent fashion by death (T_2). In the application of §4.7 $\tilde{T}_1$ would equal T_1 for individuals developing breast cancer, and would be the hypothesized time that breast cancer would have occurred for individuals dying without breast cancer. Not surprisingly, estimation proposals (e.g., Fine, Jiang, & Chappell, 2001; Barrett, Siannis, & Farewell, 2011) need to contend with identifiability issues and require additional untestable assumptions. These methods may have utility for the study of non-fatal disease processes beyond observable data modeling, but they should be viewed as fundamentally different from the methods of §4.6.

4.10 Summary

This chapter provides a brief discussion of likelihood-based copula and frailty approaches to the regression analysis of bivariate failure time data. These methods, carefully applied, can undoubtedly yield valuable insights into regression effects on the individual failure times given covariates, and on the nature of dependencies among failure types. The methods based on marginal single and dual failure hazard rates, recently proposed by the authors, substantially generalize the class of regression models, accommodate evolving covariates on the same or different follow-up axes, and allow for direct insight into covariate effects on composite (double failure) outcomes. These methods all focused on marginal hazard rate regression parameters, and they can be expected to nicely complement longer-standing counting process intensity estimation procedures that allow a focus on transitions between states and mechanistic analyses through the study of rates and regression associations conditional on the prior failure experience of the set of correlated outcomes.

In some applications one may wish to restrict baseline hazard rates, Λ_{10} and Λ_{01} in (4.8) and (4.9) or Λ_1 and Λ_2 in (4.22) to be identical, and also restrict some or all elements of corresponding regression parameters to be common. Estimation procedures that incorporate these features will be discussed in a more general context in Chapter 6.

BIBLIOGRAPHIC NOTES

The coarsening at random assumption, which essentially requires censoring rates to depend only on observed data, in relation to likelihood specification with complex data has a substantial history (Heitjan & Rubin, 1991; Heitjan, 1994; Jacobsen & Keiding, 1995) culminating in unified methods for censored longitudinal data (van der Laan & Robins, 2003) and related targeted maximum likelihood approaches (e.g., van der Laan & Rose, 2011). Research to explore whether this impressive literature can materially improve upon the plug-in empirical methods presented in Chapters 3 and 4 is highly recommended. The single and dual outcome hazard rate modeling of §4.6 follows closely a recent paper (Prentice & Zhao, 2019), where additional detail on distribution theory and additional simulation results can be found.

There is an extensive literature on copula models, and their use in bivariate failure time data analysis. A thorough inventory of copula models, and their respective properties is given by Nelsen (2007). Also see Joe (1997) for a thorough discussion of multivariate models and dependency measures, and Joe (2014) for a more recent update on copula modeling. The Clayton–Oakes copula (Clayton, 1978; Oakes, 1982, 1986, 1989) has received quite a lot of use in statistical applications. Glidden (2000) provides asymptotic theory for a two-stage approach to parameter estimation, coming from a frailty model formulation with time-independent covariates. A more general asymptotic theory with Cox model marginals does not seem to have been presented. Li, Prentice, and Lin (2008) provide a detailed development of asymptotic theory for maximum likelihood estimation under the bivariate normal transformation model (4.6) without covariates, including a demonstration of semiparametric efficiency. There is similarly an extensive literature on the use of frailty models for bivariate failure time modeling. Books on this approach include Duchateau and Janssen (2010) and Wienke (2011). Hougaard (2000) provides substantial coverage of both the frailty and copula approaches, as more recently does (Aalen et al., 2010). Frailty models with gamma mixing distributions figure prominently in this literature. Nielsen, Gill, Andersen, and Sørensen (1992) make this modeling assumption and consider an expectation-maximization (EM) algorithm for the estimation of Cox model marginal hazard rate parameters, in conjunction with likelihood profiling a cross ratio that was independent of follow-up times or covariates. Andersen et al. (1993, Chapter 9) provide a detailed account of partial likelihood estimation under this model, including giving conditions for equality of partial marginal, and marginal partial likelihoods. Nan et al. (2006) consider cross ratio models that are constant within the elements of a rectangular grid, along with Cox model marginal hazard rates, as do Bandeen-Roche and Ning (2008). See Bandeen-Roche and Liang (1996) for an approach to building multivariate survival models that combine aspects of the frailty and copula approaches in a recursive fashion. Hu, Nan, Lin, and Robins (2011) developed a regression estimation procedures for Cox model marginal hazard rates, while restricting the cross ratio to be a polynomial function of the two time components. They remark that their "pseudo-partial likelihood" procedure does not apply if the cross ratio depends on covariates.

Lin (1994) considered Cox model marginal hazard rate parameter estimation under a working independence model among two or more failure time variates, and developed asymptotic theory using empirical process methods. This work is particularly relevant if there are marginal hazard rate parameters in common across the failure time variates. See also Wei et al. (1989) and especially Spiekerman and Lin (1998) for asymptotic distribution theory in a more general context that is elaborated below (Chapter 6).

There is also a considerable literature on the use of estimating equations for bivariate failure time regression (e.g., Cai & Prentice, 1995, 1997). Prentice and Hsu (1997) consider estimating equations for hazard ratio and time-independent cross ratio regression estimation jointly. Gray and Li (2002) consider weighted logrank tests within the context of marginal Cox models and clustered failure times, noting that test efficiency may be able to be improved compared to tests based on the marginal failure time data separately. Additional research to explore the use of dual outcome hazard rate estimators (§4.6) to improve the efficiency of corresponding single outcome hazard ratio estimates through the introduction of weights in estimating equations for single outcome hazard ratio parameters, would be worthwhile.

EXERCISES AND COMPLEMENTS

Exercise 4.1

Derive the kth factor in (4.3) with external covariates for failure time variates that are everywhere absolutely continuous. Repeat this derivation for failure time variates that are everywhere discrete. Generalize to mixed continuous and discrete failure time variates.

Exercise 4.2

Show that V_1 and V_2, as defined in §4.3 have unit exponential distributions for absolutely continuous failure time variates T_1 and T_2.

Exercise 4.3

Show that the copula models (4.5) and (4.6) are "complete" in the sense that these models approach the Fréchet lower bound as θ approaches its smallest possible value, and approach the Fréchet upper bound as θ approaches its larges possible value. Show that (4.6) is everywhere absolutely continuous away from its upper and lower bounds, whereas (4.5) with $\theta \geq -0.5$ is everywhere absolutely continuous, but positive probability begins to amass along the lower boundary for $\theta < -0.5$.

Exercise 4.4

Show that the Clayton–Oakes copula model (4.5) generates a cross ratio model for (T_1, T_2) given a fixed covariate $z = z(0,0)$ that is independent of follow-up times for T_1 and T_2. How would you propose that this cross ratio be modeled as a function of z?

Exercise 4.5

Consider a fixed covariate process $Z(t_1,t_2) = z$ and suppose that the cross ratio for T_1 and T_2 given $z(0,0)$ is a constant $\alpha_{(v_1,v_2)}e^{x(v_1,v_2)\gamma}$ whenever $(t_1,t_2) \in (u_1,v_1] \times (u_2,v_2] = \Omega$. Show that the survival probability in Ω is given by

$$F\{t_1,t_2;Z\} = \{F(t_1,u_2)^{-\theta(z)} + F(u_1,t_2)^{-\theta(z)} - F(u_1,u_2)^{-\theta(z)}\}^{-1/\theta(z)} \vee 0$$

where $\theta(z) = \alpha_{(v_1,v_2)}e^{x(v_1,v_2)\gamma} - 1$ (Nan et al., 2006).

Exercise 4.6

Derive (4.14)–(4.16) from (4.11)–(4.13) by first reexpressing (4.11)–(4.13) over the follow-up period $[0,\tau_1] \times [0,\tau_2]$ in the form of (4.14)–(4.16) but with N_{1k}, N_{2k}, and $N_{1k}N_{2k}$ in place of M_{10k}, M_{01k} and M_{11k} respectively. The show that the second components of M_{10k}, M_{01k} and M_{11k} have an integrated sum of zero over $k = 1,\ldots,n$.

Exercise 4.7

Consider the survivor function (4.20) with $\beta_{10} = \beta_{01} = \gamma$. Show that the double failure hazard function in (4.21) holds. Derive the form of the double failure hazard function from (4.20) without this restriction. Could the hazard ratio in (4.10) approximate this double failure hazard rate form through the inclusion of time-dependent covariates, such as $(z, z\log t_1, z\log t_2)$, in the double failure hazard model formulation (Prentice & Zhao, 2019)?

Chapter 5

Trivariate Failure Time Data Modeling and Analysis

5.1 Introduction

The models and data analysis methods of Chapters 3 and 4 can be extended to three or more failure time variates that are subject to independent right censoring. Specifically, each of the Dabrowska, Prentice–Cai and Volterra nonparametric survivor function estimators extend to a fixed, but arbitrary, number of failure time variates on the same or different failure time axes. Semiparametric regression models for single and double failure hazard rates can be extended to marginal single, double, triple, ... failure hazard rates, and suitable estimating equations can be written for all regression parameters and for baseline hazard rates of dimension $1, 2, 3, \ldots$. The ability to precisely estimate higher dimensional survivor functions, and higher dimensional marginal hazard ratio parameters, will depend directly on the size and nature of the cohort data set. For example, even large epidemiologic cohorts will typically have few participants that experience multiple rare clinical outcomes during cohort follow-up, and most usable information on treatments or exposures in relation to such outcomes will reside in the single, and possibly the double, failure hazard rate processes. On the other hand, in a therapeutic setting, individual patients may be at high risk for experiencing each of a range of failure time events, of the same or of different types, during cohort follow-up. The baseline rates for the multiple events may all be different, or may be restricted to be common for events of the same type. The notation for these developments is somewhat awkward. Hence to fix ideas we will first consider trivariate failure time data, with the three failures being of different types. These restrictions will be relaxed in Chapter 6. In §5.2 the discrete special case of a three-dimensional version of the Dabrowska (1988) representation is used to develop a nonparametric estimator of the trivariate survivor function, and asymptotic distribution theory is sketched. Generalization of the Volterra estimator to three dimensions is also described, with an outline of related asymptotic distribution theory, and simulation evaluations and comparisons are presented. The copula approach to trivariate failure time regression is outlined in §5.3. A rather flexible trivariate regression approach that involves the modeling and estimation of marginal single, double and triple failure hazard rates is described in §5.4. A simulation evaluation of the methods of §5.4 is given in §5.5. Application to the Women's Health Initiative's postmenopausal hormone therapy trials (see §1.7.3) is briefly considered in §5.6. As mentioned above, the further generalizations of these methods to an arbitrary number of failure time variates, which may be grouped into a smaller set of failure types, will be described in some detail in Chapter 6.

5.2 Nonparametric Estimation of the Trivariate Survivor Function

5.2.1 *Dabrowska-type estimator development*

Consider an independent random sample $S_{j\ell} = T_{j\ell} \wedge C_{j\ell}$ and $\delta_{j\ell} = I[S_{j\ell} = T_{j\ell}]$, for $j = 1,2,3$ and $\ell = 1,\ldots,n$, on failure time variates (T_1,T_2,T_3) subject to independent right censoring by variates (C_1,C_2,C_3). The nonparametric likelihood for the survivor function F, where $F(t_1,t_2,t_3) = P(T_1 > t_1, T_2 > t_2, T_3 > t_3)$, under the convention that failures precede censorings in the event of tied times, can be written

$$
\begin{aligned}
L = \prod_{\ell=1}^{n} \Big[& \{-F(dS_{1\ell},dS_{2\ell},dS_{3\ell})\}^{\delta_{1\ell}\delta_{2\ell}\delta_{3\ell}} F(dS_{1\ell},dS_{2\ell},S_{3\ell})^{\delta_{1\ell}\delta_{2\ell}(1-\delta_{3\ell})} \\
& F(dS_{1\ell},S_{2\ell},dS_{3\ell})^{\delta_{1\ell}(1-\delta_{2\ell})\delta_{3\ell}} F(S_{1\ell},dS_{2\ell},dS_{3\ell})^{(1-\delta_{1\ell})\delta_{2\ell}\delta_{3\ell}} \\
& \{-F(dS_{1\ell},S_{2\ell},S_{3\ell})\}^{\delta_{1\ell}(1-\delta_{2\ell})(1-\delta_{3\ell})} \{-F(S_{1\ell},dS_{2\ell},S_{3\ell})\}^{(1-\delta_{1\ell})\delta_{2\ell}(1-\delta_{3\ell})} \\
& \{-F(S_{1\ell},S_{2\ell},dS_{3\ell})\}^{(1-\delta_{1\ell})(1-\delta_{2\ell})\delta_{3\ell}} F(S_{1\ell},S_{2\ell},S_{3\ell})\}^{(1-\delta_{1\ell})(1-\delta_{2\ell})(1-\delta_{3\ell})} \Big].
\end{aligned}
$$

Denote by $t_{11},\ldots,t_{1I}$ the ordered uncensored T_1 values in the sample, by $t_{21},\ldots,t_{2J}$ the ordered uncensored T_2 values, and by $t_{31},\ldots,t_{3K}$ the ordered uncensored T_3 values, and set $t_{10} = t_{20} = t_{30} = 0$. F is identifiable on the risk region $R = \{(t_1,t_2,t_3); X_{1\ell} \geq t_1, X_{2\ell} \geq t_2$ and $X_{3\ell} \geq t_3$ for some $\ell \in (1,\ldots,n)\}$. L can be maximized by placing positive probability within the risk region only at failure time grid points $(t_{1i},t_{2j},t_{3k}) \in R$, leading to a discrete survivor function estimator. The discrete special of a Dabrowska-type trivariate survivor function representation can be written, again using product integrals, as

$$F(t_1,t_2,t_3) = \prod_0^{t_1} \frac{F(s_1,0,0)}{F(s_1^-,0,0)} \prod_0^{t_2} \frac{F(0,s_2,0)}{F(0,s_2^-,0)} \prod_0^{t_3} \frac{F(0,0,s_3)}{F(0,0,s_3^-)}$$
$$\prod_0^{t_1}\prod_0^{t_2} \frac{F(s_1,s_2,0)F(s_1^-,s_2^-,0)}{F(s_1,s_2^-,0)F(s_1^-,s_2,0)} \prod_0^{t_1}\prod_0^{t_3} \frac{F(s_1,0,s_3)F(s_1^-,0,s_2^-)}{F(s_1,0,s_3^-)F(s_1^-,0,s_3)}$$
$$\prod_0^{t_2}\prod_0^{t_3} \frac{F(0,s_2,s_3)F(0,s_2^-,s_3^-)}{F(0,s_2,s_3^-)F(0,s_2^-,s_3)}$$
$$\prod_0^{t_1}\prod_0^{t_2}\prod_0^{t_3} \frac{F(s_1,s_2,s_3)F(s_1,s_2^-,s_3^-)F(s_1^-,s_2,s_3^-)F(s_1^-,s_2^-,s_3)}{F(s_1,s_2,s_3^-)F(s_1,s_2^-,s_3)F(s_1^-,s_2,s_3)F(s_1^-,s_2^-,s_3^-)}. \quad (5.1)$$

The validity of (5.1) follows from massive cancellations in conjunction with $F(0,0,0) = 1$. This expression decomposes $F(t_1,t_2,t_3)$ into the product of its marginal survival probabilities through the single product integrals, multiplied by its pairwise dependency components through the double product integrals, multiplied by a trivariate dependency component through the triple product integral. For example, the first of the three pairwise dependency components simplifies to $F(t_1,t_2,0)/\{F(t_1,0,0)F(0,t_2,0)\}$, and characterizes marginal dependence between T_1 and T_2. The triple product integral simplifies to

$$\frac{F(t_1,t_2,t_3)}{F(t_1,0,0)F(0,t_2,0)F(0,0,t_3)}$$
$$\left[\frac{F(t_1,t_2,0)}{F(t_1,0,0)F(0,t_2,0)} \frac{F(t_1,0,t_3)}{F(t_1,0,0)F(0,0,t_3)} \frac{F(0,t_2,t_3)}{F(0,t_2,0)F(0,0,t_3)}\right]^{-1},$$

and can be viewed as comparing $F(t_1,t_2,t_3)$ to the product of marginal survival probabilities after allowing for corresponding marginal pairwise dependencies. Expression (5.1) breaks these marginal probabilities and pairwise and trivariate dependency ratios into product integrals for ease of estimation. Specifically, each of the survival probabilities on the right side of (5.1) can be replaced by this probability divided by the same probability but with each s-value replaced by s^- (each s^- value is unchanged). The resulting conditional probabilities are readily estimated empirically to give a nonparametric trivariate survivor function estimator $\hat{F}$. This nonparametric estimator can be calculated in a recursive fashion by first calculating the KM marginal survivor function estimators, then calculating the pairwise marginal survivor function estimators recursively using (3.9) for each pair of the three failure time variates, then calculating $\hat{F}$ away from its coordinate axes, at each uncensored failure time grid point $(t_{1i},t_{2j},t_{3k}) \in R$ using the recursive expression

$$\hat{F}(t_{1i},t_{2j},t_{3k}) = \frac{\hat{F}(t_{1i},t_{2j},t_{3k}^-)\hat{F}(t_{1i},t_{2j}^-,t_{3k})\hat{F}(t_{1i}^-,t_{2j},t_{3k})\hat{F}(t_{1i}^-,t_{2j}^-,t_{3k}^-)}{\hat{F}(t_{1i},t_{2j}^-,t_{3k}^-)\hat{F}(t_{1i}^-,t_{2j},t_{3k}^-)\hat{F}(t_{1i}^-,t_{2j}^-,t_{3k})} \times$$
$$\left\{\frac{\tilde{F}(t_{1i},t_{2j},t_{3k})\tilde{F}(t_{1i},t_{2j}^-,t_{3k}^-)\tilde{F}(t_{1i}^-,t_{2j},t_{3k}^-)\tilde{F}(t_{1i}^-,t_{2j}^-,t_{3k})}{\tilde{F}(t_{1i},t_{2j},t_{3k}^-)\tilde{F}(t_{1i},t_{2j}^-,t_{3k})\tilde{F}(t_{1i}^-,t_{2j},t_{3k})}\right\} \quad (5.2)$$

where

$$\tilde{F}(u_1,u_2,u_3) = \frac{\#\{\ell; S_{i\ell} > s_i \text{ if } u_i = s_i \text{ or } S_{i\ell} \geq s_i \text{ if } u_i = s_i^-, \text{ each } i = 1,2,3\}}{\#\{\ell; S_{i\ell} \geq s_i, \text{ each } i = 1,2,3\}}$$

for $u_i = s_i$ or s_i^- for $i = 1,2,3$. The final factor in (5.2) is undefined if one or more of the denominator $\tilde{F}$ terms takes value zero, as can occur on the boundary of the risk region. The specification of $\hat{F}$ can be completed by setting the final factor equal to zero in these circumstances.

Empirical process methods can be used to show the Dabrowska-type estimator $\hat{F}$ to be strongly consistent for F, to show $n^{1/2}(\hat{F} - F)$ to converge in distribution to a mean zero Gaussian process, and to show the applicability of bootstrap procedures over a follow-up region $[0,\tau_1] \times [0,\tau_2] \times [0,\tau_3]$ where $P(S_1 > \tau_1, S_2 > \tau_2, S_3 > \tau_3) > 0$. For $s_i \geq 0$, and $i = 1,2,3$ one can express the factors in (5.1) in terms of hazard rates. For example, in an obvious hazard rate notation

$$\begin{aligned}
&F(s_1,s_2^-,s_3^-)/F(s_1^-,s_2^-,s_3^-) = 1 - \Lambda_{100}(ds_1,s_2^-,s_3^-),\\
&F(s_1,s_2,s_3^-)/F(s_1^-,s_2^-,s_3^-) =\\
&1 - \Lambda_{100}(ds_1,s_2^-,s_3^-) - \Lambda_{010}(s_1^-,ds_2,s_3^-) + \Lambda_{110}(ds_1,ds_2,s_3^-), \text{ and}\\
&F(s_1,s_2,s_3)/F(s_1^-,s_2^-,s_3^-) = 1 - \Lambda_{100}(ds_1,s_2^-,s_3^-) - \Lambda_{010}(s_1^-,ds_2,s_3^-)\\
&- \Lambda_{001}(s_1^-,s_2^-,ds_3) + \Lambda_{110}(ds_1,ds_2,s_3^-) + \Lambda_{101}(ds_1,s_2^-,ds_3)\\
&+ \Lambda_{011}(s_1^-,ds_2,ds_3) - \Lambda_{111}(ds_1,ds_2,ds_3).
\end{aligned} \tag{5.3}$$

Substituting these expressions, along with corresponding expressions interchanging the roles of s_1, s_2 and s_3, gives an expression for the discrete $F(t_1,t_2,t_3)$ as a function of single, double and triple failure hazard rates at $s_i \leq t_i, i = 1,2,3$. Also from the triple product integral in (5.1) one sees that there will be no trivariate dependency among the three failure time variates at (s_1,s_2,s_3) if $F(s_1,s_2,s_3)/F(s_1^-,s_2^-,s_3^-) = F(s_1,s_2,s_3^-)F(s_1,s_2^-,s_3)F(s_1^-,s_2,s_3)/\{F(s_1,s_2^-,s_3^-)F(s_1^-,s_2,s_3^-)F(s_1^-,s_2^-,s_3)\}$. Setting the left side of (5.3) equal to this quantity uniquely defines a triple failure hazard rate

$$\begin{aligned}
\Lambda_{111}^0(ds_1,ds_2,ds_3) = &1 - \Lambda_{100}(ds_1,s_2^-,s_3^-) - \Lambda_{010}(s_1^-,ds_2,s_3^-) - \Lambda_{001}(s_1^-,s_2^-,ds_3)\\
&+ \Lambda_{110}(ds_1,ds_2,s_3^-) + \Lambda_{101}(ds_1,s_2^-,ds_3) + \Lambda_{011}(s_1^- ds_2,ds_3)\\
&- \frac{F(s_1,s_2,s_3^-)F(s_1,s_2^-,s_3)F(s_1^-,s_2,s_3)}{F(s_1,s_2^-,s_3^-)F(s_1^-,s_2,s_3^-)F(s_1^-,s_2^-,s_3)}
\end{aligned} \tag{5.4}$$

for which the trivariate dependency factor in (5.1) takes value one at (s_1,s_2,s_3). The survival probability (5.1) can be re-expressed in terms of product integrals of standardized form as

$$F(t_1,t_2,t_3) =$$
$$\prod_0^{t_1}\{1-\Lambda_{100}(ds_1,0,0)\}\prod_0^{t_2}\{1-\Lambda_{010}(0,ds_2,0)\}\prod_0^{t_3}\{1-\Lambda_{001}(0,0,ds_3)\}$$
$$\prod_0^{t_1}\prod_0^{t_2}\{1+L_{110}(ds_1,ds_2,0)\}\prod_0^{t_1}\prod_0^{t_3}\{1+L_{101}(ds_1,0,ds_3)\}$$
$$\prod_0^{t_2}\prod_0^{t_3}\{1+L_{011}(0,ds_2,ds_3)\}\prod_0^{t_1}\prod_0^{t_2}\prod_0^{t_3}\{1-L_{111}(ds_1,ds_2,ds_3)\} \quad (5.5)$$

where, for example,

$$L_{110}(ds_1,ds_2,s_3^-) = \frac{\Lambda_{110}(ds_1,ds_2,s_3^-)-\Lambda_{100}(ds_1,s_2^-,s_3^-)\Lambda_{010}(s_1^-,ds_2,s_3^-)}{\{1-\Lambda_{100}(\Delta s_1,s_2^-,s_3^-)\}\{1-\Lambda_{010}(s_1^-,\Delta s_2,s_3^-)\}},$$

and where

$$L_{111}(ds_1,ds_2,ds_3) =$$
$$\frac{\{\Lambda_{111}(ds_1,ds_2,ds_3)-\Lambda_{111}^0(ds_1,ds_2,ds_3)\}}{\{1-\Lambda_{100}(\Delta s_1,s_2^-,s_3^-)\}\{1-\Lambda_{010}(s_1^-,\Delta s_2,s_3^-)\}\{1-\Lambda_{001}(s_1^-,s_2^-,\Delta s_3)\}}$$
$$\times[\{1+L_{110}(\Delta s_1,\Delta s_2,s_3^-)\}\{1+L_{101}(\Delta s_1,s_2^-,\Delta s_3)\}\{1+L_{011}(s_1^-,\Delta s_2,\Delta s_3)\}]^{-1}. \quad (5.6)$$

In fact, this decomposition of F in terms of single, double and triple failure hazard rates applies also to absolutely continuous or mixed failure time variates and (5.5) provides a representation for the trivariate survivor function. Now define counting processes $N_{100},N_{010},N_{001},N_{110},N_{101},N_{011}$, and N_{111}, and "at-risk" process Y, for example, by

$$N_{100}(t_1,t_2,t_3) = n^{-1}\#\{\ell;S_{1\ell}\le t_1,S_{2\ell}>t_2,S_{3\ell}>t_3,\delta_{1\ell}=1\},$$
$$N_{110}(t_1,t_2,t_3) = n^{-1}\#\{\ell;S_{1\ell}\le t_1,S_{2\ell}\le t_2,S_{3\ell}>t_3,\delta_{1k}=1,\delta_{2k}=1\},$$
$$N_{111}(t_1,t_2,t_3) = n^{-1}\#\{\ell;S_{1\ell}\le t_1,S_{2\ell}\le t_2,S_{3\ell}\le t_3,\delta_{1\ell}=1,\delta_{2\ell}=1,\delta_{3\ell}=1\} \text{ and}$$
$$Y(t_1,t_2,t_3) = n^{-1}\#\{\ell;S_{1\ell}\ge t_1,S_{2\ell}\ge t_2,S_{3\ell}\ge t_3\}.$$

The Glivenko–Cantelli and Donsker theorems (see Appendix A) apply to $(N_{100},N_{010},N_{001},N_{110},N_{101},N_{011},N_{111},Y)$ over $[0,\tau_1]\times[0,\tau_2]\times[0,\tau_3]$ to show these processes to be supremum norm consistent for, and weakly convergent to their targets as $n\to\infty$. The corresponding hazard process estimators $(\hat\Lambda_{100},\hat\Lambda_{010},\hat\Lambda_{001},\hat\Lambda_{110},\hat\Lambda_{101},\hat\Lambda_{011},\hat\Lambda_{111})$ defined, for example, by

$$\hat\Lambda_{100}(t_1,t_2,t_3) = \int_0^{t_1} Y(s_1,t_2,t_3)^{-1}N_{100}(ds_1,t_2,t_3)$$
$$\hat\Lambda_{110}(t_1,t_2,t_3) = \int_0^{t_1}\int_0^{t_2} Y(s_1,s_2,t_3)^{-1}N_{110}(ds_1,ds_2,t_3), \text{ and}$$
$$\hat\Lambda_{111}(t_1,t_2,t_3) = \int_0^{t_1}\int_0^{t_2}\int_0^{t_3} Y(s_1,s_2,s_3)^{-1}N_{111}(ds_1,ds_2,ds_3),$$

with the usual convention that $0/0 = 0$, are then strongly consistent for, and weakly convergent to, their single, double and triple hazard function targets as $n \to \infty$, based on the continuity and (weakly continuous) compact differentiability of the hazard process transformations. These properties also apply to the further transformed empirical processes $(\hat{\Lambda}_{100}, \hat{\Lambda}_{010}, \hat{\Lambda}_{001}, \hat{L}_{110}, \hat{L}_{101}, \hat{L}_{011}, \hat{L}_{111})$, where each L process arises by replacing hazard rates in (5.5) by corresponding empirical hazard rates, on the basis of the continuity and compact differentiability of the transformations to these L processes. Finally, the continuity and compact differentiability of the product integral transformations from $(\hat{\Lambda}_{100}, \hat{\Lambda}_{010}, \hat{\Lambda}_{001}, \hat{L}_{110}, \hat{L}_{101}, \hat{L}_{011}, \hat{L}_{111})$ to $\hat{F}$ via (5.5) shows

$$\sup_{(t_1,t_2,t_3)\in[0,\tau_1]\times[0,\tau_2]\times[0,\tau_3]} |\hat{F}(t_1,t_2,t_3) - F(t_1,t_2,t_3)| \xrightarrow{P} 0$$

and shows $n^{1/2}(\hat{F} - F)$ to converge in distribution to a mean zero Gaussian process over $[0,\tau_1] \times [0,\tau_2] \times [0,\tau_3]$. The Donsker theorem and (weakly continuous) compact differentiability of each of the sequence of transformations listed above also leads to justification for bootstrap procedures as applied to $\hat{F}$, for example, for confidence interval or confidence band estimation.

Note that (5.5) simplifies considerably for absolutely continuous (T_1, T_2, T_3). Specifically Λ^0_{111} is then given by

$$\begin{aligned}
\Lambda^0_{111}(ds_1,ds_2,ds_3) &= \Lambda_{100}(ds_1,s_2^-,s_3^-)\Lambda_{010}(s_1^-,ds_2,s_3^-)\Lambda_{001}(s_1^-,s_2^-,ds_3) \\
&\quad + \Omega_{110}(ds_1,ds_2,s_3^-)\Lambda_{001}(s_1^-,s_2^-,ds_3) \\
&\quad + \Omega_{101}(ds_1,s_2^-,ds_3)\Lambda_{010}(s_1^-,ds_2,s_3^-) + \Omega_{011}(s_1^-,ds_2,ds_3)\Lambda_{100}(ds_1,s_2^-,s_3^-)
\end{aligned}$$

where, for example, Ω_{110} simplifies to

$$\Omega_{110}(ds_1,ds_2,s_3^-) = \Lambda_{110}(ds_1,ds_2,s_3^-) - \Lambda_{100}(ds_1,s_2^-,s_3^-)\Lambda_{010}(s_1^-,ds_2,s_3^-),$$

and each product integral in (5.5) can be written in exponential form giving expression (1.8).

5.2.2 *Volterra estimator*

The Prentice–Cai and Volterra plug-in estimators considered in Chapter 3 also can be extended to define nonparametric estimators of the trivariate survivor function. For the latter, one can write, for any $t_1 \geq 0, t_2 \geq 0$ and $t_3 \geq 0$,

$$F(t_1,t_2,t_3) = \Psi(t_1,t_2,t_3) - \int_0^{t_1}\int_0^{t_2}\int_0^{t_3} F(s_1^-,s_2^-,s_3^-)\Lambda_{111}(ds_1,ds_2,ds_3),$$

where

$$\begin{aligned}
\Psi(t_1,t_2,t_3) =& 1 - F(t_1,0,0) - F(0,t_2,0) - F(0,0,t_3) \\
&+ F(t_1,t_2,0) + F(t_1,0,t_3) + F(0,t_2,t_3),
\end{aligned}$$

which is an inhomogeneous Volterra integral equation in F having a unique solution in a Péano series form. This shows that F is uniquely specified by its lower dimensional marginal survivor functions and the triple failure hazard rates away from the coordinate planes. The continuity and compact differentiability of the Péano series transformation, in conjunction with asymptotic properties for marginal and pairwise marginal survivor function estimators can be used to show the Volterra-type estimator $\hat{F}$ arising from KM estimators, Volterra–type pairwise marginal survivor functions, and empirical triple failure hazard rates to be strongly consistent for F, and to show $n^{1/2}(\hat{F}-F)$ to be weakly convergent to a mean zero Gaussian process, and to show applicability of bootstrap procedures for variance estimation and other purposes.

The trivariate step function Volterra estimator $\hat{F}$ at grid point (t_{1i},t_{2j},t_{3k}) can be calculated recursively, after calculating marginal and pairwise marginal survivor function estimators using

$$\begin{aligned}\hat{F}(t_{1i},t_{2j},t_{3k}) =& \hat{F}(t_{1i},t_{2j},t_{3k}^-)+\hat{F}(t_{1i},t_{2j}^-,t_{3k})+\hat{F}(t_{1i}^-,t_{2j},t_{3k})\\ &-\hat{F}(t_{1i},t_{2j}^-,t_{3k}^-)-\hat{F}(t_{1i}^-,t_{2j},t_{3k}^-)-\hat{F}(t_{1i}^-,t_{2j}^-,t_{3k})\\ &+\hat{F}(t_{1i}^-,t_{2j}^-,t_{3k}^-)\{1-\hat{\Lambda}_{111}(\Delta t_{1i},\Delta t_{2j},\Delta t_{3k})\}\end{aligned} \tag{5.7}$$

where the empirical estimator $\hat{\Lambda}_{111}$ is given by

$$\hat{\Lambda}_{111}(\Delta t_{1i},\Delta t_{2j},\Delta t_{3k}) = d_{ijk}^{111}/r_{ijk},$$

the ratio of the number of triple failures to the size of the risk set, for any $(t_{1i},t_{2j},t_{3k}) \in R$.

5.2.3 *Trivariate dependency assessment*

In an analogous fashion to (3.7) for bivariate dependency assessment, one can define a local trivariate dependency measure at (t_1,t_2,t_3) by $\alpha_{111}(t_1,t_2,t_3) = \Lambda_{111}(dt_1,dt_2,dt_3)/\Lambda_{111}^0(dt_1,dt_2,dt_3)$, which compares the trivariate hazard rate at (t_1,t_2,t_3) to that under no trivariate dependence, on a relative scale. An average trivariate dependency ratio $C_{111}(\tau_1,\tau_2,\tau_3)$ over a region $[0,\tau_1]\times[0,\tau_2]\times[0,\tau_3]$ where (τ_1,τ_2,τ_3) is in the support of the observed times (S_1,S_2,S_3) can be defined by

$$C_{111}(\tau_1,\tau_2,\tau_3)^{-1} = \frac{\int_0^{\tau_1}\int_0^{\tau_2}\int_0^{\tau_3}\{\Lambda_{111}^0(dt_1,dt_2,dt_3)/\Lambda_{111}(dt_1,dt_2,dt_3)\}F(dt_1,dt_2,dt_3)}{\int_0^{\tau_1}\int_0^{\tau_2}\int_0^{\tau_3}F(dt_1,dt_2,dt_3)}.$$

This measure can be estimated nonparametrically by

$$\begin{aligned}\hat{C}_{111}(\tau_1,\tau_2,\tau_3) = & \int_0^{\tau_1}\int_0^{\tau_2}\int_0^{\tau_3}\hat{F}(t_1^-,t_2^-,t_3^-)\hat{\Lambda}_{111}(\Delta t_1,\Delta t_2,\Delta t_3)/\\ & \int_0^{\tau_1}\int_0^{\tau_2}\int_0^{\tau_3}\hat{F}(t_1^-,t_2^-,t_3^-)\hat{\Lambda}_{111}^0(\Delta t_1,\Delta t_2,\Delta t_3),\end{aligned}$$

where $\hat{\Lambda}_{111}^0$ is obtained by everywhere inserting $\hat{F}$ for F in (5.4), and where $\hat{F}$ can be any of the nonparametric survivor function estimators mentioned above.

Note that $\hat{C}_{111}$ as a process over $[0,\tau_1]\times[0,\tau_2]\times[0,\tau_3]$ inherits strong consistency, weak convergences and bootstrap applicability properties as an estimator of C_{111} from these same properties for $\hat{F}$.

5.2.4 *Simulation evaluation and comparison*

As with the bivariate survivor function estimators from (3.6) or (3.9), the trivariate survivor function estimator arising from (5.2) or (5.7) can incorporate negative mass. Nevertheless these estimators can be expected to have good moderate sample size properties, and to be a suitable choice for many applications. To evaluate the moderate sample size properties of $\hat{F}$ from (5.2) and (5.7) failure times were generated from the specialized survivor function model

$$F(t_1,t_2,t_3)=\{F(t_1,0,0)^{-\theta}+F(0,t_2,0)^{-\theta}+F(0,0,t_3)^{-\theta}-2\}^{-1/\theta}\vee 0, \quad (5.8)$$

which has bivariate and trivariate dependency controlled by the single parameter θ. Straightforward calculations from (5.8) show, at any continuity point (s_1,s_2,s_3), that

$$\Lambda_{110}(ds_1,ds_2,s_3)=(1+\theta)\Lambda_{100}(ds_1,s_2,s_3)\Lambda_{010}(s_1,ds_2,s_3)$$

so that the cross ratio function for (T_1,T_2) at $T_3=s_3$ equals $(1+\theta)$, independently of (s_1,s_2,s_3). The corresponding pairwise covariance rates are simply

$$\Omega_{110}(ds_1,ds_2,s_3)=\theta\Lambda_{100}(ds_1,s_2,s_3)\Lambda_{010}(s_1,ds_2,s_3), \quad (5.9)$$

with corresponding expressions for Ω_{101} and Ω_{001}. One can also calculate

$$\Lambda_{111}(ds_1,ds_2,ds_3)=(1+\theta)(1+2\theta)\Lambda_{100}(ds_1,s_2,s_3)\Lambda_{010}(s_1,ds_2,s_3)\Lambda_{001}(s_1,s_2,ds_3)$$

from which the trivariate dependency function Ω_{111} (see §1.4) is given by

$$\Omega_{111}(ds_1,ds_2,ds_3)=2\theta^2\Lambda_{100}(ds_1,s_2,s_3)\Lambda_{010}(s_1,ds_2,s_3)\Lambda_{001}(s_1,s_2,ds_3). \quad (5.10)$$

Failure times (t_1,t_2,t_3) under (5.8) with $\theta\geq -1/3$ are everywhere absolutely continuous and can be generated from independent uniform $(0,1)$ variates (u_1,u_2,u_3) by probability integral transformations of the marginal density for T_1, the conditional density for T_2 given $T_1=t_1$, and the conditional density for T_3 given $(T_1,T_2)=(t_1,t_2)$. Without loss of generality the marginal survivor functions can each be taken to be unit exponential leading to

$t_1=-\log u_1,$

$t_2=\theta^{-1}\log\{1-u_1^{-\theta}(1-u_2^{-\theta(1+\theta)^{-1}})\}$ if $\theta\neq 0$ and $t_2=-\log u_2$ if $\theta=0$, and

$t_3=\theta^{-1}\log\{1-u_1^{-\theta}u_2^{-\theta(1+\theta)^{-1}}(1-u_3^{-\theta(1+2\theta)^{-1}})\}$ if $\theta\neq 0$ and $t_3=-\log u_3$ if $\theta=0$.

Failure times were generated for sample sizes of $n=30,60$ and 120 at θ values of 0 (independence), 2 (moderate positive dependence), and 5 (strong positive dependence). Censoring times c_1,c_2 and c_3 were generated from independent exponential

Table 5.1 *Simulation mean and standard deviation estimates** *for trivariate Dabrowska* ($\hat{F}_0$) *and Volterra* ($\hat{F}_v$) *survivor function estimators* (5.2) *and* (5.7) *under the specialized Clayton–Oakes model* (5.8), *at* $n = 60$, *with unit exponential marginal survivor functions and with censoring times that were independent of each other, each having expectation 0.5. Survivor function estimators presented at arguments of 0.163, 0.357 and 0.598, which are the values at which marginal survival probabilities equal 0.85, 0.70 and 0.55 for each of* T_1, T_2 *and* T_3.

Claton–Oakes Parameter	$\theta = 0$			$\theta = 2$		
Marginal Survival Probabilities	F	$\hat{F}_D$	$\hat{F}_v$	F	$\hat{F}_D$	$\hat{F}_v$
0.85 0.85 0.85	0.614	0.614 (0.070)	0.615 (0.069)	0.682	0.683 (0.066)	0.683 (0.066)
0.85 0.85 0.70	0.506	0.503 (0.077)	0.504 (0.077)	0.597	0.598 (0.074)	0.598 (0.074)
0.85 0.85 0.55	0.397	0.395 (0.087)	0.396 (0.088)	0.495	0.495 (0.090)	0.496 (0.091)
0.85 0.70 0.70	0.417	0.416 (0.081)	0.415 (0.083)	0.537	0.539 (0.079)	0.540 (0.080)
0.85 0.70 0.55	0.327	0.327 (0.088)	0.325 (0.092)	0.640	0.460 (0.093)	0.461 (0.096)
0.85 0.55 0.55	0.257	0.265 (0.097)	0.254 (0.111)	0.408	0.414 (0.105)	0.410 (0.109)
0.70 0.70 0.70	0.343	0.342 (0.086)	0.340 (0.087)	0.493	0.494 (0.081)	0.494 (0.082)
0.70 0.70 0.55	0.270	0.274 (0.091)	0.270 (0.096)	0.431	0.436 (0.091)	0.434 (0.097)
0.70 0.55 0.55	0.212	0.225 (0.096)	0.212 (0.111)	0.388	0.402 (0.101)	0.396 (0.105)
0.55 0.55 0.55	0.166	0.188 (0.091)	0.161 (0.116)	0.355	0.381 (0.123)	0.367 (0.114)

*Based on 1000 simulated samples at each configuration. All samples in the risk region at a failure time grid point contributed to summary statistics. Tabular entries are sample mean and sample standard deviation.

distributions each with expectation of $0 \cdot 5$, so that there is a 2/3rds probability of censoring for each observed $s_i = t_i \wedge c_i$ value, for $i = 1,2,3$.

Table 5.1 presents simulation summary statistics for the Dabrowska and Volterra estimators at selected values of the marginal survival probabilities $F(t_1,0,0)$, $F(0,t_2,0)$ and $F(0,0,t_3)$, at $n = 60$ and for $\theta = 0$ and $\theta = 2$. Note that the expected number of triply uncensored failures in the sample is only $60(1/3)^3 = 2 \cdot 22$ at $\theta = 0$. Nevertheless the nonparametric trivariate survivor function estimators both appear to be fairly accurate under these simulation conditions.

Table 5.2 shows simulation summary statistics for these estimators at $n = 180$ with censoring times having independent unit exponential distributions each with expectation 2.0, so that there is a 1/3rd probability of censoring for each observed s_i value, $i = 1,2,3$ at $\theta = 2$. Some overestimation of targeted dependency function values is evident under these sampling configurations. See Prentice and Zhao (2018) for additional simulations for $\hat{F}$, $\hat{C}_{110}$ and $\hat{C}_{111}$ under a trivariate normal transformation model. These simulations show similar estimation properties to those under (5.8).

Table 5.2 *Simulation summary statistics* for the average pairwise marginal cross ratio estimator $\hat{C}_{110}$ and for the average trivariate dependency estimator $\hat{C}_{111}$ under the survivor function* (5.8) *with $\theta = 2$ and $n = 180$, with each failure time having a one-third probability of censoring, using either the Dabrowska or Volterra nonparametric survivor function estimators.*

t_1	t_2	C_{110}	$\hat{C}_{110}$ (SD)-Dabrowska	$\hat{C}_{110}$ (SD)-Volterra
0.163	0.163	3	3.142 (1.366)	3.148 (1.398)
0.163	0.357	3	3.102 (1.121)	3.123 (1.230)
0.163	0.598	3	3.138 (1.308)	3.277 (1.435)
0.357	0.357	3	3.087 (0.917)	3.115 (1.068)
0.357	0.598	3	3.101 (0.946)	3.172 (1.302)
0.598	0.598	3	3.120 (0.910)	3.226 (1.448)

t_1	t_2	t_3	C_{111}	$\hat{C}_{111}$ (SD)-Dabrowska	$\hat{C}_{111}$ (SD)-Volterra
0.163	0.163	0.163	2.143	2.341 (1.343)	2.334 (1.377)
0.163	0.163	0.357	2.143	2.276 (1.095)	2.286 (1.207)
0.163	0.163	0.598	2.143	2.351 (1.180)	2.446 (1.592)
0.163	0.357	0.357	2.143	2.291 (0.929)	2.306 (1.072)
0.163	0.357	0.598	2.143	2.338 (1.051)	2.671 (8.865)
0.163	0.598	0.598	2.143	2.397 (1.341)	2.525 (3.529)
0.357	0.357	0.357	2.143	2.280 (1.744)	2.278 (0.864)
0.357	0.357	0.598	2.143	2.338 (1.016)	2.353 (1.066)
0.357	0.598	0.598	2.143	2.373 (1.964)	2.393 (1.324)
0.598	0.598	0.598	2.143	2.510 (2.354)	2.470 (1.818)

*Tabular entries are sample mean (sample standard deviation) based on all simulations out of 1000 for which the point $(t_1,t_2,0)$ for C_{110}, or the point (t_1,t_2,t_3) for C_{111} is in the risk period for the data. Note that 0.163, 0.357 and 0.598 are the values giving marginal survival probabilities of 0.85, 0.70 and 0.55 respectively, for each of T_1, T_2 and T_3.

5.3 Trivariate Regression Analysis via Copulas

The copula approach of §4.3 extends readily to three failure time variates. Let $z(t_1,t_2,t_3) = \{z_1(t_1,t_2,t_3), z_2(t_1,t_2,t_3),\ldots\}$ denote covariate values at follow-up times $t_i \geq 0, i = 1,2,3$ for failure time variates T_1,T_2,T_3, and let $Z(t_1,t_2,t_3) = \{z(s_1,s_2,s_3); s_j = 0 \text{ if } t_j = 0 \text{ and } s_j < t_j \text{ if } t_j > 0 \text{ for each } j = 1,2,3\}$ denote the corresponding history prior to (t_1,t_2,t_3) for covariates that are time-independent or external to the failure time process. A copula approach proceeds by defining marginal hazard rate models $\Lambda_{100}, \Lambda_{010}$ and Λ_{001}, and standardized variates

$$
\begin{aligned}
V_1 &= \int_0^{T_1} \Lambda_{100}\{dt_1,0,0;Z(t_1,0,0)\}, V_2 = \int_0^{T_2} \Lambda_{010}\{0,dt_2,0;Z(0,t_2,0)\},\\
V_3 &= \int_0^{T_3} \Lambda_{001}\{0,0,dt_3;Z(0,0,t_3)\},
\end{aligned}
$$

which are assumed to have a joint survivor function F_0 given $z = z(0,0,0)$, that is specified up to a parameter vector θ. For example, one could specify a trivariate Clayton–Oakes model (1.9) with parameter $\theta_{111}(z)$, in conjunction with bivariate Clayton–Oakes models with parameters $\theta_{110}(z), \theta_{101}(z)$ and $\theta_{011}(z)$ for $F_0(t_1,t_2,0), F_0(t_1,0,t_3)$ and $F_0(0,t_2,t_3)$ respectively. Alternatively one could consider a trivariate standardized normal distributions with pairwise correlation parameters $\theta_{110}(z), \theta_{101}(z)$ and $\theta_{011}(z)$ respectively for $\Phi^{-1}(1-e^{-V_i}), i = 1,2,3$ for F_0.

Application of a copula model to absolutely continuous censored failure time regression data can proceed through maximization of the likelihood function for F given Z; namely,

$$
\begin{aligned}
L = \prod_{k=1}^{n} \Big(& [-F\{dS_{1k},dS_{2k},dS_{3k};Z_k(S_{1k},S_{2k},S_{3k})\}]^{\delta_{1k}\delta_{2k}\delta_{3k}} \\
& F\{dS_{1k},dS_{2k},S_{3k};Z_k(S_{1k},S_{2k},S_{3k})\}^{\delta_{1k}\delta_{2k}(1-\delta_{3k})} \\
& F\{dS_{1k},S_{2k},dS_{3k};Z_k(S_{1k},S_{2k},S_{3k})\}^{\delta_{1k}(1-\delta_{2k})\delta_{3k}} \\
& F\{S_{1k},dS_{2k},dS_{3k};Z_k(S_{1k},S_{2k},S_{3k})\}^{(1-\delta_{1k})\delta_{2k}\delta_{3k}} \\
& [-F\{dS_{1k},S_{2k},S_{3k};Z_k(S_{1k},S_{2k},S_{3k})\}]^{\delta_{1k}(1-\delta_{2k})(1-\delta_{3k})} \\
& [-F\{S_{1k},dS_{2k},S_{3k};Z_k(S_{1k},S_{2k},S_{3k})\}]^{(1-\delta_{1k})\delta_{2k}(1-\delta_{3k})} \\
& [-F\{S_{1k},S_{2k},dS_{3k};Z_k(S_{1k},S_{2k},S_{3k})\}]^{(1-\delta_{1k})(1-\delta_{2k})\delta_{3k}} \\
& [F\{S_{1k},S_{2k},S_{3k};Z_k(S_{1k},S_{2k},S_{3k})\}]^{(1-\delta_{1k})(1-\delta_{2k})(1-\delta_{3k})} \Big). \qquad (5.11)
\end{aligned}
$$

The elements of (5.11) are given, for example, by

$$
\begin{aligned}
F\{t_1,t_2,t_3;Z(t_1,t_2,t_3)\} &= F_0\{v_1,v_2,v_3;\theta(z)\} \\
F\{dt_1,t_2,t_3;Z(t_1,t_2,t_3)\} &= F_0\{dv_1,v_2,v_3;\theta(z)\}dt_1/dv_1, \\
F\{dt_1,dt_2,t_3;Z(t_1,t_2,t_3)\} &= F_0\{dv_1,dv_2,v_3;\theta(z)\}(dt_1/dv_1)(dt_2/dv_2), \text{ and} \\
F\{dt_1,dt_2,dt_3;Z(t_1,t_2,t_3)\} &= F_0\{dv_1,dv_2,dv_3;\theta(z)\}(dt_1/dv_1)(dt_2/dv_2)(dt_3/dv_3),
\end{aligned}
$$

where

$$v_1 = \int_0^{t_1} \Lambda_{100}\{ds_1;0,Z(s_1,0,0)\}, \text{ and } dt_1/dv_1 = \Lambda_{100}\{dt_1,0,0;Z(t_1,0,0)\}^{-1}$$

along with corresponding expressions for $v_2, dt_2/dv_2, v_3$ and dt_3/dv_3.

As with copula models for bivariate failure time data (§4.3) the derivatives of $\log L$ with respect to parameters in the marginal hazard rates may be sensitive to the choice of copula function F_0. In addition, with a parameter θ of low dimension a particular copula model may embrace only a limited class of two- and three-variable dependency models for the failure time variates. Also these dependencies can depend on baseline covariate values $z(0,0,0)$, but not on stochastic covariates that evolve over the study follow-up period. Nevertheless, if carefully applied, the copula approach can be expected to provide useful inferences on marginal hazard rates and on the dependency parameter θ. Furthermore, standard asymptotic likelihood procedure can be applied if marginal hazard rates are specified parametrically. To avoid biases in marginal hazard rate estimation on the basis of inappropriate modeling of bivariate and trivariate dependencies one can combine estimating equations of the types discussed in Chapter 2 for marginal hazard rates, with likelihood-based equations as described above, at specified values for marginal hazard rate parameters, for θ. This type of approach is described by Glidden (2000) under the specialized Clayton–Oakes model where $\theta_{110}(z) = \theta_{101}(z) = \theta_{011}(z) = \theta_{111}(z) = \theta$. This approach can undoubtedly be generalized to the larger class of models (1.9), and may yield quite useful inferences when (1.9) provides an adequate data description. Such generalization, however, has yet to appear in the literature.

5.4 Regression on Marginal Single, Double and Triple Failure Hazard Rates

The semiparametric marginal single failure hazard rate and double failure hazard rate regression methods of §4.6 can be extended to yield a flexible class of regression models for the analysis of trivariate failure time data even if the regression variable includes internal time-varying components. Consider Cox models for the marginal single failure hazard functions $\Lambda_{100}, \Lambda_{010}$ and Λ_{001} given Z, so that

$$\begin{aligned}
\Lambda_{100}\{dt_1,0,0;Z(t_1,0,0)\} &= \Lambda_{100}(dt_1,0,0)\exp\{x(t_1,0,0)\beta_{100}\},\\
\Lambda_{010}\{0,dt_2,0;Z(0,t_2,0)\} &= \Lambda_{010}(0,dt_2,0)\exp\{x(0,t_2,0)\beta_{010}\},\\
\Lambda_{001}\{0,0,dt_3;Z(0,0,t_3)\} &= \Lambda_{001}(0,0,dt_3)\exp\{x(0,0,t_3)\beta_{001}\}.
\end{aligned} \tag{5.12}$$

Analogous to (4.10) one can also specify multiplicative form regression models for each of the marginal double failure hazard rates given Z, so that, in an obvious notation,

$$\begin{aligned}
\Lambda_{110}\{dt_1,dt_2,0;Z(t_1,t_2,0)\} &= \Lambda_{110}(dt_1,dt_2,0)\exp\{x(t_1,t_2,0)\beta_{110}\},\\
\Lambda_{101}\{dt_1,0,dt_3;Z(t_1,0,t_3)\} &= \Lambda_{101}(dt_1,0,dt_3)\exp\{x(t_1,0,t_3)\beta_{101}\},\\
\Lambda_{011}\{0,dt_2,dt_3;Z(0,t_2,t_3)\} &= \Lambda_{011}(0,dt_2,dt_3)\exp\{x(0,t_2,t_3)\beta_{011}\},
\end{aligned} \tag{5.13}$$

with unspecified "baseline" double failure hazard rates, and data-analyst-defined fixed-length regression variables.

Similarly, one can specify a Cox-type model for the marginal triple failure hazard rates away from the coordinate planes so that

$$\Lambda_{111}\{dt_1,dt_2,dt_3;Z(t_1,t_2,t_3)\} = \Lambda_{111}(dt_1,dt_2,dt_3)\exp\{x(t_1,t_2,t_3)\beta_{111}\} \quad (5.14)$$

with fixed-length row regression variable $x(t_1,t_2,t_3)$ and corresponding column vector parameter β_{111}.

The single failure hazard rate parameters can each be estimated as in Chapter 2 using only the marginal data for each of the three failure times. The double failure hazard rate parameters can be estimated as in Chapter 4 using only the marginal bivariate data for each failure time pair. Similarly the triple failure hazard rate regression parameter can be estimated by $\hat{\beta}_{111}$ solving

$$\sum_{i=1}^{I}\sum_{j=1}^{J}\sum_{k=1}^{K}\Bigg\{\sum_{\ell\in D(\Delta t_{1i},\Delta t_{2j},\Delta t_{3k})} x_\ell(t_{1i},t_{2j},t_{3k}) - d_{ijk}^{111}\frac{\sum_{\ell\in R(t_{1i},t_{2j},t_{3k})} x_\ell(t_{1i},t_{2j},t_{3k})e^{x_\ell(t_{1i},t_{2j},t_{3k})\beta_{111}}}{\sum_{\ell\in R(t_{1i},t_{2j},t_{3k})} e^{x_\ell(t_{1i},t_{2j},t_{3k})\beta_{111}}}\Bigg\} = 0, \quad (5.15)$$

where $D(\Delta t_{1i},\Delta t_{2j},\Delta t_{3k})$ denotes the set of individuals experiencing a triple failure at failure time grid point (t_{1i},t_{2j},t_{3k}) with $d_{ijk}^{111} = \#D(\Delta t_{1i},\Delta t_{2j},\Delta t_{3k})$ and $R(t_{1i},t_{2j},t_{3k})$ is the set of individuals at risk for a triple failure at this grid point. The baseline (cumulative) triple failure hazard rate function can be estimated by the step function $\hat{\Lambda}_{111}$ where

$$\hat{\Lambda}_{111}(t_1,t_2,t_3) = \sum_{t_{1i}\le t_1}\sum_{t_{2j}\le t_2}\sum_{t_{3k}\le t_3} d_{ijk}^{111} \Big/ \sum_{\ell\in R(t_{1i},t_{2j},t_{3k})} e^{x_\ell(t_{1i},t_{2j},t_{3k})\hat{\beta}_{111}}$$

for all $(t_1,t_2,t_3) \in R$.

Corresponding to the marginal single, double, and triple failure hazard rate processes, one can define a process F given Z that, away from the coordinate planes, uniquely solves the inhomogeneous Volterra integral equation

$$F\{t_1,t_2,t_3;Z(t_1,t_2,t_3)\} = \Psi\{t_1,t_2,t_3;Z(t_1,t_2,t_3)\} - \int_0^{t_1}\int_0^{t_2}\int_0^{3} F\{s_1^-,s_2^-,s_3^-;Z(s_1,s_2,s_3)\}\Lambda_{111}\{ds_1,ds_2,ds_3;Z(s_1,s_2,s_3)\},$$

at any covariate history Z with Ψ defined as in §5.2.2 at any specific Z. The process will have a survivor function interpretation for covariates that are fixed or are external to the failure time variates (T_1,T_2,T_3).

At any covariate history Z one can calculate a semiparametric estimator $\hat{F}$ given

Z recursively, under (5.12)–(5.14), using

$$\begin{aligned}
\hat{F}\{t_{1i},t_{2j},t_{3k};Z(t_{1i},t_{2j},t_{3k})\} &= \hat{F}\{t_{1i},t_{2j},t_{3k}^-;Z(t_{1i},t_{2j},t_{3k})\} \\
&+\hat{F}\{t_{1i},t_{2j}^-,t_{3k};Z(t_{1i},t_{2j},t_{3k})\}+\hat{F}\{t_{1i}^-,t_{2j},t_{3k};Z(t_{1i},t_{2j},t_{3k})\} \\
&-\hat{F}\{t_{1i},t_{2j}^-,t_{3k}^-;Z(t_{1i},t_{2j},t_{3k})\}-\hat{F}\{t_{1i}^-,t_{2j},t_{3k}^-;Z(t_{1i},t_{2j},t_{3k})\} \\
&-\hat{F}\{t_{1i}^-,t_{2j}^-,t_{3k};Z(t_{1i},t_{2j},t_{3k})\}+\hat{F}\{t_{1i}^-,t_{2j}^-,t_{3k}^-;Z(t_{1i},t_{2j},t_{3k})\} \\
&[1-\hat{\Lambda}_{111}\{t_{1i},t_{2j},t_{3k};Z(t_{1i},t_{2j},t_{3k})\}], \qquad (5.16)
\end{aligned}$$

where $\hat{\Lambda}_{111}\{t_{1i},t_{2j},t_{3k};Z(t_{1i},t_{2j},t_{3k})\} = \hat{\Lambda}_{111}(t_{1i},t_{2j},t_{3k})\exp\{x(t_{1i},t_{2j},t_{3k})\hat{\beta}_{111}\}$.

To apply (5.16), one first estimates $\hat{F}$ given Z along the three failure time axes, then estimates $\hat{F}$ given Z for each of the coordinate planes, then uses (5.16) to estimate $\hat{F}$ given Z away from the coordinate planes throughout the risk region of the data.

After estimating $\hat{F}$ given Z with fixed or external covariates, one can readily calculate estimators of bivariate dependency or trivariate dependency given Z. For example an average trivariate dependency function C_{111} given Z can be defined over a region $[0,\tau_1\times[0,\tau_2]\times[0,\tau_3]$, with (τ_1,τ_2,τ_3) in the support of (S_1,S_2,S_3), by

$$C_{111}\{\tau_1,\tau_2,\tau_3;Z(\tau_1,\tau_2,\tau_3)\} = \frac{\int_0^{\tau_1}\int_0^{\tau_2}\int_0^{\tau_3} F\{t_1^-,t_2^-,t_3^-;Z(t_1,t_2,t_3)\}\Lambda_{111}\{dt_1,dt_2,dt_3;Z(t_1,t_2,t_3)\}}{\int_0^{\tau_1}\int_0^{\tau_2}\int_0^{\tau_3} F\{t_1^-,t_2^-,t_3^-;Z(t_1,t_2,t_3)\}\Lambda_{111}^0\{dt_1,dt_2,dt_3;Z(t_1,t_2,t_3)\}} \qquad (5.17)$$

where the "no trivariate dependency" hazard rate process Λ_{111}^0 given Z is specified recursively by

$$\begin{aligned}
\Lambda_{111}^0\{dt_1,dt_2,dt_3;Z(t_1,t_2,t_3)\} &= 1-\Lambda_{100}\{dt_1,t_2^-,t_3^-;Z(t_1,t_2,t_3)\} \\
&-\Lambda_{010}\{t_1^-,dt_2,t_3^-;Z(t_1,t_2,t_3)\}-\Lambda_{001}\{t_1^-,t_2^-,dt_3;Z(t_1,t_2,t_3)\} \\
&+\Lambda_{110}\{dt_1,dt_2,t_3^-;Z(t_1,t_2,t_3)\}+\Lambda_{101}\{dt_1,t_2^-,dt_3;Z(t_1,t_2,t_3)\} \\
&+\Lambda_{011}\{t_1^-,dt_2,dt_3;Z(t_1,t_2,t_3)\} \\
&-\frac{F\{t_1,t_2,t_3^-;Z(t_1,t_2,t_3)\}F\{t_1,t_2^-,t_3;Z(t_1,t_2,t_3)\}F\{t_1^-,t_2,t_3;Z(t_1,t_2,t_3)\}}{F\{t_1,t_2^-,t_3^-;Z(t_1,t_2,t_3)\}F\{t_1^-,t_2,t_3^-;Z(t_1,t_2,t_3)\}F\{t_1^-,t_2^-,t_3;Z(t_1,t_2,t_3)\}}.
\end{aligned} \qquad (5.18)$$

Hence trivariate dependencies given Z over $[0,\tau_1]\times[0,\tau_2]\times[0,\tau_3]$ for (τ_1,τ_2,τ_3) in the risk region of the data can be estimated semiparametrically by $\hat{C}_{111}\{\tau_1,\tau_2,\tau_3;$ $Z(\tau_1,\tau_2,\tau_3)\}$ obtained by everywhere inserting $\hat{F}$ for F in (5.17).

Asymptotic distribution theory for marginal single, double and triple failure hazard rate parameter estimates under an independent and identically distributed assumption for failure, censoring and covariate processes, and under (5.12)–(5.14), can undoubtedly be obtained using empirical process methods, as is also the case for the related estimators $\hat{F}$ given Z and $\hat{C}_{111}$ given Z. These results will include the usual strong consistency and asymptotic mean zero Gaussian weak convergence for all parameters, as well as a sandwich-type analytic variance estimator for the combined single, double and triple failure hazard ratio regression parameters. Proofs for some of these results will be sketched in a more general context in Chapter 6.

Analogous to Chapter 4 the single, double and triple failure hazard rate models (5.12)–(5.14) need not be mutually consistent in their regression dependencies. Biases in parameter estimates and in related survival process estimates may occur under departures from the specified models, as usual in statistical estimation. However, any such biases can be minimized by exercising the time-dependent covariate features, and corresponding time-dependent baseline hazard rate stratification features, of the hazard ratio regression models.

5.5 Simulation Evaluation of Hazard Ratio Estimators

The trivariate failure time model (5.8) was generalized to

$$F(t_1,t_2,t_3;z) = \{F_0(t_1,0,0)^{-\theta} + F_0(0,t_2,0)^{-\theta} + F_0(0,0,t_3)^{-\theta} - 2\}^{-e^{z\gamma}/\theta} \vee 0 \quad (5.19)$$

to include a baseline regression variable $z = z(0,0,0)$; where F_0 denotes the trivariate survivor function at $z = 0$. The marginal single failure hazard rates from (5.19) have the form $\Lambda_{100}(dt_1,0,0;z) = \Lambda_{100}(dt_1,0,0)e^{z\gamma}, \Lambda_{010}(0,dt_2,0;z) = \Lambda_{010}(0,dt_2,0)e^{z\gamma}$, and $\Lambda_{001}(0,0,dt_3;z) = \Lambda_{001}(0,0,dt_3)e^{z\gamma}$. The marginal double failure hazard rates have the form

$$\begin{aligned}
&\Lambda_{110}(dt_1,dt_2,0;z) = \Lambda_{110}(dt_1,dt_2,0)e^{z\gamma}(e^{z\gamma}+\theta)/(1+\theta),\\
&\Lambda_{101}(dt_1,0,dt_3;z) = \Lambda_{101}(dt_1,0,dt_3)e^{z\gamma}(e^{z\gamma}+\theta)/(1+\theta), \text{ and}\\
&\Lambda_{011}(0,dt_2,dt_3;z) = \Lambda_{011}(0,dt_2,dt_3)e^{z\gamma}(e^{z\gamma}+\theta)/(1+\theta),
\end{aligned}$$

and the triple failure hazard rates have the form

$$\Lambda_{111}(dt_1,dt_2,dt_3;z) = \Lambda_{111}(dt_1,dt_2,dt_3)\frac{e^{z\gamma}(e^{z\gamma}+\theta)(e^{z\gamma}+2\theta)}{(1+\theta)(1+2\theta)}.$$

For a one-dimensional binary covariate z these hazard rates conform to the multiplicative model forms of §5.4 with regression variables $x(t_1,0,0) = x(0,t_2,0) = x(0,0,t_3) = x(t_1,t_2,0) = x(t_1,0,t_3) = x(0,t_2,t_3) = x(t_1,t_2,t_3) = z$ and with regression parameters $\beta_{100} = \beta_{010} = \beta_{001} = \gamma$, $\beta_{110} = \beta_{101} = \beta_{011} = \log\{e^{\gamma}(e^{\gamma}+\theta)/(1+\theta)\}$ and $\beta_{111} = \log[e^{\gamma}(e^{\gamma}+\theta)(e^{\gamma}+2\theta)/\{(1+\theta)(1+2\theta)\}]$. Failure times under this model can be generated as in 5.2.4 at $z = 0$, as is also the case for failure times divided by e^{γ} at $z = 1$. Table 5.3 shows simulation summary statistics for estimation of β_{111} with data generated under this model with z taking values 0 or 1 with probability 0.5 and with unit exponential marginal failure times at $z = 0$, at some choices for n, θ and γ with censoring times independent exponential variates with expectation 2.0. There is little evidence of bias in regression parameter estimates under these sampling configurations and approximate 95% confidence intervals appear to be quite accurate.

Table 5.3 *Simulation sample mean and sample standard deviation, and corresponding average of sandwich standard deviation estimators and related asymptotic 95% confidence interval (CI) coverage probability, for marginal single, double and triple failure regression parameters under (5.19) with binary covariate z taking values 0 and 1 with probability 0.5.*

Regression	True		$\theta = 2, \gamma = 0$ Sandwich	Sample	95% CI	True		$\theta = 2, \gamma = \log 2$ Sandwich	Sample	95% CI
Parameter	Value	Mean*	SD	SD	coverage	Value	Mean	SD	SD	coverage
					$n = 250$					
β_{100}	0	0.007	0.217	0.221	0.955	0.693	0.706	0.201	0.204	0.958
β_{010}	0	0.003	0.225	0.221	0.959	0.693	0.705	0.205	0.203	0.958
β_{001}	0	0.001	0.231	0.220	0.943	0.693	0.697	0.211	0.203	0.944
β_{110}	0	0.008	0.355	0.346	0.957	0.981	1.004	0.323	0.317	0.949
β_{101}	0	0.009	0.349	0.346	0.951	0.981	1.002	0.324	0.317	0.959
β_{011}	0	0.003	0.369	0.346	0.938	0.981	0.991	0.332	0.316	0.942
β_{111}	0	0.012	0.500	0.471	0.945	1.163	1.194	0.447	0.424	0.954
					$n = 500$					
β_{100}	0	−0.007	0.154	0.156	0.947	0.693	0.693	0.141	0.143	0.947
β_{010}	0	−0.004	0.156	0.156	0.954	0.693	0.690	0.142	0.143	0.954
β_{001}	0	−0.008	0.158	0.155	0.948	0.693	0.693	0.146	0.143	0.954
β_{110}	0	−0.009	0.247	0.244	0.942	0.981	1.981	0.229	0.223	0.953
β_{101}	0	−0.015	0.247	0.243	0.934	0.981	1.973	0.225	0.223	0.942
β_{011}	0	−0.013	0.242	0.244	0.947	0.981	0.976	0.225	0.223	0.947
β_{111}	0	−0.016	0.334	0.329	0.951	1.163	1.163	0.303	0.297	0.952

* Summary statistics based on 1000 simulations at each sampling configuration.

5.6 Postmenopausal Hormone Therapy in Relation to CVD and Mortality

Consider again the Women's Health Initiative postmenopausal hormone therapy randomized trial described in §1.7.3. Early adverse effects were observed in the combined estrogen plus progestin (CEE + MPA) trial for each of CHD, stroke and venous thromboembolism (VT), with similar but smaller hazard ratio elevations for the estrogen-alone (CEE) trial. For CHD and VT the risk elevations were relatively larger earlier compared to later post-randomization, while estimated hazard ratios for stroke showed little time dependence and were of similar magnitude (about 1.4) for both CEE and CEE + MPA.

There were too few women experiencing each of CHD, stroke and VT during trial follow-up to support a triple failure hazard ratio comparison of active and placebo groups during the intervention period in either trial. This was also the situation for the marginal double failure hazard ratio analyses involving VT. For CHD and stroke the numbers of double failures in the CEE trial were 14 in the active group compared to 17 in the placebo group, giving a double failure hazard ratio estimate of 0.92 with approximate 95% confidence interval of (0.44, 1.89). The corresponding numbers were 15 and 5 in the CEE + MPA group with double failure hazard ratio estimate of 2.87 and 95% confidence interval of (1.05, 7.89). Hence there is some indication of elevated double failure risk with CEE + MPA, which is not at all suggested for CEE. However, the numbers of double failures is quite small and a cautious interpretation is needed. Related to this, special efforts would be needed to justify the use of asymptotic approximations in this context, primarily because of the small numbers of double failures. Marginal single outcome hazard ratio analyses for these and other outcomes were shown in Figure 2.2.

There are, of course, many other outcomes of interest in these large clinical trials, including the incidence of gallbladder disease, diabetes and hypertension, for which there was evidence for departure from the null in marginal single outcome hazard ratio analyses. We defer consideration of this larger set of outcomes to Chapter 6, which focuses on hazard ratio regression methods for higher dimensional failure time data.

BIBLIOGRAPHIC NOTES

There is only a limited literature on the modeling and analysis of trivariate failure time data. The trivariate Dabrowska estimator discussed in §5.2 was considered recently by the present authors (Prentice & Zhao, 2018). The trivariate copula model (1.9) was introduced in Prentice (2016). The more specialized Clayton–Oakes copula model (5.8) has been considered by several authors. For example, Glidden (2000) considers a model that extends (5.8) to an arbitrary number of failure times with Cox model marginal hazard rates, and consider a two-stage model for estimation of the dependence parameter θ. Glidden and Self (1999) and Pipper and Martinussen (2003) consider this same model with joint estimation of marginal hazard rate and cross ratio parameters. The regression analysis of trivariate failure time data via the semiparametric models (5.12)–(5.14) was proposed recently by the present authors (Prentice & Zhao, 2019).

EXERCISES AND COMPLEMENTS

Exercise 5.1

Show that the right side of (5.1) reduces to $F(t_1,t_2,t_3)$, for any (t_1,t_2,t_3) value with discrete failure time variates (T_1,T_2,T_3).

Exercise 5.2

Develop the recursive relationship (5.2) at a general uncensored failure time grid point (t_{1i},t_{2j},t_{3k}) away from the coordinate planes (where one or more of t_{1i},t_{2j}, and t_{3k} take value zero).

Exercise 5.3

Develop the hazard rate–based expression (5.5) using (5.3). Provide an argument as to why (5.5) holds even if the failure time variates may include both continuous and discrete components.

Exercise 5.4

Show that (5.5) reduces to (1.8) for absolutely continuous failure times (T_1,T_2,T_3).

Exercise 5.5

Using empirical process convergence results, particularly the Glivenko–Cantelli and Donsker theorems, show the Volterra estimator $\hat{F}$ described in §5.2.2 to converge to a Gaussian process over a region $[0,\tau_1]\times[0,\tau_2]\times[0,\tau_3]$ where $P(S_1>\tau_1,S_2>\tau_2,S_3>\tau_3)>0$ under IID conditions.

Exercise 5.6

Derive expressions (5.9) and (5.10) from (5.8). Show that failure times under (5.8), for $\theta\geq 1/3$ can be generated from independent uniform $(0,1)$ variables (u_1,u_2,u_3) via the transformation given in §5.2.4. Can you generalize this result to the generation of failure times $(t_1,\ldots,t_m)$ from independent uniform $(0,1)$ variates $(u_1,\ldots,u_m)$ under the model $F(t_1,\ldots,t_m)=\{F(t_1,0\ldots,0)^{-\theta}+\ldots+F(0,\ldots,0,t_m)^{-\theta}-(m-1)\}^{-1/\theta}\vee 0$ for an arbitrary number, m, of failure time variates?

Exercise 5.7

Discuss, based on the application in §5.6, whether or not the copula model (1.9), with each marginal survival probability allowed to depend arbitrarily on randomization assignment, would provide an adequate description of the Women's Health Initiative hormone therapy trial data. Does this copula model lead to convenient inferences about hormone therapy effects on the composite outcome of CHD and stroke?

Exercise 5.8

Consider a trivariate survivor function model

$$\begin{aligned}F(t_1,t_2,t_3) =&\{F(t_1,t_2,0)^{-\theta}+F(t_1,0,t_3)^{-\theta}+F(0,t_2,t_3)^{-\theta} \\ &-F(t_1,0,0)^{-\theta}-F(0,t_2,0)^{-\theta}-F(0,0,t_3)^{-\theta}+1\}^{-1/\theta}\vee 0.\end{aligned}$$

Using L'Hôpital's rule show that $F(t_1,t_2,t_3)$ approaches

$$F(t_1,t_2,0)F(t_1,0,t_3)F(0,t_2,t_3)/\{F(t_1,0,0)F(0,t_2,0)F(0,0,t_3)\}$$

as $\theta \to 0$, approaches the upper bound

$$F(t_1,t_2,0)\wedge F(t_1,0,t_3)\wedge F(0,t_2,t_3)$$

as $\theta \to \infty$, and approaches the lower bound

$$0\vee\{F(t_1,t_2,0)+F(t_1,0,t_3)+F(0,t_2,t_3)-F(t_1,0,0)-F(0,t_2,0)-F(0,0,t_3)+1\}$$

as $\theta \to -1$, and that all points (t_1,t_2,t_3) away from this lower bound are continuity points for (T_1,T_2,T_3) for any $\theta \in [-1,\infty)$ (Prentice, 2016).

Consider the special case where the three bivariate survivor functions adhere to Clayton–Oakes models (1.7) with respective parameters θ_{12},θ_{13} and θ_{23}. Show that (5.8) is the much more restrictive model with $\theta_{12}=\theta_{13}=\theta_{23}=\theta$, and therefore comment on the utility of (5.8) as a general model for trivariate failure time data.

Exercise 5.9

Consider a regression generalization of the above model to

$$\begin{aligned}F(t_1,t_2,t_3;z) =&\{F(t_1,t_2,0;z)^{-\theta}+F(t_1,0,t_3;z)^{-\theta|}+F(0,t_2,t_3;z)^{-\theta} \\ &-F(t_1,0,0;z)^{-\theta}-F(0,t_2,0;z)^{-\theta}-F(0,0,t_3;z)^{-\theta}+1\}^{-e^{z\gamma}/\theta}\vee 0.\end{aligned}$$

Further consider Cox models

$$\begin{aligned}F(t_1,0,0;z) =&F_0(t_1,0,0)^{e^{z\beta_{100}}}, F(0,t_2,0;z)=F_0(0,t_2,0)^{e^{z\beta_{010}}}, \\ &\text{and } F(0,0,t_3;z)=F_0(0,0,t_3)^{e^{z\beta_{001}}}\end{aligned}$$

for marginal survivor functions, and Clayton–Oakes models

$$\begin{aligned}F(t_1,t_2,0;z) &= \{F(t_1,0,0;z)^{-\theta_{12}}+F(0,t_2,0;z)^{-\theta_{12}}-1\}^{-e^{z\beta_{110}}/\theta_{12}}\vee 0, \\ F(t_1,0,t_3;z) &= \{F(t_1,0,0;z)^{-\theta_{13}}+F(0,0,t_3;z)^{-\theta_{13}}-1\}^{-e^{z\beta_{101}}/\theta_{13}}\vee 0, \text{ and} \\ F(0,t_2,t_3;z) &= \{F(0,t_2,0;z)^{-\theta_{23}}+F(0,0,t_3;z)^{-\theta_{23}}-1\}^{-e^{z\beta_{011}}/\theta_{23}}\vee 0,\end{aligned}$$

for pairwise survivor functions. Show for a binary covariate z that the single, double and triple failure hazard rates conform to the multiplicative models (5.12)–(5.14) under this model. Can you develop an approach to generating failure times under this model for F given z? In what ways might the data analysis methods of §5.4 add valuable flexibility to parametric or semiparametric data analysis methods under this model? In what ways might the regression model of this exercise have comparative advantages for summarizing data from, say, a genetic epidemiology study of breast cancer that includes index cases (probands) as well as their female siblings and daughters.

Chapter 6

Higher Dimensional Failure Time Data Modeling and Estimation

6.1 Introduction

This chapter extends the regression methods of Chapters 4 and 5 in two important respects: First, the number of possibly correlated failure time variates is extended to a fixed, but arbitrary, number m. Secondly, the baseline rates in the multiplicative (Cox-type) models are allowed to be shared by failure times of the same "type," with failure times uniquely classified into $K \leq m$ types. This latter feature allows "individuals" to contribute multiple times to risk sets that arise in regression parameter estimation, thereby leading also to a marginal modeling approach to recurrent event data that will be elaborated in Chapter 7. The methods of this chapter provide a culmination of the marginal modeling approach for correlated outcomes that is central to this monograph. Regression methods for marginal single outcome hazard rates will be presented in §6.3, while those for marginal single and dual outcome hazard rates will be given in §6.5. As previously, the multivariate failure times may be on the same or different time axes, though failures of the same type will be required to be on the same time axis. Before entertaining these regression methods, for completeness, the nonparametric survivor function estimators of Chapters 3 and 5 will be extended to an arbitrary number of failure time variates (§6.2). Also, the copula approach to higher dimensional failure time data will be discussed (§6.4).

As mentioned above, in this chapter the survivor function and regression estimation procedures of Chapters 3–5 will be generalized to an arbitrary number, m, of failure time variates, denoted by $T_1,\ldots,T_m$. Suppose that $(T_1,\ldots,T_m)$ is subject to censoring by a variate $(C_1,\ldots,C_m)$, and let $Z(t_1,\ldots,t_m) = \{z(s_1,\ldots,s_m); s_j = 0$ if $t_j = 0$ and $s_j < t_j$ if $t_j > 0$, for $j = 1,\ldots,m\}$ denote the history of a corresponding covariate process, Z, up to $(t_1,\ldots,t_m)$. A marginal hazard process can be defined for any subset of the m failure time variates given Z. For example, for $(T_1,\ldots,T_j), j \leq m$ one can define a marginal j-dimensional failure hazard rate process $\Lambda_{1\cdots10\cdots0}$ by

$$\Lambda_{1\cdots10\cdots0}\{dt_1,dt_2,\ldots,dt_j,0\cdots0;Z(t_1,\ldots,t_j,0\cdots0)\} =$$
$$\mathrm{pr}\{T_1 \in [t_1,t_1+dt_1),\ldots,T_j \in [t_j,t_j+dt_j); T_1 \geq t_1,\ldots,T_j \geq t_j, Z(t_1,\ldots,t_j,0,\ldots,0)\},$$

where the first j subscripts of Λ are 1 and the remainder 0.

A global independent censoring assumption given Z specifies that $C_1 \geq t_1,\ldots,C_j \geq t_j$ can be added to the conditioning event without changing the value of this hazard rate for all $(t_1,\ldots,t_j)$ and $Z(t_1,\ldots,t_j,0,\ldots,0)$, and similarly for hazard rates for each of the $2^m - 1$ non-empty subsets of $(T_1,\ldots,T_m)$. This independent censoring assumption can be weakened to only single failure, or to only single and double failure hazard rates if estimation is restricted to these marginal hazard rates. Note that a different modeling approach may be needed if marginal hazard rates given Z depend on the preceding values of the companion failure time variates. Counting process intensity modeling may be useful in that context, but regression parameter interpretation and assumptions differ substantially between these two modeling approaches, as will be elaborated in §6.6.

6.2 Nonparametric Estimation of the *m*-Dimensional Survivor Function

6.2.1 *Dabrowska-type estimator development*

Consider an arbitrary number of failure time variates $(T_1,\ldots,T_m)$ subject to independent right censoring by variate $(C_1,\ldots,C_m)$ and suppose that statistically independent and identically distributed replicates $S_{j\ell} = T_{j\ell} \wedge C_{j\ell}$ and $\delta_{j\ell} = I[S_{j\ell} = T_{j\ell}]$ for $j = 1,\ldots,m$ are obtained, for $\ell = 1,\ldots,n$.

The nonparametric likelihood function, L, for the joint survivor function F, where $F(t_1,\ldots t_m) = P(T_1 > t_1,\ldots,T_m > t_m)$ can be readily specified, and can be seen to be maximized by placing probability within the risk region of the data only at grid points formed by the uncensored observations for each of the m failure time variates. In fact L is maximized by a discrete survivor function with "point mass" assignments within $R = \{(t_1,\ldots,t_m); S_{j\ell} \geq t_j$ for each $j = 1,\ldots,m$, for some $\ell \in (1,\ldots,n)\}$ only at these grid points.

Building on Dabrowska (1988), Gill (1994) and Prentice and Zhao (2018), one can represent the discrete survivor function F by

$$F(t_1,\dots,t_m) = \prod_{j=1}^{m} Q_j(t_1,\dots,t_m), \tag{6.1}$$

where $Q_1(t_1,\dots,t_m)$ is the product of the m single product integrals of the form $\prod_0^{t_1} F(s_1,0,\dots,0)/F(s_1^-,0,\dots,0)$ for the marginal survival probabilities; $Q_2(t_1,\dots,t_m)$ is the product of the $\binom{m}{2}$ double product integrals of the form

$$\prod_0^{t_1}\prod_0^{t_2}[F(s_1,s_2,0,\dots,0)F(s_1^-,s_2^-,0,\dots,0)/\{F(s_1,s_2^-,0,\dots,0)F(s_1^-,s_2,0,\dots,0)\}]$$

for the marginal pairwise dependencies; and for $j=3,\dots,m$ $Q_j(t_1,\dots,t_m)$ is the product of the $\binom{m}{j}$ j-dimensional product integrals of the form

$$\prod_0^{t_1}\prod_0^{t_2}\cdots\prod_0^{t_j}\frac{A(s_1,\dots,s_j,0,\dots,0)}{B(s_1,\dots,s_j,0,\dots,0)}, \tag{6.2}$$

for marginal j-variate dependencies.

In (6.2) $A(s_1,\dots,s_j,0,\dots,0)$ is composed of the product of the 2^{j-1} factors $F(u_1,\dots,u_j,0,\dots,0)$ having $u_j = s_i^-$ for an even number of u_j's and the remaining u_j's equal to s_i, for $i=1,\dots,j$; and $B(s_1,\dots,s_j,0,\dots,0)$ is the product of the complementary 2^{j-1} factors $F(u_1,\dots,u_j,0,\dots,0)$ having an odd number of u_j's equal to s_i^- and the remainder of the u_j's equal to s_i, for $i=1,\dots,j$.

The decomposition (6.1) follows from massive cancellations, in conjunction with $F(0,\dots,0)=1$. The jth factor $Q_j(t_1,\dots,t_m)$ characterizes the j-variate dependencies among the m-variates for $j=2,\dots,m$. Because of the equal number of factors in $A(s_1,\dots,s_j,0,\dots,0)$ and $B(s_1,\dots,s_j,0,\dots,0)$ one can divide each such factor by $F(s_1^-,\dots,s_j^-,0,\dots,0)$ without altering (6.2), giving an expression for F in terms of conditional survival probabilities at each potential mass point for the discrete survivor function. The conditional survival probabilities at each uncensored failure time grid point in the risk region for the data are readily estimated empirically via

$$\tilde{F}(u_1,\dots,u_j,0,\dots,0) = \frac{\#\{\ell; S_{i\ell} > s_i \text{ if } u_i = s_i, \text{ or } S_{i\ell} \geq s_i \text{ if } u_i = s_i^-, \text{ for all } i=1,\dots,j\}}{\#\{\ell; S_{i\ell} \geq s_i, \text{ all } i=1,\dots,j\}},$$

giving a nonparametric estimator $\hat{F}$ of the m-dimensional survivor function.

This estimator can be calculated in a recursive fashion. Specifically, $\hat{F}$ can be calculated by first calculating the m marginal KM estimators, then recursively calculating the $\binom{m}{2}$ pairwise marginal survival function estimators using (3.6), then recursively calculating the $\binom{m}{3}$ trivariate marginal survivor function estimators using (5.2), continuing through the recursive calculation of the m marginal survivor function estimators of dimension $m-1$, and finally calculating $\hat{F}$ away from its coordinate axes where one or more arguments are equal to zero, recursively by equating the m-variate dependency factor at uncensored failure time grid point $(t_1,\ldots,t_m)$ to its corresponding empirical estimator, giving

$$\hat{F}(t_1,\ldots,t_m) = \frac{\hat{B}(t_1,\ldots,t_m)}{\hat{A}_{\text{-}}(t_1,\ldots,t_m)} \frac{\tilde{A}(t_1,\ldots,t_m)}{\tilde{B}(t_1,\ldots,t_m)}, \tag{6.3}$$

where $\hat{B}(t_1,\ldots,t_m)$ is $B(t_1,\ldots,t_m)$ with all survival probability factors $F(u_1,\ldots,u_m)$ replaced by $\hat{F}(u_1,\ldots,u_m)$ from preceding calculations, where each u_i equals t_i or t_i^-. $\hat{A}_{\text{-}}(t_1,\ldots,t_m)$ similarly replaces each $F(u_1,\ldots,u_m)$ in $A(t_1,\ldots,t_m)$ by $\hat{F}(u_1,\ldots,u_m)$ after dropping $F(t_1,\ldots,t_m)$ from this product; and $\tilde{A}(t_1,\ldots,t_m)$ and $\tilde{B}(t_1,\ldots,t_m)$ equal $A(t_1,\ldots,t_m)$ and $B(t_1,\ldots,t_m)$ respectively with each survival probability replaced by its empirical conditional survival probability $\tilde{F}$ estimator, with $\hat{F}$ defined to take value zero at any grid point (only on the boundary of the risk region) where $\tilde{B} = 0$.

Using this recursive procedure it will be practical to calculate $\hat{F}$ for fairly large data sets, at least for a moderate number of failure time variates. Also note that from the decomposition (6.1) one sees that a nonparametric estimator of F under the restriction of no dependencies of dimension higher than i among the m-variates is readily obtained as $\prod_{j=1}^{i} \hat{Q}_j(t_1,\ldots,t_m)$, where $\hat{Q}_j(t_1,\ldots,t_m)$ everywhere inserts survivor function estimates $\hat{F}$ for F for $i \leq m$, which simply truncates the recursive procedure described above following the ith step.

Asymptotic distributional results for this m-dimensional estimator follow from empirical process theory with little change from §5.2.1, so only a brief account will be given here: The discrete failure time representation (6.1)–(6.2), following re-expression in terms of conditional survival probabilities, can be further expressed in terms of single, double, $\ldots, m$ variate hazard functions each of which has an empirical estimator with asymptotic distribution determined by empirical process theory. For example one can write

$$\begin{aligned}
&\frac{F(s_1,\ldots,s_i,0,\ldots,0)}{F(s_1^-,\ldots,s_i^- 0,\ldots,0)} = \\
&1 - \Lambda_{10\cdots0}(ds_1,s_2^-,\ldots,s_i^-,0,\ldots,0) - \cdots - \Lambda_{0\cdots010\cdots0}(s_1^-,\ldots,s_{i-1}^-,ds_i,0,\ldots,0) \\
&+ \Lambda_{110\cdots0}(ds_1,ds_2,s_3^-,\ldots,s_i^-,0,\ldots,0) + \cdots \\
&+ \Lambda_{0\cdots0110\ldots0}(s_1^-,\ldots,s_{i-2}^-,ds_{i-1},ds_i,0,\ldots,0) \\
&- \Lambda_{1110\cdots0}(ds_1,ds_2,ds_3,s_4^-,\ldots s_i^-,0,\ldots,0) - \cdots \\
&- \Lambda_{0\cdots01110\cdots0}(s_1^-,\ldots,s_{i-3}^-,ds_{i-2},ds_{i-1},ds_i,0,\ldots,0) \\
&+ \cdots (-1)^i \Lambda_{1\ldots10\cdots0}(ds_1,\ldots,ds_i,0,\ldots,0).
\end{aligned} \tag{6.4}$$

Also (6.4) can be used to define a j-variate hazard rate function $\Lambda^0_{1\cdots10\cdots0}$ such that, given lower dimensional hazard rate functions,

$$\begin{aligned}
\Lambda^0_{1\cdots10\cdots0}(s_1\ldots,s_j,0,\ldots,0) = B(s_1,\ldots,s_j,0,\ldots,0)/ \\
\{A_{\text{-}}(s_1,\ldots,s_j,0,\ldots,0)F(s_1^-,\ldots,s_j^-,0,\ldots,0)\}.
\end{aligned} \tag{6.5}$$

Note that there will be no j-variate dependency among $(T_1,\ldots,T_j)$ under the hazard rate function $\Lambda^0_{1\cdots10\cdots0}$. One can rewrite (6.2) in standard product integral format as

$$\prod_0^{t_1}\cdots\prod_0^{t_j}\Big[1+\{\Lambda_{1\cdots10\cdots0}(ds_1,\ldots,ds_j,0,\ldots,0)-\Lambda^0_{1\cdots10\cdots0}(ds_1,\ldots,ds_j,0,\ldots,0)\}$$
$$F(t_1^-,\ldots,t_j^-,0\cdots0)\frac{A_-(t_1,\ldots,t_j,0,\ldots,0)}{B(t_1,\ldots,t_j,0,\ldots,0)}\Big]. \tag{6.6}$$

Similarly each of the conditional survival probabilities in (6.1) can be re-expressed in terms of standard-form product integrals. In fact, after doing so, the resulting hazard-based representation for F applies not only to discrete, but also to absolutely continuous and mixed failure time variates.

One can define 2^m-1 single, double,$\cdots$,m-variate counting processes $(N_{10\cdots0},\ldots,N_{0\cdots01},N_{110\cdots0},\ldots,N_{0\cdots011},N_{1110\cdots0},\ldots,N_{1\cdots1})$ and at-risk process Y over a region $[0,\tau_1]\times\cdots\times[0,\tau_m]$ where $P(S_1>\tau_1,\ldots,S_m>\tau_m)>0$. The strong consistency, weak Gaussian convergence, and bootstrap applicability for these 2^m processes, based on the Glivenko–Cantelli and Donsker theorems, imply these same properties for the 2^m-1 single, double,$\ldots$,m-variate empirical hazard function processes on the basis of the continuity and (weakly continuous) compact differentiability of the hazard process transformations. These same properties also hold for the further product integral transformations for the 2^m-1 hazard processes to the 2^m-1 estimated (conditional) probability factors on the right side of (6.1) on the basis of the continuity and compact differentiability of factors of the form (6.6), and for $\hat F$ itself, based on the continuity and compact differentiability of the transformation (6.1). Hence one sees (informally) that

$$\sup_{[0,\tau_1]\times\cdots\times[0,\tau_m]}|\hat F(t_1,\ldots,t_m)-F(t_1,\ldots,t_m)|\xrightarrow{P}0,$$

$n^{1/2}(\hat F-F)$ converges in distribution to a mean zero Gaussian process, and bootstrap procedures apply to the nonparametric estimator $\hat F$ over the region $[0,\tau_1]\times\cdots\times[0,\tau_m]$.

6.2.2 *Volterra nonparametric survivor function estimator*

The Volterra bivariate survivor function estimators described in Chapters 3 and 5 can also be generalized to an arbitrary number of failure time variates. In particular, the survivor function F is the unique solution to the inhomogeneous Volterra integral equation

$$F(t_1,\ldots,t_m)=\psi(t_1,\ldots,t_m)+\int_0^{t_1}\cdots\int_0^{t_m}F(s_1^-,\ldots s_m^-)\Lambda_{11\cdots1}(ds_1,\ldots,ds_m), \tag{6.7}$$

where

$$\psi(t_1,\ldots,t_m) =$$
$$F(t_1,\ldots,t_{m-1},0)+\cdots+F(0,t_2,\ldots,t_m)-F(t_1,\ldots,t_{m-2},0,0)-\cdots-F(0,0,t_3,\ldots,t_m)$$
$$+F(t_1,\ldots,t_{m-3},0,0,0)+\cdots+F(0,0,0,t_4,\ldots t_m)-\cdots+(-1)^{m-2}F(t_1,0,\ldots,0)+$$
$$\cdots+(-1)^{m-2}F(0,\ldots,0,t_m)+(-1)^{m-1}$$

is a function of marginal survivor probabilities of dimension less than m.

The Péano series solution to (6.7) can be written

$$F(t_1,\ldots,t_m) = \psi(t_1,\ldots,t_m)+\sum_{k=1}^{\infty}\int\int_{0<s_{11}<\cdots<s_{1k}=t_1}\cdots\int \cdots \int\int_{0<s_{m1}<\cdots<s_{mk}=t_m}\cdots\int$$
$$\psi(s_{11}^-,\ldots,s_{m1}^-)\prod_{\ell=1}^{k}\Lambda_{11\cdots 1}(ds_{1\ell},\ldots,ds_{m\ell}). \tag{6.8}$$

The corresponding Volterra estimator, $\hat{F}$, is obtained by plugging empirical hazard rate estimators into (6.8) and into each of its lower dimensional marginal survivor functions. Empirical process theory, in conjunction with the continuity and weakly continuous compact differentiability of each of the pertinent Péano series transformations are then the key elements needed to show $\hat{F}$ to be strongly consistent and asymptotically Gaussian with bootstrap applicability.

A simple recursive procedure can be used to calculate the step function $\hat{F}$ at uncensored failure grid points in the risk region of the data, starting with the KM marginal estimators that arise from plugging Nelson–Aalen estimators into (6.8). Specifically, following the calculation of lower dimensional marginals, the Volterra estimator at an uncensored data grid point $(t_1,\ldots,t_m)$ away from the coordinate axes is given by

$$\begin{aligned}\hat{F}(t_1,\ldots,t_m) =& \hat{F}(t_1,\ldots,t_{m-1},t_m^-)+\cdots+\hat{F}(t_1^-,t_2,\ldots,t_m)\\ &-\hat{F}(t_1,\ldots,t_{m-2},t_{m-1}^-,t_m^-)-\cdots-\hat{F}(t_1^-,t_2^-,t_3,\ldots t_m)\\ &+\hat{F}(t_1,\ldots,t_{m-3},t_{m-2}^-,t_{m-1}^-,t_m^-)+\cdots+\hat{F}(t_1^-,t_2^-,t_3^-,t_4,\ldots,t_m)-\cdots\\ &+(-1)^{m-2}\hat{F}(t_1,t_2^-,\ldots,t_m^-)+\cdots+(-1)^{m-2}\hat{F}(t_1^-,\ldots,t_{m-1}^-,t_m)\\ &+(-1)^{m-1}\hat{F}(t_1^-,\ldots,t_m^-)\{1-\hat{\Lambda}_{11\cdots 1}(\Delta t_1,\ldots,\Delta t_m)\},\end{aligned} \tag{6.9}$$

where $\hat{\Lambda}_{11\cdots 1}(\Delta t_1,\ldots,\Delta t_m) = \#\{\ell; S_{j\ell}=t_j, \delta_{j\ell}=1, \text{all } j=1,\ldots,m\}/\#\{\ell; S_{j\ell}\geq t_j, \text{all } j=1,\ldots,m\}$.

6.2.3 *Multivariate dependency assessment*

A local measure of i-variate dependency, for $i=2,\ldots,m$ can be defined for $(T_1,\ldots,T_i)$ at $(t_1,\ldots,t_i)$ by

$$\Lambda_{1\cdots 10\cdots 0}(dt_1,\ldots dt_i,0,\ldots,0)/\Lambda^0_{1\cdots 10\cdots 0}(dt_1,\ldots,dt_i,0,\ldots,0)$$

which compares the i-variate hazard rate to that under no i-variate dependency at $(t_1,\ldots,t_i,0,\ldots,0)$ on a relative scale. A corresponding average i-variate dependency ratio $C(\tau_1,\ldots,\tau_i,0,\ldots,0)$, for $(\tau_1,\ldots,\tau_i,0,\ldots,0)$ in the support of $(S_1,S_2,\ldots,S_m)$ can be defined by

$$C_{1\cdots 10\cdots 0}(\tau_1,\ldots\tau_i,0,\ldots,0)^{-1} = \int_0^{\tau_1}\cdots\int_0^{\tau_i}\{\Lambda^0_{1\cdots 10\cdots 0}(dt_1,\ldots,dt_i,0,\ldots,0)/ \Lambda_{1\cdots 10\cdots 0}(dt_1,\ldots,dt_i,0,\ldots,0)\}F(dt_1,\ldots dt_i,0,\ldots,0)\Big/ \int_0^{\tau_1}\cdots\int_0^{\tau_i}F(dt_1,\ldots,dt_i,0,\ldots,0).$$

This i-variate dependency ratio can be estimated nonparametrically by

$$\hat{C}_{1\cdots 10\cdots 0}(\tau_1,\ldots,\tau_i,0,\ldots,0) = \int_0^{\tau_1}\cdots\int_0^{\tau_i}\hat{F}(t_1^-,\ldots,t_i^-,0,\ldots 0)\hat{\Lambda}_{1\cdots 10\cdots 0}(\Delta t_1,\ldots,\Delta t_i,0,\ldots 0)\Big/ \int_0^{\tau_1}\cdots\int_0^{\tau_i}\hat{F}(t_1^-,\ldots,t_i^-,0,\ldots,0)\hat{\Lambda}^0_{1\cdots 10\cdots 0}(\Delta t_1,\ldots,\Delta t_i,0,\ldots,0).$$

As a process $\hat{C}_{1\cdots 10\cdots 0}$ inherits strong consistency, weak Gaussian convergence, and bootstrap applicability properties as an estimator of $C_{1\cdots 10\cdots 0}$ from those for $\hat{F}$; for example, using the Dabrowska- or Volterra-nonparametric estimators.

More specifically, the bootstrap procedures alluded to above involve random sampling from the data $\{(S_{jk},\delta_{j\ell}), j=1,\ldots,n\}$ with replacement until a new sample of size n has been drawn. A joint survivor function estimator, say $\hat{F}_*$, is then developed using one of the estimation procedures described above. This process is repeated independently for a large number of replicates (e.g., 100 or more) giving a set of $\hat{F}_*$ values that in large samples act like a random sample from the distribution of $\hat{F}$ from the original data, providing the basis for the estimation of confidence intervals or bands for $\hat{F}$ and for functions thereof such as $\hat{C}_{1\cdots 10\cdots 0}$, or for other purposes. Some care may be needed in using bootstrap estimators of $\hat{F}$ near the boundary of the risk region of the data, since bootstrap samples may have a slightly reduced risk region compared to the original data.

6.3 Regression Analysis on Marginal Single Failure Hazard Rates

Consider an independent and identically distributed sample $\{S_{ji} = T_{ji}\wedge C_{ji}\ \delta_{ji} = I[T_{ji}=C_{ji}]$ for $j=1,\ldots,m; Z_i(S_{1i},\ldots,S_{mi})\}$, for $i=1,\ldots,n$ with possible dependencies among the m failure times $(T_{1i},\ldots,T_{mi})$ for each i, and with censoring variates $(C_{1i},\ldots,C_{mi})$ independent of $(T_{1i},\ldots,T_{mi})$, given a possibly evolving covariate Z. One can consider any of the regression models of Chapter 2 for the marginal hazard rates for each of the m failure time variates, conditional on pertinent covariate histories. For example, one could specify a Cox model for the jth marginal single failure hazard rate by

$$\Lambda_{0\cdots010\cdots0}\{0,\ldots,0,dt_j,0,\ldots0;Z(0,\ldots,0,t_j,0\cdots0)\} = \Lambda_{0\cdots010\cdots0}(0,\ldots,0,dt_j,0,\ldots0)\exp\{x(0,\ldots,0,t_j,0,\ldots,0)\beta_{0\cdots010\cdots0}\} \quad (6.10)$$

for each $j = 1,\ldots,m$. The regression parameters in these models, as well as the corresponding baseline hazard functions can be readily estimated simply by restricting the analysis to the censored failure times and marginal covariate histories for each T_j, for $j = 1,\ldots,m$ separately. To explore models, for example, that place restrictions (e.g., some common values) among the regression parameters in (6.10) requires somewhat more complex analyses to accommodate dependencies among the m failure time variates. Procedures for doing so can be embedded in a class of models that also allows baseline hazard models to be shared among certain of the correlated failure times. Such models will be natural in some settings, for example in studies of failure time among littermates in animal experiments, or studies including multiple generation kindreds in genetic epidemiology.

In the terminology of Spiekerman and Lin (1998) suppose that the jth failure time variable is assigned a unique "failure type" $k = M(j)$, for each $j = 1,\ldots,m$ with failures of the same type on the same time axis. Suppose also that failure times of the same type, k, have marginal single failure hazard rates modeled with a common baseline hazard function Γ_k for each failure type $k = 1,\ldots,K \leq m$. Denote the regression vector formed from $\{t_j;Z(0,\ldots,t_j,0,\ldots,0)\}$ by $x_k(t_j)$, so that Γ_k is the single failure hazard rate for T_j given its corresponding covariate history at $x_k(t_j) \equiv 0$.

With these specifications the Cox-type model marginal single failure hazard rate models for each T_j given Z can be written

$$\Lambda_{0\cdots010\cdots0}\{0,\ldots,0,dt_j,0,\ldots,0;Z(0,\ldots,0,t_j,0,\ldots,0)\} = \Gamma_k(dt_j)\exp\{x_k(t_j)\beta\}, \quad (6.11)$$

with $k = M(j)$ for each $j = 1,\ldots,m$. The fixed-length modeled regression vector $x_k(t_j) = \{x_{1k}(t_j),x_{2k}(t_j),\ldots\}$ in (6.11) is defined to include the same elements for each j such that $M(j) = k$. These models have been written with a single regression parameter β. Hazard ratio functions that, for example, have distinct regression parameters for each $k = 1,\ldots,K$ can be included in (6.11) by appropriate specifications of the modeled regression variable $x_k(t_j)$. That is, $x_k(t_j)$ can include interaction terms that allow distinct parameter vectors for each k. The methods of Chapter 2 do not immediately apply to the estimation of model parameters $(\beta,\Gamma_1,\ldots,\Gamma_K)$ because of dependencies among the m failure time variates, given corresponding covariate histories. However, useful and convenient estimation is possible using estimating equations derived under (6.11).

It is convenient to express estimators for parameters in (6.11) using counting process notation, as in §2.9. Consider $\hat{\beta}$ that solves

$$\sum_{i=1}^{n}\left[\sum_{j=1}^{m}\sum_{k=1}^{K} I\{M(j)=k\}\int_0^{\tau_k}\{x_{ki}(t_k)-E_k(t_k;\beta)\}N_{ji}(dt_k)\right] = 0 \quad (6.12)$$

where

$$\begin{aligned} Y_{ji}(t) &= \{1 \text{ if } t \leq S_{ji}; 0 \text{ otherwise}\}, \\ N_{ji}(t) &= \{1 \text{ if } t \geq S_{ji}, \delta_{ji} = 1; 0 \text{ otherwise}\}, \\ \text{and} \tau_k &= \max_{(j,i)}\{S_{ji}; M(j) = k\}. \end{aligned}$$

Also in (6.12)

$$\begin{aligned} E_k(t_k;\beta) =& n^{-1} \sum_{\ell=1}^{n} \sum_{j=1}^{m} I\{M(j)=k\} Y_{j\ell}(t_k) x_{k\ell}(t_k) e^{x_{k\ell}(t_k)\beta} \Big/ \\ & \left[n^{-1} \sum_{\ell=1}^{n} \sum_{j=1}^{m} I\{M(j)=k\} Y_{j\ell}(t_k) e^{x_{k\ell}(t_k)\beta} \right]. \end{aligned} \tag{6.13}$$

Simple conditioning arguments can be used to show the integrand in (6.12) to have mean zero at any t_k if the m failure time variates are of distinct types, but otherwise "individuals" may contribute multiple times to the type k risk set at t_k complicating the distribution theory emanating from the centering variables in (6.12). However, under IID sampling for failure, censoring and covariate processes, $\hat{\beta}$ quite generally still provides a consistent estimator of the true β value in (6.11), which will now be denoted as β_0.

To see this property, consider the centered counting processes $L_{ji}(\cdot,\beta)$ defined by

$$L_{ji}(t;\beta) = N_{ji}(t) - \int_0^t \sum_{k=1}^{K} I\{M(j)=k\} Y_{ji}(s) e^{x_{ki}(s)\beta} \Gamma_k(ds) \tag{6.14}$$

for all $i = 1,\ldots,n; j = 1,\ldots,m$. Though typically not having the martingale properties enjoyed by the centered counting processes in §2.9, these are zero mean processes under (6.11) at $\beta = \beta_0$, and a simple exercise shows that (6.12) can be rewritten as

$$\sum_{i=1}^{n} \left[\sum_{j=1}^{m} \sum_{k=1}^{K} I\{M(j)=k\} \int_0^{\tau_k} \{x_{ki}(t_k) - E_k(t_k;\beta)\} L_{ji}(dt_k;\beta) \right] = 0. \tag{6.15}$$

Under IID conditions the numerator and denominator of (6.13) each approach their expectation almost surely as $n \to \infty$, and some careful analysis by Spiekerman and Lin (1998) shows that this convergence is sufficiently rapid that $E_k(t_k;\beta)$ in (6.15) can be replaced by the ratio of these expectations, which we denote by $e_k(t_k;\beta)$, without changing the asymptotic distribution of the left side of (6.15), under quite general conditions. It then follows that $n^{-1/2}$ times the left side of (6.12) at $\beta = \beta_0$ has the same asymptotic distribution as the IID summation

$$n^{-1/2} \sum_{i=1}^{n} \left[\sum_{j=1}^{m} \sum_{k=1}^{K} I\{M(j)=k\} \int_0^{\tau_k} \{x_{ki}(t_k) - e_k(t_k;\beta_0)\} L_{ji}(dt_k;\beta_0)\} \right]$$

which under the central limit theorem typically converges weakly, under (6.11) as $n \to \infty$, to a mean zero Gaussian distribution with variance matrix

$$A(\beta_0) = \varepsilon \left\{ \sum_{j=1}^{m} w_j(\beta_0)^{\otimes 2} \right\},$$

where ε denotes expectation and

$$w_j(\beta_0) = \sum_{k=1}^{K} I\{M(j) = k\} \int_0^{\tau_k} \{x_k(t_k) - e_k(t_k;\beta_0)\} L_j(dt_k;\beta_0).$$

For example, this asymptotic distribution obtains under IID conditions when region of integration $[0,\tau_1] \times \cdots \times [0,\tau_K]$ is restricted so that τ_k is in the support of the type k follow-up times for each $k = 1,\ldots,K$, if the modeled covariates in (6.11) have bounded total variation, if $A(\beta_0)$ is positive definite, and some additional mild regularity conditions hold.

The consistency of $\hat{\beta}$ as estimator of β under these conditions can be shown from the fact that $\hat{\beta}$ maximizes

$$\ell(\beta) = \sum_{i=1}^{n} \left[\sum_{j=1}^{m} \sum_{k=1}^{K} I\{M(j) = k\} \right.$$
$$\left. \int_0^{\tau_k} \left\{ x_{ki}(t_k)\beta - \log[\sum_{\ell=1}^{n} \sum_{j=1}^{m} I\{M(j) = k\} Y_{j\ell}(t_k) e^{x_{k\ell}(t_k)\beta}] \right\} N_{j\ell}(dt_k) \right],$$

which can be shown to be maximized at β_0 with probability tending to one, using arguments that are essentially the same as those used by Andersen and Gill (1982).

Not surprisingly the baseline hazard rates $\Gamma_k, k = 1,\ldots,K$ can be conveniently estimated by $\hat{\Gamma}_k(\cdot;\hat{\beta})$ where

$$\hat{\Gamma}_k(t;\beta) = \int_0^t \sum_{i=1}^{n} \sum_{j=1}^{m} I\{M(j) = k\} N_{ji}(ds) \Big/ \left\{ \sum_{\ell=1}^{n} \sum_{j=1}^{m} I\{M(j) = k\} Y_{j\ell}(s) e^{x_{k\ell}(s)\beta} \right\}.$$

A Taylor series expansion of the left side of (6.12) about $\beta = \beta_0$ can be used to show $n^{1/2}(\hat{\beta} - \beta_0)$ to converge to a mean zero Gaussian variate, under (6.11) and the regularity conditions just mentioned, with variance matrix that is consistently estimated by the sandwich form estimator

$$I(\hat{\beta})^{-1} \hat{A}(\hat{\beta}) I(\hat{\beta})^{-1}, \tag{6.16}$$

where

$$\hat{A}(\hat{\beta}) = n^{-1} \sum_{i=1}^{n} \left\{ \sum_{j=1}^{m} \hat{w}_{ji}(\hat{\beta}) \right\}^{\otimes 2}$$

$$\text{and } \hat{w}_{ji}(\hat{\beta}) = \sum_{k=1}^{K} I\{M(j) = k\} \int_0^{\tau_k} \{x_{ki}(t_k) - E_k(t_k;\hat{\beta})\} \hat{L}_{ji}(t_k;\hat{\beta})$$

with $\hat{L}_{ji}$ given by (6.14) with $\hat{\beta}$ substituted for β and with $\hat{\Gamma}_k(ds;\hat{\beta})$ substituted for $\Gamma_k(ds)$. Also in (6.16) $I(\beta)$ is the negative derivative of the left side of (6.12) with respect to β' and can be written

$$
\begin{aligned}
I(\beta) = & n^{-1}\sum_{i=1}^{n}\left[\sum_{j=1}^{m}\sum_{k=1}^{K} I\{M(j)=k\}\right. \\
& \int_0^{\tau_k}\left\{\sum_{\ell=1}^{n}\sum_{j=1}^{m} I\{M(j)=k\}Y_{j\ell}(t_k)x_{k\ell}(t_k)'x_{k\ell}(t_k)e^{x_{k\ell}(t_k)\beta}\Big/\right. \\
& [\sum_{\ell=1}^{n}\sum_{j=1}^{m}\{M(j)=k\}Y_{j\ell}(t_k)e^{x_{k\ell}(t_k)\beta}] - \left(\sum_{\ell=1}^{n}\sum_{j=1}^{m}\{M(j)=k\}Y_{j\ell}(t_k)x_{k\ell}(t_k)e^{x_{k\ell}(t_k)\beta}\right. \\
& \left.\left.\left.\Big/[\sum_{\ell=1}^{n}\sum_{j=1}^{m}\{M(j)=k\}Y_{j\ell}(t_k)x_{k\ell}(t_k)e^{x_{k\ell}(t_k)\beta}]\right)^{\otimes 2}\right\}N_{ji}(dt_k)\right].
\end{aligned}
$$

Spiekerman and Lin (1998) go on to show that $n^{1/2}(\hat{\Gamma}_k - \Gamma_k), k = 1,\ldots,K$ converge jointly to a mean zero Gaussian field under the conditions already mentioned, and they develop a perturbation resampling procedure for estimating confidence intervals and confidence bands for the type-specific baseline hazard rates. These are results of considerable generality and importance for inference on marginal single failure hazard rates. As outlined above these results can be developed without relying on an independence working model, or any other working model, concerning the joint distribution of $(T_1,\ldots,T_m)$ given Z.

It may be possible to improve on the efficiency of β estimation by introducing some form of weighting in (6.12) to take advantage of dependencies among $T_1,\ldots,T_m$ given Z, though the impact is likely to be small unless the dependencies are strong and censoring is light.

A copula modeling approach could augment the marginal single failure hazard rate analyses of this section, to include parameters that reflect the nature of dependencies among the failure times given Z, as will be discussed in §6.4. A more flexible modeling approach that focuses on regression associations for both marginal single, and marginal double, failure hazard rates using semiparametric Cox-type models for each will be described in §6.5.

6.4 Regression on Marginal Hazard Rates and Dependencies

6.4.1 Likelihood specification

The likelihood function for failure distribution parameters with m-dimensional failure time regression data, under a global independent censoring assumption given Z, which we now assume is composed of time-independent or external covariates only, has the rather complex form

$$L = \tag{6.17}$$

$$\prod_{i=1}^{n}\Big((-1)^m F\{dS_{1i},\ldots,dS_m;Z_i(S_{1k},\ldots,S_{mi})\}^{\delta_{1i}\cdots\delta_{mi}}$$

$$[(-1)^{m-1}F\{dS_{1i},\ldots,dS_{m-1,i},S_{mi};Z_i(S_{1i},\ldots,S_{mi})\}]^{\delta_{1i}\cdots\delta_{m-1,i}(1-\delta_{mi})} \quad \ldots$$

$$[(-1)^{m-1}F\{S_{1i},dS_{2i},\ldots,dS_{mi};Z_i(S_{1i},\ldots,S_{mi})\}]^{(1-\delta_{1i})\delta_{2i}\cdots\delta_{mi}}$$

$$[(-1)^{m-2}F\{dS_{1i},\ldots,dS_{m-1,i},S_{m-1,i},S_{mi};Z(S_{1i},\ldots,S_{mi})\}^{\delta_{1i}\cdots\delta_{m-2,i}(1-\delta_{m-1,i})(1-\delta_{mi})}]\ldots$$

$$[(-1)^{m-2}F\{S_{1i},S_{2i},dS_{3i},\ldots,dS_{mi};Z(S_{1i},\ldots,S_{mi})\}^{(1-\delta_{1i})(1-\delta_{2i})\delta_{3i}\cdots\delta_{mi}}]$$

$$\ldots$$

$$[(-1)F\{dS_{1i},S_{2i},\ldots,S_{mi};Z_i(S_{1i},\ldots,S_{mi})\}^{\delta_{1i}(1-\delta_{2i})\cdots(1-\delta_{mi})}]\ldots$$

$$[(-1)F\{S_{1i},\ldots,S_{m-1},dS_{mi};Z_i(S_{1i},\ldots,S_{mi})\}^{(1-\delta_{1i})\cdots(1-\delta_{m-1,i})\delta_{mi}}]$$

$$F\{S_{1i},\ldots,S_{mi};Z_i(S_{1i},\ldots S_{mi})\}^{(1-\delta_{1i})\cdots(1-\delta_{mi})}\Big), \tag{6.18}$$

involving derivatives of F with respect to each (non-empty) subset of its time arguments. A copula approach can be considered for a specification of L.

6.4.2 *Estimation using copula models*

A copula approach to the regression analysis of the m-variate failure time data proceeds by defining standardized variates

$$V_1 = \int_0^{T_1} \Lambda_{10\cdots 0}\{dt_1,0\ldots,0;Z(t_1,0,\ldots,0)\},\ldots,$$
$$V_m = \int_0^{T_m} \Lambda_{0\cdots 01}\{0,\ldots,0,dt_m;Z(0,\ldots,0,t_m)\},$$

and assuming these variates to have a joint survivor function F_0, with parameter θ that can depend on baseline covariates $z = z(0,\ldots,0)$. Suppose that each of $T_1,\ldots,T_m$ is absolutely continuous marginally, given corresponding covariate histories, so that $V_1,\ldots,V_m$ have unit exponential marginal distributions. For example, an

m-dimensional Clayton–Oakes model

$$
\begin{aligned}
&F_0(v_1,\ldots,v_m)\\
&=\Big\{F_0(v_1,\ldots,v_{m-1},0)^{-\theta}+F_0(v_1,\ldots,v_{m-2},0,v_m)^{-\theta}+\cdots+F_0(0,v_2,\ldots,v_m)^{-\theta}\\
&\quad+(-1)F_0(v_1,\ldots,v_{m-2},0,0)^{-\theta}+\cdots+(-1)F_0(0,0,v_3,\ldots,v_m)^{-\theta}\\
&\quad+(-1)^2F_0(v_1\ldots,v_{m-3},0,0,0)^{-\theta}+\cdots+(-1)^2F_0(0,0,0,v_4,\ldots,v_m)^{-\theta}\\
&\quad+\cdots+\\
&\quad+(-1)^{m-2}F_0(v_1,0,\ldots,0)^{-\theta}+\cdots+(-1)^{m-2}F_0(0,\ldots,0,v_m)^{-\theta}\\
&\quad+(-1)^{m-1}\Big\}^{-1/\theta}\vee 0, \qquad (6.19)
\end{aligned}
$$

specifies F_0 in terms of lower dimensional survivor functions and a parameter $\theta=\theta(z)\in[-1,\infty)$ that controls the m-variate dependency for $(V_1,\ldots,V_m)$. The first m terms on the right side of (6.19) are the $(m-1)$ dimensional marginal survivor functions, the next $m(m-1)/2$ terms are the $(m-2)$ dimensional marginal survivor functions,$\cdots$, until finally there are the 1-dimensional marginal survivor functions and a constant term. Expression (6.19) approaches the upper bound of $F(v_1,\ldots,v_{m-1},0)\wedge F(v_1,\ldots,v_{m-2},0,v_m)\wedge\cdots\wedge F(0,v_2,\ldots,v_m)$ as $\theta\to\infty$, while the lower bound is given by (6.19) evaluated at $\theta=-1$. As $\theta\to 0$ (6.19) approaches the product of all survival probabilities having a positive coefficient divided by the product of all survival probabilities having a negative coefficient on the right side of this expression. All points away from the lower boundary are continuity points for $(T_1,\ldots,T_m)$.

To apply (6.19) one needs to further specify marginal survivor function models for the survivor functions of dimension $2,\ldots,m-1$. For example Clayton–Oakes models of the form (6.19) could be considered for each of these marginal survivor functions, each with its own θ-parameter. Doing so would allow differential strengths of dependency among each subset of the failure time variates, but would lead to rather cumbersome likelihood-based estimation procedures.

There are some nice reproductive properties under a model of the form (6.19) with the same θ value for all marginal survivor functions of dimension q or larger, for $1\le q<m$. For example, if $q=2$ (6.19) reduces to

$$
\begin{aligned}
F_0(v_1,\ldots,v_m)=\{&F_0(v_1,v_2,0,\ldots,0)^{-\theta}+\cdots+F_0(0,\ldots,0,v_{m-1},v_m)^{-\theta}\\
&-(m-2)F_0(v_1,0,\ldots,0)^{-\theta}-\cdots-(m-2)F_0(0,\ldots,0,v_m)^{-\theta}\\
&+(m-1)(m-2)/2\}^{-1/\theta}\vee 0. \qquad (6.20)
\end{aligned}
$$

If one additionally assumes each pairwise marginal survivor function to be of Clayton–Oakes model form with its own dependency parameter one obtains, at continuity point $(v_1, \ldots, v_m)$

$$\begin{aligned} F_0(v_1,\ldots,v_m) =& \{(e^{v_1\theta_{12}} + e^{v_2\theta_{12}} - 1)^{\theta/\theta_{12}} + \cdots \\ &+ (e^{v_{m-1}\theta_{m-1,m}} + e^{v_m\theta_{m-1,m}} - 1)^{\theta/\theta_{m-1,m}} \\ &- (m-2)e^{v_1\theta} - \cdots - (m-2)e^{v_m\theta} + (m-1)(m-2)/2\}^{-1/\theta}, \end{aligned} \tag{6.21}$$

where $1+\theta_{ij} = 1+\theta_{ij}(z)$ is the pairwise marginal cross ratio between V_i and V_j for any $i < j$. If one additionally lets $\theta \to 0$, so that there are no third- or higher-order dependencies among the V_i's, $i = 1, \ldots, m$, one obtains

$$F_0(v_1,\ldots,v_m) = \prod_{i=1}^{m} e^{(m-2)v_i} \prod_{h<j} (e^{v_h\theta_{hj}} + e^{v_j\theta_{hj}} - 1)^{-1/\theta_{hj}}. \tag{6.22}$$

Expression (6.22) provides a rather convenient copula model for likelihood-based estimation of marginal hazard rate regression parameters, and pairwise cross ratio parameters for the standardized variates $(V_1, \ldots, V_m)$, under a working model with no trivariate or higher-order dependencies among the standardized variates.

Likelihood-based inference under a copula model such as (6.21) or (6.22) is conceptually straightforward. For example, standard asymptotic likelihood formulae will generally apply if a parametric form is assumed for each of the m baseline hazard functions in Cox model marginal hazard rate specifications. In particular one could model marginal hazard rates using (6.11) with parametric specifications of $\Gamma_1, \ldots, \Gamma_K$, and with pairwise cross ratio parameters θ_{hj} restricted to $\theta_{hj} = \eta_{gk}$ where $g = M(h)$ is the failure type for T_h and $k = M(j)$ is the failure type for T_j, for each $h < j$, with β, parameters in $\Gamma_1, \ldots, \Gamma_K$, and η_{gk} for $l \leq g \leq k \leq K$ as parameters to be estimated.

Typically such a model would be considered with $\Gamma_1, \ldots, \Gamma_K$ as arbitrary baseline hazard functions, rather than parametric functions. Corresponding estimation could proceed by an extension of the work of Pipper and Martinussen (2003) to allow pairwise cross ratios to differ among failure types. Though presumably having good efficiency properties the consequent estimators of marginal hazard ratio parameters could be biased because of departures from the fairly limited class of pairwise dependencies allowed under (6.21) or (6.22). Hence one could instead use the marginal hazard rate estimators of §6.3, in a two-stage estimation procedure with estimators of cross ratio parameters that characterize pairwise dependencies in the second stage. Such analyses can proceed using an extension of the work of Glidden (2000). In spite of cross ratios that are independent of their respective time variates this form of data analysis may be adequate for many multivariate failure time regression problems, and fleshing out the estimation procedure just alluded to in a rigorous fashion would be useful. The emergent methodology could be well suited, for example, to the analysis of family study cohort data in genetic epidemiology with estimators of $1+\eta_{gk}$ characterizing pairwise cross ratios between family members of type g and k. Of course $\eta_{gk} = 0$ implies independence between type g and k failure times given Z under this model, so that a convenient test for independence could be based on $\hat{\eta}_{gk}$

and its corresponding estimated standard error. Estimators of these dependency parameters (given Z) could also be considered for the introduction of weights into the estimating equations (6.12). See Spiekerman and Lin (1998) for distributional results with weighted estimating equations for β.

6.5 Marginal Single and Double Failure Hazard Rate Modeling

Now consider Cox models (6.11) for marginal single failure hazard rates in conjunction with corresponding semiparametric models for marginal double failure hazard rates for pairs of the m failure times $T_1,\ldots,T_m$ given Z. Related estimation may allow additional information on covariate associations with failure rates to be extracted by considering dual outcomes in addition to individual outcomes. This approach allows a flexible modeling of time-varying covariates in relation to both single and dual hazard failure rates, and with fixed or external covariates resulting estimators can be used to develop estimators of other quantities of interest, such as pairwise average cross ratios, and pairwise average concordance functions.

In addition to (6.11) for marginal single failure hazard rates, consider semiparametric multiplicative models for double failure hazard rates, for the (h,j) pair, according to

$$\Lambda_{0\cdots010\cdots010\cdots0}\{0,\ldots,0,dt_h,0,\ldots,0,dt_j,0\cdots0;Z(0,\ldots,0,t_h,0,\ldots,0,t_j,0\cdots0)\}$$
$$= \Gamma_{gk}(dt_h,dt_j)\exp\{x_{gk}(t_h,t_j)\gamma\} \tag{6.23}$$

for $1 \le h < j \le m$, where $g = M(h)$ and $k = M(j)$ denote unique failure types for T_h and T_j respectively, and $x_{gk}(t_h,t_j)$ is a fixed-length regression vector formed from $\{t_h,t_j,Z(0,\ldots,t_h,0,\ldots,t_j,0\ldots0)\}$ that can be defined, for example, to allow distinct double failure hazard ratio parameters for each (g,k) pair, and γ is a double failure hazard ratio parameter to be estimated.

Estimation of marginal single and double failure hazard rate parameters under (6.11) and (6.23) can combine the estimating equation (6.12) for β with a corresponding equation

$$\sum_{i=1}^{n}\left[\sum_{h=1}^{m}\sum_{j=h+1}^{m} I\{M(h)=g,M(j)=k\}\right.$$
$$\left.\int_0^{\tau_g}\int_0^{\tau_k}\{x_{gki}(t_g,t_k)-E_{gk}(t_g,t_k;\gamma)\}N_{hi}(dt_g)N_{ji}(dt_k)=0\right. \tag{6.24}$$

for γ. In this expression $E_{gk}(t_g,t_j;\gamma)$ is

$$n^{-1}\sum_{\ell=1}^{n}\sum_{h=1}^{m}\sum_{j=h+1}^{m} I\{M(h)=g,M(j)=k\}\}Y_{h\ell}(t_g)Y_{j\ell}(t_k)x_{gk\ell}(t_g,t_k)e^{x_{gk\ell}(t_g,t_k)\gamma} \tag{6.25}$$

divided by

$$n^{-1}\sum_{\ell=1}^{n}\sum_{h=1}^{m}\sum_{j=h+1}^{m} I\{M(h)=g,M(j)=k\}Y_{h\ell}(t_g)Y_{j\ell}(t_k)e^{x_{gk\ell}(t_g,t_k)\gamma}. \tag{6.26}$$

One can define centered counting processes $L_{hji}(\cdot,\cdot;\gamma)$ by

$$L_{hji}(t_g,t_k;\gamma) = N_{hi}(t_g)N_{ji}(t_k) - \int_0^{t_g}\int_0^{t_k} Y_{hi}(s_g)Y_{ji}(s_k)e^{x_{gki}(s_g,s_k)\gamma}\Gamma_{gk}(ds_g,ds_k)$$

for all (h,j,i), which will be zero mean processes at $\gamma=\gamma_0$, the "true" γ value, under (6.23). One can rewrite (6.24) as

$$\sum_{i=1}^{n}\left[\sum_{h=1}^{m}\sum_{j=h+1}^{m} I\{M(h)=g,M(j)=k\}\right.$$
$$\left.\int_0^{\tau_g}\int_0^{\tau_k}\{x_{gki}(t_g,t_k)-E_{gk}(t_g,t_k;\gamma)\}L_{hji}(dt_g,dt_k;\gamma)\right]=0. \quad (6.27)$$

Under IID conditions (6.25) and (6.26), each approach their expectations almost surely for any t_g and t_k in the support of the type g and type k follow-up times. The arguments of Spiekerman and Lin (1998) generalize to allow $E_{gk}(t_g,t_k;\gamma)$ to be everywhere replaced by the ratio $e_{gk}(t_g,t_k;\gamma)$ of these expectations without changing the asymptotic distribution of $n^{-1/2}$ times the left side of (6.27), at γ_0, under (6.23).

It follows under (6.11) and (6.23) that the left sides of (6.12) and (6.24), at $\beta=\beta_0$ and $\gamma=\gamma_0$ respectively, have asymptotic distribution equal to the sum of n mean zero IID variates to which the central limit theorem applies. In fact the product of $n^{-1/2}$ and the left sides of (6.12) and (6.24) converge jointly to a zero mean Gaussian distribution with variance matrix

$$A(\beta_0,\gamma_0)=\varepsilon\begin{pmatrix}\sum_{j=1}^{m} w_j(\beta_0)\\ \sum_{h=1}^{m}\sum_{j=h+1}^{m} w_{hj}(\gamma_0)\end{pmatrix}^{\otimes 2},$$

where

$$w_{hj}(\gamma_0)=\sum_{g=1}^{K}\sum_{k=g+1}^{K} I\{M(h)=g,M(j)=k\}$$
$$\int_0^{\tau_g}\int_0^{\tau_k}\{x_{gk}(t_g,t_k)-e_{gk}(t_g,t_k)\}L_{hj}(dt_g,dt_k;\gamma_0),$$

and ε again denotes expectation. The consistency of $(\hat\beta,\hat\gamma)$ solving (6.12) and (6.23) for (β_0,γ_0) again follows from arguments of the type used by Andersen and Gill (1982), and each baseline double failure hazard rate function Γ_{gk} is readily consistency estimated by $\hat\Gamma_{gk}(\cdot,\cdot;\hat\gamma)$ where

$$\hat\Gamma_{gk}(t_g,t_k;\gamma)=\int_0^{t_g}\int_0^{t_k}\sum_{i=1}^{n}\left[\sum_{h=1}^{m}\sum_{j=h+1}^{m} I\{M(h)=g,M(j)=k\}N_{hi}(ds_g)N_{ji}(ds_k)\right/$$
$$\left.\left\{\sum_{\ell=1}^{n}\sum_{h=1}^{m}\sum_{j=h+1}^{m} I\{M(h)=g,M(j)=k\}Y_{h\ell}(s_g)Y_{j\ell}(s_k)e^{x_{gk\ell}(s_g,s_k)\gamma}\right\}\right].$$

Taylor series expansions for the left sides of (6.12) and (6.23) about (β_0,γ_0) then lead to an asymptotic mean zero Gaussian distribution for $n^{1/2}\begin{pmatrix}\hat{\beta}_0-\beta_0\\ \hat{\gamma}-\gamma_0\end{pmatrix}$ with variance matrix consistently estimated by

$$\begin{pmatrix} I_\beta(\hat{\beta}) & 0 \\ 0 & I_\gamma(\hat{\gamma}) \end{pmatrix}^{-1} \hat{A}(\hat{\beta},\hat{\gamma}) \begin{pmatrix} I_\beta(\hat{\beta}) & 0 \\ 0 & I_\gamma(\hat{\gamma}) \end{pmatrix}^{-1}, \tag{6.28}$$

where

$$\hat{A}(\hat{\beta},\hat{\gamma}) = n^{-1}\sum_{i=1}^{n} \begin{pmatrix} \sum_{j=1}^{m} & \hat{w}_{ji}(\hat{\beta}) \\ \sum_{h=1}^{m}\sum_{j=h+1}^{m} & \hat{w}_{hji}(\hat{\gamma}) \end{pmatrix}^{\otimes 2}$$

where $\hat{w}_{ji}$ and $\hat{w}_{hji}$ substitute estimated values for marginal single and double failure hazard rate parameters in expressions for w_{ji} and w_{hji} respectively. Also in (6.28) I_β and I_γ are the Hessian-type matrices that derive from differentiating the negative of the left sides of (6.12) and (6.23) with respect to β' and γ' respectively. The arguments of Spiekerman and Lin (1998) generalize to show a joint mean zero asymptotic Gaussian distribution for $[n^{1/2}(\hat{\beta}-\beta_0), n^{1/2}\{\hat{\Gamma}_k(\cdot,\hat{\beta})-\Gamma_k(\cdot)\}, k = 1,\ldots,K, n^{1/2}(\hat{\gamma}-\gamma_0)$ and $n^{1/2}\{\hat{\Gamma}_{gk}(\cdot,\hat{\gamma})-\Gamma_{gk}(\cdot)\}, g<k]$ under (6.11) and (6.23). A perturbation resampling procedure can be used for confidence interval/confidence band calculation, for marginal single and double failure baseline hazard function estimation.

The asymptotic results just asserted arise under IID conditions along with conditions of total variation boundedness of the modeled covariates in (6.23) and positive definiteness of $I_\gamma(\gamma_0)$ in addition to conditions for marginal single failure hazard rate parameters as mentioned in §6.3, and some additional mild regularity conditions.

An interesting aspect of the estimation procedure just outlined is the typical lack of complete agreement between the single and double failure rate models (6.11) and (6.23). The central limit theorem will apply simultaneously to the estimating equations (6.12) and (6.24) but, as usual, some asymptotic bias can be expected in the estimation of single hazard rate parameters under departure from (6.11) and in doubled hazard failure rate parameters under departure from (6.23). If these models have been applied in a manner that provides a good fit to these respective hazard rates, then (6.11) and (6.22) will hold simultaneously to a good approximation, and related constructs such as bivariate survivor function estimators, and pairwise dependency measures, assuming time-independent or external covariates only in Z, can also be expected to be well estimated. An attractive feature of (6.11) and (6.23) is that their semiparametric nature, in conjunction with time-varying hazard ratio options provide the context for ensuring a simultaneous good fit of both (6.11) and (6.23) in any particular application context, as was illustrated with $m = 2$ in Chapter 4. Prentice and Zhao (2019) provide further detail on the asymptotic developments just sketched, and also provide simulations under a model having marginal single failure hazard rates that adhere to (6.11) but with marginal double failure hazard that differs from (6.23). Joint survivor function estimators were shown to have related bias much reduced by exercising some simple time-dependent features in marginal hazard rate modeling.

The above presentation assumed that marginal double failure hazard rates (6.23) are specified for each pair (h, j), with $h < j$, of the m failure time variates. A simple modification allows double failure hazard rate models to be specified only for selected composite pairwise outcomes of interest, thereby somewhat reducing modeling assumptions, including that of independent censorship, to the set of modeled marginal single and double failure hazard rate processes.

The efficiency of the marginal single failure hazard ratio parameter estimate $\hat{\beta}$ may be able to be improved by including weights in (6.12) that reflect dependencies among the m failure times given Z. The marginal double failure hazard rate parameter estimates described in this section have potential to provide a source of information for such weighting without introducing bias into β estimation. This possibility merits further statistical development.

It is also conceptually direct to extend models (6.11) and (6.23) to include semiparametric models for higher-order marginal hazard rates, as was illustrated in Chapter 5 for marginal single, double and triple failure hazard rates. This topic too merits further development for use, for example, in therapeutic contexts where individual patients may have a high rate of multiple health events of various types.

The applicability of an independent censoring assumption is an important consideration when applying marginal hazard rate models to correlated failure time data. Specifically if the censoring rates for the failure times under study depend on the emerging counting process data for other failure time variates in a correlates set $(T_1,\ldots,T_m)$, given Z, then an independent censoring assumption will typically be inappropriate. Depending on the structure of the collective data, a counting process intensity modeling approach may then provide a practical data analytic option.

6.6 Counting Process Intensity Modeling and Estimation

Expanding upon the discussion in §4.8 one can see that counting process intensity modeling of the form (4.22) may be applicable for failure times $T_1,\ldots,T_m$, assuming that these failure times fall on the same time axis, along which covariates may also evolve, in conjunction with a common censoring variate $C_1 = \cdots = C_m = C$. The relationship of regression variates to the rates of various types of failure can be conveniently estimated in such models using a simple extension of results summarized in §2.9, as will be elaborated in Chapter 7. The interpretation of regression parameters in such models is, however, conditional on the evolving counting process data for the set of correlated failure times given covariates, and hence can be quite different from the marginal methods described in this chapter. The intensity modeling approach also does not allow the m failure times to have separate censoring patterns, and generalizations to allow a more general censoring variate $(C_1,\ldots,C_m)$ may require a complex missing data approach.

However, when conditions for the marginal modeling approaches of §6.3 and §6.5 and counting process intensity modeling are both met the two methods can each provide powerful insight into regression influences, and failure time dependencies, and they should be regarded as both being useful and substantially complementary.

6.7 Women's Health Initiative Hormone Therapy Illustration

Consider again the WHI randomized controlled hormone therapy trials introduced in §1.7.3. Univariate (marginal single outcome) analyses for multiple clinical outcomes from both the estrogens alone (CEE) trial, and from the combined estrogens and progestin (CEE + MPA) trial were considered in §2.8, over trial intervention periods with median of 7.2 years in the CEE trial and 5.6 years in the CEE + MPA trial, and over extended follow-up periods with a median of about 13 years. Dual outcome hazard ratio analyses for certain cardiovascular diseases were also considered briefly in §5.6.

Here we present dual outcome hazard ratio analyses for pairs of some broad non-fatal disease categories, and for these non-fatal outcomes in conjunction with death from any cause. These analyses are presented for methodologic illustration only, and dual outcome analyses with more specific outcomes with substantive interpretation will be presented elsewhere.

The non-fatal outcomes considered are all CVD (earliest cardiovascular disease event), all Cancer (earliest invasive cancer, excluding non-melanoma skin cancer), all Fracture (earliest fracture of any site), along with self-reported outcomes of diabetes, gallbladder disease and hypertension. Women who had experienced these later outcomes prior to enrollment were excluded from corresponding the dual outcome analyses.

Dual outcome hazard ratio estimates (e^{γ}) and corresponding sandwich estimator–based 95% CIs based on data through the hormone trial intervention phases are presented in Figure 6.1 for the CEE trial and in Figure 6.2 for the CEE + MPA trial. The lower left of Figures 6.1 and 6.2 shows the number of participants experiencing the dual outcome in the active and placebo groups, in addition to the intervention versus placebo dual outcome hazard ratio estimate and 95% CI. These analyses arise from application of (6.11) and (6.23) with baseline hazard rates stratified as baseline age (10-year categories), prior outcome status (if appropriate), and randomization status in the companion WHI dietary modification trial (intervention, comparison, not randomized) described in §1.7.5. Follow-up times were from randomization to the earliest of first relevant outcome, death, withdrawal from active follow-up or stoppage of the trial intervention phase, whichever came first, for each outcome variable.

The upper right of Figures 6.1 and 6.2 shows the same dual outcome hazard ratio information in the form of "platter plots." This graphical technique, developed by our colleague Aaron Aragaki, has intensity on the right side scale determined by the significance level of a test of HR=1, and with areas within circles determined by the absolute value of the logHR(γ) estimator and by the corresponding lower and upper approximate 95% CI limits.

Figure 6.1 provides evidence for a reduction in the rate of the dual outcome of cancer and fractures, as well as evidence for an increase in gallbladder disease with hypertension or with total CVD, in the active CEE group during the trial intervention period. Perhaps not surprisingly, since there was not a significant effect of CEE on all-case mortality (Fig 2.2), none of the paired non-fatal outcome/total mortality outcomes showed evidence of intervention influence. Figure 6.2 does not show a

Figure 6.1 *Number of double failures (CEE-alone v placebo) and estimated dual outcome hazard ratios (95%confidence interval) for non-overlapping non-fatal endpoints, self-reported events, and deaths from all-causes that occurred in the WHI CEE-alone trial during the intervention phase.*

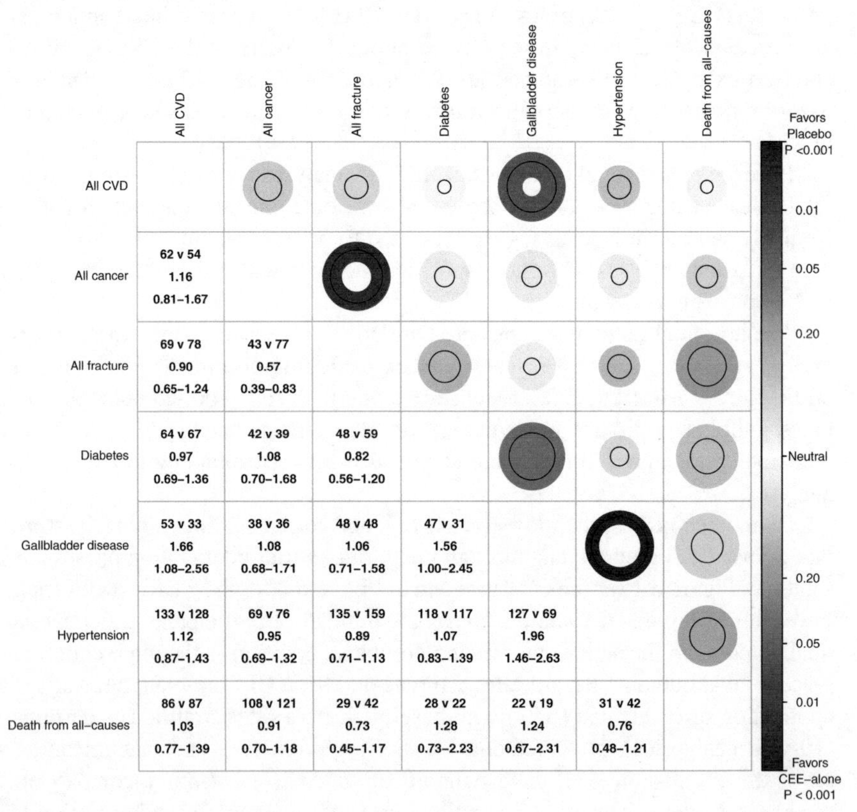

significant reduction in the dual outcome of cancer and fracture with CEE + MPA, but does provide evidence of a reduction in the risk of experiencing both cancer and CVD during the intervention period, along with evidence for increased risk of gallbladder disease with hypertension or CVD, and increased risk of the dual outcome of hypertension and CVD. Also, in spite of a lack of evidence for an influence of CEE + MPA on total mortality (Fig 2.2) there is an elevation in the risk of developing hypertension and subsequently dying during the intervention period.

The dual outcome hazard ratios considered above can, for course, depend on follow-up times (t_1, t_2) for the two outcomes in various ways. We relaxed the hazard ratio models to allow separate values according to whether $t_1 < t_2$ or $t_1 \geq t_2$ for the paired non-fatal outcomes by setting $x(t_1, t_2) = \{zI(t_1 < t_2), zI(t_1 \geq t_2)\}$ with z, a randomization indicator variable. It is natural to give priority to the dual outcomes for which there was overall evidence of an intervention effect. With CEE one ob-

Figure 6.2 *Number of double failures (CEE + MPA v placebo) and estimated dual outcome hazard ratios (95% confidence interval) for non-overlapping non-fatal endpoints, self-reported events, and deaths from all-causes that occurred in the WHI CEE + MPA trial during the intervention phase.*

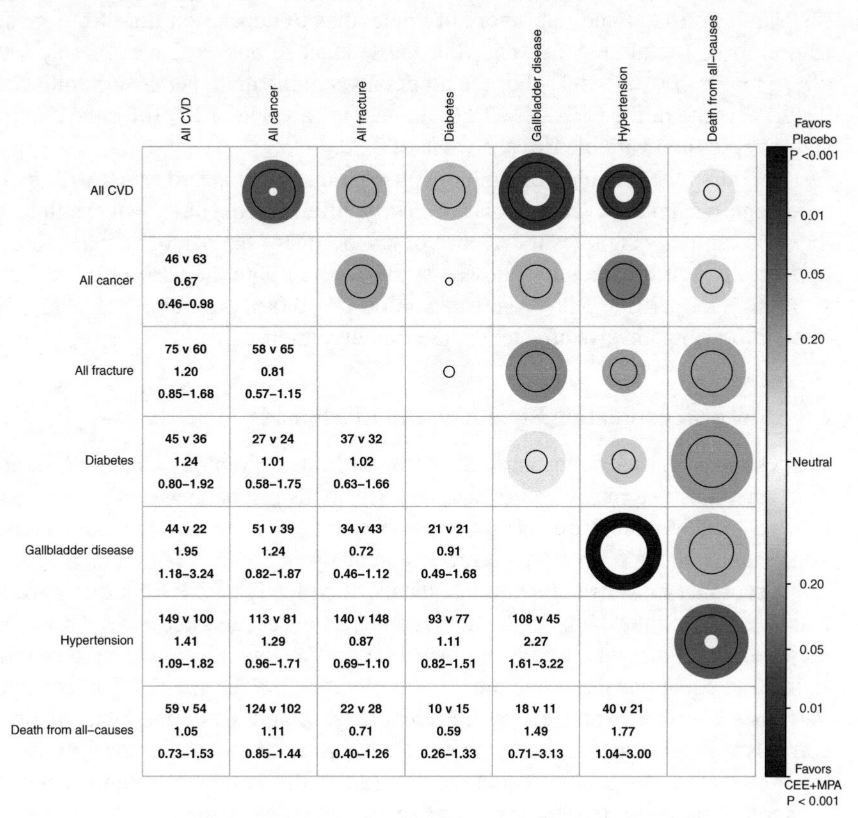

tains HR(95% CI) of 0.71(0.39, 1.29) for the dual outcome of fracture followed by cancer based on 18 and 26 dual outcomes in active and placebo groups, compared to an HR(95% CI) of 0.51(0.31, 0.82) for the dual outcome cancer followed by fracture based on 25 and 51 dual outcomes in the two randomization groups, with an intervention p-value of 0.39 for comparing the two HRs. Similarly there was little evidence of differential HRs according to which outcome occurred first for the dual outcomes of gallbladder disease and hypertension (interaction $p = 0.62$) or the dual outcomes of gallbladder disease and CVD (interaction $p = 0.45$). Similarly in the CEE + MPA trial there was no evidence of dual outcome HR variation with the ordering of the two outcomes for cancer and CVD (interaction $p = 0.41$), gallbladder disease and hypertension (interaction $p = 0.53$), gallbladder disease and CVD (interaction $p = 0.93$), but the ordering may be relevant for the dual hypertension and CVD outcome. Specifically the dual outcome HR(95% CI) for hypertension followed by CVD was 2.03 (1.35,3.05) versus 1.09 (0.79,1.52) for non-fatal CVD followed by a hypertension diagnosis (interaction $p = 0.02$) providing possible mechanistic insight into CEE + MPA influence on cardiovascular disease risk factors and events. Analyses were also conducted that allowed the (upper wedge) dual outcome HRs for paired non-fatal and total mortality outcomes to depend on time from randomization to non-fatal outcome, and time subsequent to non-fatal outcome by setting $x(t_1,t_2) = \{z, zt_1, z(t_2 - t_1)\}$. For the nominally significant hypertension followed by death outcome in the CEE + MPA trial a test for a value of $(0,0)$ for the two interaction regression variable had a p-value of 0.50.

Of course there could be variations in dual outcome hazard ratios with its time arguments even if the overall HR is not clearly different from unity. For example, here there is nominally significant evidence of lower HR for the risk of diabetes followed by fracture than for fracture followed by diabetes in both the CEE trial (interaction $p = 0.05$) and CEE + MPA trial (interaction $p = 0.09$), providing potential insight into biological pathways affected by these interventions.

6.8 More on Estimating Equations and Likelihood

This chapter continues our emphasis on hazard rates given covariates. With failure time outcomes that may be correlated these methods can be viewed as aiming to extract information about treatments, exposures, or general covariate associations beyond that available from separate regression analysis for each failure time outcome. We expect that most useful additional data will typically derive from the analysis of pairwise failure time data. While multivariate response data more generally are often modeled using marginal means and pairwise dependencies, often using generalized estimating equations that avoid the need to specify a full data model, the fact that the outcomes considered here are events supports an emphasis on marginal single outcome as well as marginal dual outcome hazard rates, the latter augmenting relevant regression association information, while additionally leading to semiparametric estimation of pairwise dependency with fixed or external covariates.

With a focus on single and dual outcome hazard rates one can impose an independent censoring assumption that allows these hazard rates to be estimated using available data. In comparison a coarsening at random assumption would presumably entail the quite different requirement that censoring rates for a multivariate censoring variate depend only on observable aspects of corresponding failure and covariate data. This assumption evidently has implications for marginal hazard rates for dimensions higher than single and dual outcomes.

The estimating equation procedure described here for single and dual outcomes under independent censoring are conceptually and computationally fairly simple. It can be viewed as an advantage that modeled regression variables can be disassociated for the single and dual outcomes for ease of calculation and interpretation, with modeling inaccuracies for some such hazard rates having little influence on inferences for the other modeled hazard rates. Corresponding disadvantages include the lack of a likelihood framework for simulation evaluation of proposed estimation procedures if the modeled single and dual hazard rates are not consistent with some overarching probability model, and lack of much study to date of the efficiency of the proposed single and dual outcome hazard rate estimation procedures.

Experience with the methods of this chapter to explore how to best use marginal double failure hazard rate analyses to augment findings from marginal single failure (i.e., univariate) hazard rate analyses in this type of setting will be needed in upcoming years. Note that use of the defined time-dependent covariate feature in (6.11) and (6.23) in a randomized controlled setting of this type can be used to compare marginal double failure HRs according to which of the two outcomes occurs first, and for non-fatal outcomes followed by death, to examine double failure HRs in relation to time from randomization to non-fatal outcome, and time from non-fatal outcome to death, while retaining the intention-to-treat interpretation for HR estimates.

BIBLIOGRAPHIC NOTES

The Dabrowska generalization in §6.2 was alluded to in Dabrowska (1988) and Gill (1994), and more explicitly by Prentice and Zhao (2018), where simulations were presented and dependency estimators were considered. The representation leading to the higher dimensional Volterra estimator was noted in Kalbfleisch and Prentice (2002, Chapter 10).

Much of the material of §6.3–6.5 has recently been assembled to provide a measure of completeness to the marginal modeling approach emphasized in this monograph. The m-dimensional Clayton–Oakes model (6.19) was presented in Prentice (2016), where the reproductive property leading to (6.20) was given in a more general form. The special case (6.21) is novel, and may provide a convenient framework for estimation, for example in genetic epidemiology family study contexts. The methods of §6.3 were given in a rigorous fashion in Spiekerman and Lin (1998), which build upon earlier work by Wei et al. (1989), Lee, Wei, Amato, and Leurgans (1992) and Lin (1994). The methods of §6.5 have only recently been proposed by the present authors (Prentice & Zhao, 2019) where additional detail is provided on the asymptotic distribution theory developments sketched in §6.3 and §6.5.

EXERCISES AND COMPLEMENTS

Exercise 6.1

For the special case $m = 4$, derive an explicit expression for the joint survivor function F, where $F(t_1,t_2,t_3,t_4) = P(T_1 > t_1, T_2 > t_2, T_3 > t_3, T_4 > t_4)$ in terms of single, double, triple and quadruple failure hazard rates using (6.6). Provide a justification for this expression when the failure time variates may include continuous components.

Exercise 6.2

Show that (6.15) follows from (6.12) thereby showing that the left side of (6.12) is in the form of the sum of stochastic integrals with respect to zero mean processes under

(6.11) at $\beta = \beta_0$. Similarly show that (6.27) follows from (6.24) thereby showing the left side of (6.24) to be the sum of stochastic integrals with respect to zero mean processes under (6.23) at $\gamma = \gamma_0$.

Exercise 6.3

Derive a general expression for F_0 in (6.19) in terms of marginal survivor functions of j or fewer of the failure time variates $(j = 1, \ldots, m)$ upon assuming that all marginal survival probabilities among $j+1, \ldots, m$ variates adhere to a Clayton–Oakes model of the form (6.19) with the same θ value. Does (6.20) follow from your more general result if $j = 2$?

Exercise 6.4

Develop a likelihood-based estimation procedure under Cox models for the standardized variates $V_1, \ldots, V_m$ in §6.3 and the copula model (6.19) assuming the baseline marginal hazard rates for each of $T_1, \ldots T_m$ given Z are specified parametrically. Can you extend this procedure to include unspecified baseline marginal hazard rates with Breslow-type empirical estimators?

Exercise 6.5

Write expressions for estimators of average cross ratios, and average concordance rates of the type shown in §4.6.3 for failure times T_h and T_j given $\{t_h, t_j, ; Z(0, \ldots, t_h, 0, \ldots, 0, t_j, 0, \ldots, 0\}$ under (6.11) and (6.23). Are assumptions about marginal single and double failure hazard rates other than those for T_h and T_j needed for these estimators to have good behavior? What conditions on the bivariate survivor function for T_h and T_j given their corresponding (fixed or external) covariate histories may be needed for (6.11) and (6.23) to simultaneously hold?

Exercise 6.6

Consider the platter plots of Figures 6.1 and 6.2. Describe potential insights into health risks and benefits that may be derived from these analyses, and from related analyses using time-dependent hazard ratio features of (6.11) and (6.23), which may not be apparent from marginal single failure analyses alone. Develop an estimation procedure for comparing marginal double failure HRs between CEE and CEE + MPA and discuss possible issues with the interpretation of this comparison.

Chapter 7

Recurrent Event Data Analysis Methods

7.1 Introduction

We now provide additional attention to an important class of multivariate failure time data analysis contexts where individual study subjects may continue follow-up beyond a first failure to second and subsequent failures on the same time axis. Moreover, such failures may be of the same or different types. The "point process" of failure times for an individual may be right censored with censoring rates independent of the individual's preceding failure time history, or censoring rates may be more complex. Furthermore, there could be multiple failure time axes for each study subject, with the possibility of multiple failure times and multiple failure types, for each. We will focus attention on settings in which there tends to be rather few failures per individual, with asymptotic distribution theory that applies as the number of study subjects becomes large.

One can view the methods discussed in the chapter as primarily elucidating those of preceding chapters. The extensions will involve the modeling and estimation of various types of failure rates that differ in their extent of conditioning on the individual's prior failure history. The counting process intensity modeling approach described in Chapter 2 conditions at any follow-up time t on the individual's entire prior history of failures. As such intensity models can allow right censoring rates to depend in a complex fashion on this preceding history, provided failure rates at any follow-up time are independent of prior censoring information for the study cohort given the prior failure histories and the prior covariate histories. The interpretation of the associated regression parameters may be complicated by the conditioning on the individual's prior failure time history. Marginal models for the successive failure times on a study subject may often have a useful "population averaged" interpretation for associated regression parameters, but apply under a more restrictive set of censoring requirements. Furthermore, there may be additional useful regression information from marginal hazard rate models for composite outcomes, where two or more failure times on an individual are simultaneously considered. These latter analyses may be of interest, for example, for the joint occurrence of recurrent events of different types.

The presentation here mainly focuses on the estimation of regression associations for relative failure rates. In many applications absolute failure rates, and such related quantities as the mean number of failures in a specified follow-up period, may be of central interest. Assumptions and estimation procedures for these parameters will be described briefly in §7.6.

The intensity process and marginal hazard rate modeling approaches are both quite powerful and useful for identifying and elucidating regression and failure rate associations. Moreover these approaches can be regarded as largely complementary, with marginal hazard rates providing insights into relationships between covariate histories and failure rates in the overall study population, with counting process intensity analyses valuable for elucidating pathways and mechanisms for regression associations with failure rates, after accounting for the evolving prior failure time experience for the individual study subject.

7.2 Intensity Process Modeling on a Single Failure Time Axis

7.2.1 *Counting process intensity modeling and estimation*

Consider a cohort of n study subjects, and now denote failure times relative to a defined time origin ($t = 0$) for the ith individual by $0 < T_{i1} < T_{i2} < \cdots$. Suppose that this "point process" of failures is subject to right censoring during cohort follow-up. One can define a counting process N_i and an "at-risk" process Y_i for the ith individual, $i = 1, \ldots, n$ such that N_i has right-continuous sample paths and $N_i(\Delta t) \geq 1$ if one or more failures is observed on the ith individual at time t and $N_i(\Delta t) = 0$ otherwise, and Y_i has left-continuous sample paths such that $Y_i(t) = 1$ if the ith individual is under active follow-up to observe failure occurrence at time t and $Y_i(t) = 0$ otherwise.

The failure intensity process Λ_i for the ith individual is defined by

$$\Lambda_i(dt) = E\{N_i(dt); \mathscr{H}_t\}$$

for $t \geq 0$, where $\mathscr{H}_t$ is the collective counting, at risk, and covariate histories for the cohort prior to time t. It is often assumed that the probability of two or more failures in $[t, t+dt]$ approaches zero as $dt \to 0$ but here we retain the possibility of tied failure times on individual study subjects, as in §2.9. An independent censoring requirement implies that

$$\Lambda_i(dt) = Y_i(t)\Lambda[dt; \{N_j(t^-), Z_j(t)\}, j = 1, \ldots, n], \tag{7.1}$$

for all (i,t), where Λ without a subscript denotes failure rate, and as usual $Z_j(t)$ denotes a covariate history for the jth study subject prior to time t. Note that (7.1) may hold even if censoring rates depend on the prior counting process history for other cohort members. Typically, it will be natural to make the slightly stronger modeling assumption

$$\Lambda_i(dt) = Y_i(t)\Lambda\{dt; N_i(t^-), Z_i(t)\}. \tag{7.2}$$

all (i,t), in which case the failure intensity for subject i depends only on that individual's preceding counting and covariate histories. The further, more substantial, modeling specification

$$\Lambda_i(dt) = Y_i(t)\Lambda_0(dt)\exp\{x_i(t)\beta\}, \tag{7.3}$$

gives the intensity model (2.15) considered in §2.9, where asymptotic distribution theory appropriate to recurrent event data was sketched. In (7.3) $x_i(t) = \{x_{i1}(t), x_{i2}(t), \ldots\}$ is a fixed-length regression vector with corresponding (hazard ratio) parameter $\beta = (\beta_1, \beta_2, \ldots)'$. The parametric hazard ratio factor, $\exp\{x_i(t)\beta\}$ aims to fully capture the ith subject's failure rate dependence on that individual's preceding covariate history, as well as on the number and timing of the subject's preceding failures. To do so may pose a considerable modeling challenge. Furthermore, to apply the partial likelihood estimators solving (2.16) and (2.19) for (β, Λ_0) the regression model should include all aspects of the prior counting and covariate processes that are needed to justify the model specifications (7.2) and (7.3).

If these modeling challenges have been met then the solutions $(\hat{\beta}, \hat{\Lambda}_0)$ to (2.16) and (2.19) provide a valuable approach to recurrent event regression data analysis. The powerful martingale convergence results mentioned in Chapter 2 require only modest regularity and stability conditions that ensure that data pertinent to each parameter accumulates in an orderly fashion as sample size becomes large, and to ensure that the influence of any specific individual's data on the estimation becomes trivial as $n \to \infty$. Note that the discrete form of the covariation process for the estimating function $U(\beta, t)$ as given in §2.9, will be required for consistent variance estimation if the intensity model incorporates tied failure times.

As noted in Andersen and Gill (1982) these estimation procedures extend readily if the baseline failure rate Λ_0 is allowed to differ arbitrarily among a finite number of baseline strata. This is undoubtedly the case also if a finite number of time-dependent strata $s = s\{t; N(t^-), Z(t)\}$ are defined, and the failure rate in (7.3) is modeled as

$$\Lambda\{dt; N(t^-), Z(t)\} = \Lambda_{0s}(dt)\exp\{x(t)\beta\}, \tag{7.4}$$

for $s = 1, 2, \ldots$, subject to the condition that a non-zero fraction of failures accrue to each stratum at every $t > 0$ as $n \to \infty$. Note that the subscript i has been dropped from (7.4) for notational convenience.

For example, if $s = N(t^-) + 1$, and $x(t)$ doesn't depend on $N(t^-)$, then in each stratum (7.4) has the form of a stratified inhomogeneous Poisson process that is modulated by covariates via the hazard ratio factor $\exp\{x(t)\beta\}$. With this same stratification one can alternatively consider a class of models

$$\Lambda\{dt; N(t^-), Z(t)\} = \Lambda_{0s}(t - T_{N(t^-)}) \exp\{x(t)\beta\}, \tag{7.5}$$

which expresses the failure rate as an unspecified function of time since the individual's most recent failure, with $T_{N(t^-)} = 0$ if $N(t^-) = 0$. This model can be regarded as a stratified semiparametric renewal model that is modulated by covariates through its exponential factor.

Partial likelihood–based estimating procedures apply to data arising from (7.4) quite generally, and under (7.5) also if the stratification is at least as fine as $s = N(t^-) + 1$ so that individuals contribute at most once to the risk set at time $t - T_{N(t^-)}$ from the subject's immediately preceding failure, in each stratum. The estimating equations for (β, Λ_0) under (7.4) or (7.5) are then given by (2.16), augmented by a summation over strata, and (2.19) for each stratum, with appropriate specifications of failures and risk sets in each stratum. It follows that these models can be applied using standard Cox model software simply by regarding each failure period for a study subject as if it were a separate observation. The "at-risk" period for the $(j+1)$st failure on individual i begins immediately following the jth failure (or zero) and extends to the earlier of the jth failure or censoring under (7.4), while that under (7.5) extends from zero to the earlier of the gap time to the $j+1$th failure or censoring. The hazard ratio function in (7.4) or (7.5) can be allowed to depend on aspects of the prior failure history beyond that used to define strata via $s = N(t^-) + 1$. For example, $x(t)$ may include a component equal to the length of time from the immediately preceding failure in order to include a renewal component to (7.4), or may include a component equal to the subject's total follow-up duration in (7.5). As another example, $x(t)$ in (7.4) or (7.5) could include interactions of a basic model regression vector with $N(t^-)$ to allow separate regression parameters for each value $0, 1, 2, \ldots$ for $N(t^-)$.

7.2.2 *Bladder tumor recurrence illustration*

Table 1.2 in §1.7.4 lists some data from a Veterans Administration randomized trial of thiotepa versus placebo for reducing bladder tumor recurrence risk. There were 38 patients assigned to thiotepa at 48 patients assigned to placebo, with a total 45 and 87 post-randomization recurrences respectively over a follow-up period that averaged about 31 months. There was grouping of follow-up times into months, yielding some tied recurrence times among patients, but ties were not so common as to have much influence on the interpretation of regression parameter estimates. Following analyses described in Kalbfleisch and Prentice (2002, pp. 291–299) we first note that an oversimplified model (7.3) with a single stratum and with time-independent regression vector comprised of a treatment indicator variable (x_1), a variable (x_2) equal to the number of initial tumors (that were each removed at baseline), and a variable (x_3) equal to the size in centimeters of the patient's largest baseline tumor. The partial likelihood estimator solving (2.16) then gives $\hat{\beta}_1 = -0.524$ with estimated standard error of 0.187, and a logrank significance level $p = 0.005$ for testing $\beta_1 = 0$. The corresponding coefficient (estimated standard deviation) for the other two regression variables were 0.201(0.044) and −0.040(0.065). At face value these analyses suggest a benefit for treatment with recurrence rate reduced by an estimated factor $\exp(-0.524) = 0.59$, with higher recurrence rates among patients having a larger number of tumors at baseline.

This simple model (7.3) implicitly assumes that recurrence rates do not depend on the patient's post-randomization history of recurrence. Relaxing the regression model to include time-dependent indicator variables for one, two, three, or four or more, post-randomization recurrences gives a more flexible model. The partial likelihood estimators (estimated standard error) of the treatment indicator is then −0.301(0.195) with significance level of $p = 0.12$ for testing $\beta_1 = 0$. The regression coefficient here estimates the log-hazard ratio for thiotepa use among patients who have experienced the same number of post-randomization recurrences. The four time-dependent regression variables each have strongly positive regression coefficients, and a partial likelihood ratio test that these coefficients are simultaneously equal to zero has value 37.76, which is very extreme in relation to a χ_4^2 distribution. Dropping these time-dependent indicator variables, while retaining the original three regression variables in a model (7.4) that has time-dependent stratification $s = N(t^-) + 1$ gives a more flexible modeling provision for the dependencies of the recurrence rate on the number of prior post-randomization recurrences. This analysis yields regression parameter estimates (estimated standard errors) of −0.324 (0.211), 0.118 (0.052), −0.007 (0.072) for the original three regression variables, giving only modest evidence for treatment benefit ($p = 0.12$) during follow-up, after accounting for the patient's number of prior recurrences.

One can also use Cox models of the form (2.5) to examine how the (univariate) censoring rates depend on the history of bladder tumor recurrences during trial follow-up. A model with the same three regression variables as in the recurrence analyses just described, along with a time-dependent indicator variable for whether or not the patient experienced a recurrence in the preceding month shows lower censoring rates among patients having a large number of pre-randomization tumors, as well as higher censoring rates among patients having a recurrence during the immediately preceding month during follow-up, the latter with coefficient (estimated standard error) of 1.017 (0.375). This analysis suggests that a careful modeling of the dependence of recurrence intensity ratio on post-randomization recurrence history may be necessary to justify an independent censoring assumption in this clinical trial. See Kalbfleisch and Prentice (2002, pp. 291–299) for additional analyses of these data, including examination of dependence of recurrence rate on gap time from the patient's most recent recurrence, and on an indicator for whether or not there was a recurrence within the previous month. These analyses give an estimated treatment hazard ratio of about 0.70 for treatment with significance level of $p = 0.05$ for testing $\beta_1 = 0$. Some application of accelerated failure time models of the form (2.20), rather than Cox models, is also included in these further analyses. These intensity rate analyses may be of interest to patients, for example to inform their recurrence risk compared to other patients who are at the same length of time from randomization with the same number of post-randomization recurrences, if assigned to thiotepa versus placebo. The dependent censorship mentioned above may be able to accommodated by the inclusion of inverse censoring probability weights in the estimating functions for the recurrence ratio regression parameter, as will be elaborated in a more general context in §8.2.

However, these analyses will not provide a summary assessment of the utility of thiotepa for reducing recurrence risk in this patient population. Marginal hazard rate estimation for recurrent events provide the potential for estimating a summary treatment occurrence ratio that averages appropriately over the patient's preceding counting process history. These models will be discussed in §7.3.

7.2.3 *Intensity modeling with multiple failure types*

Suppose that failure time variates $0 < T_{i1} < T_{i2} < \cdots$ are each accompanied by a failure type variate, taking values in $\{1,2,\ldots,K\}$ as in Chapter 6. Let $m_i(T_{ij})$ denote the failure type for $T_{ij}, j = 1,2,\ldots$ with all failures at a specific follow-up time t for the ith individual required to be of the same type. One can define a failure type process M_i having right-continuous sample paths for the ith subject so that

$$M_i(dt) = \begin{cases} k & \text{if } N_i(dt) > 0 \text{ and } m_i(t) = k \\ 0 & \text{otherwise} \end{cases}$$

that equals the failure type of the most recent failure on this subject, or zero prior to a first failure, jumping to the new failure type whenever a failure occurs for the individual. The counting process intensity Λ_{ik} for a type k failure at follow-up time t is given by

$$\Lambda_{ik}(dt) = E\{N_i(dt) \text{ and } M_i(dt) = k; \mathscr{H}_t\}$$

where $\mathscr{H}_t$ has been augmented to include counting, at-risk and covariate histories, as well as failure type histories for the study cohort prior to time t. In this notation the failure type process $M_i(t) = \int_0^t M_i(ds)$ is a right-continuous step function that takes value equal to the sum of failure types prior to time t, at any follow-up time t, for the ith individual. Hence $M_i(t)$ complements $N_i(t)$ by providing the entire history of failure types for failures at or before time t on the ith study subject. Assumptions like (7.2) and (7.3) but with failure type histories included the conditioning event can be entertained, along with Cox-type models (again dropping subscript i)

$$\Lambda_k\{dt; N(t^-), M(t^-), Z(t)\} = \Gamma_k(dt)\exp\{x_k(t)\beta\} \tag{7.6}$$

for each (t,k), with Γ_k an unspecified failure rate for failure type k, and with regression vector specifications that can, for example, allow a distinct hazard ratio regression parameter for each $k = 1,\ldots,K$ through the inclusion of interaction terms with $N(t^-)$ in $x_k(t)$. The model (7.6) is formally the same as model (6.11), but the conditioning event in (7.6) includes the number and timing of prior failures on the study subject along with the failure type for each such failure, affecting the interpretation of the regression parameter β. Nevertheless, with suitable regression modeling $\{\beta,\Gamma_1,\Gamma_2,\ldots\}$ can be estimated using partial likelihood and martingale procedures as in §2.9.

As in the preceding subsection the baseline rates in (7.6) can be further stratified, with little complication for parameter estimation. For example one could stratify Γ_k in (7.6) on the preceding number of type k failures for the individual along the lines of (7.4), or with this same stratification could allow the time argument in Γ_k to be time from the most recent type k failure, or time from the most recent failure of any type for the study subject. Clearly there are a plethora of intensity models that can be entertained, with stratified Poisson and stratified renewal processes that are modulated by covariates, sometimes having particular appeal. Some care needs to be taken in defining detailed stratification in such models for reliable corresponding baseline hazard estimation. However for regression parameter estimation in large cohorts where only a small fraction of study subjects experience failures of any of the study types, one can expect to have little efficiency loss for β estimation, as a result of baseline hazard rate stratification that is somewhat finer than necessary.

Intensity modeling approaches are not suited to censoring patterns that differ among the failure times on an individual. For example, the first but not subsequent outcomes were centrally adjudicated by expert committees for certain clinical outcomes in the Women's Health Initiative, for reasons of cost. Furthermore, different types of outcomes, such as cancers, cardiovascular disease and diabetes had quite different outcome ascertainment and adjudication processes that could lead to differing type-specific censoring. Along the same lines, the ascertainment of mortality outcomes had National Death Index matching as a source of information, beyond that arising from internal outcomes data collection efforts in this research program. Importantly, the defining feature of intensity models for recurrent events is the inclusion of all prior counting, "at-risk," and covariate data in the conditioning event for the hazard rate. In comparison, marginal hazard rate methods may allow estimation of simpler regression associations with failure rates that pertain to the study population as a whole, averaging over individual-level prior failure histories.

7.3 Marginal Failure Rate Estimation with Recurrent Events

In §6.3 methods for the estimation of regression associations based on marginal failure rate models were considered. The methods described there can be applied to recurrent events of a single or multiple types on a single failure time axis, as well as to recurrent events of one or more types on multiple unrelated failure time axes. There are some necessary details for modeling recurrent event data in the notation of §6.3: Since marginal single failure hazard rates (6.10) in this context do not condition, at follow-up time t, on the individual's preceding failure time and failure type histories one can analyze the recurrent event data separately for each of the K failure types, using (6.11) with modeled covariate dependent only on the prior covariate history. Hence one can consider a specific failure type (k) and define T_{i1} to be follow-up time to first type k recurrence, T_{i2} to be time to second type k recurrence,.... One can allow T_{ij} to have multiplicity greater than one to accommodate tied recurrence times of a specific type on individual i.

With these designations the methods of 6.3 apply to each failure type $k = 1,\ldots,K$, and are readily extended to the failure types combined, while allowing failures of different types to fall on unrelated time axes. Note that in spite of a common model format in (7.3) and (6.11), the associated regression parameters may have quite different interpretations because of the different conditioning events; specifically the need to model failure rate dependencies on the individual's prior counting process history in (7.3) but not (6.11). Because of this simplification in the marginal single failure hazard rate modeling approach, there is a need for a sandwich-type variance estimator for $\hat{\beta}$, rather than the second derivative–based estimator from the log-partial likelihood that applies under well-specified intensity models (without tied failure times). Also there are some related constraints on the censoring processes that can be allowed.

This estimation procedure, using (6.12), has been criticized in the recurrent event context since a working independence model was used in estimating equation development (e.g., Spiekerman & Lin, 1998). Such a working assumption is not a fit to recurrent events on a study subject, since the time to the second event is necessarily larger than the time to the first, the time to the third event is necessarily larger than the time to the second, and so forth. However, this working model was used only as a tool to develop the estimation equation (6.12) for β, and distribution theory for the solution $\hat{\beta}$ to (6.12), and the related estimators $\hat{\Gamma}_1, \hat{\Gamma}_2, \ldots$ made no use of this assumption, and is appropriate under the specified marginal single failure rate regression models. Hence these estimators can be expected to behave well for the estimation of regression effects on marginal hazard rates, at least under the random censorship model discussed in §6.1, and under the assumed model form for the marginal hazard rates. This random censorship model allows censoring times to differ among the failure times on an individual, allowing the issue mentioned above where there are differing censoring schemes for different failure types to be addressed, but does not allow censoring times to depend on the individual's preceding failure times during cohort follow-up, given pertinent covariate histories. Hence these methods may not immediately apply to the bladder tumor recurrences data discussed above, since censoring rates for the point process of events for the ith patient showed some dependence, for example on the length of time from the patient's recent recurrence.

In that context one may need to include some aspect of the patient's post-randomization recurrence history in the conditioning event for the rate of the next recurrence, complicating the parameter interpretation. The distribution theory developed in Lin et al. (2000) for recurrent events (of a single type) allows the flexibility to include aspects of the previous counting process history, as necessary, to justify an independent censoring assumption. An alternate approach could retain the marginal hazard rate models while introducing inverse non-censoring probability weights into each term of the summation (6.12). This later approach would retain the simple regression association interpretation, though the intent-to-treat property of the test for zero coefficient for the treatment indicator in the bladder tumor clinical trial would be lost if the censoring rates differs by treatment group. Inverse censoring probability weighted methods will be elaborated in Chapter 8.

7.4 Single and Double Failure Rate Models for Recurrent Events

As described in §6.5 one may be able to extract additional useful regression information from multivariate failure time outcome data by examining not just single failure hazard rates, but also double failure hazard rates. The double failure hazard rate analyses may be of interest here primarily for events of different types. A marginal double failure hazard rate model (6.23) leads to (6.24) as estimating equation for double failure hazard ratio parameters, which can be used in conjunction with estimating equation (6.12) for single failure hazard ratio parameters, even though the regression models for single and double failure hazard rates may not be fully compatible. The joint asymptotic Gaussian distribution for these regression parameters will obtain regardless of the nature of trivariate and higher-order hazard rate dependencies on their pertinent regression histories, and either of the single or double failure regression parameters will be consistently estimated by the solutions to (6.12) or (6.24) under the validity of the corresponding specific regression model and related independent censoring. If single and double failure hazard rates have both been well modeled, then quantities that combine the two, such as marginal bivariate survival probability estimators, and their associated average cross ratio and average concordance measures with fixed or external covariates, can also be expected to be well estimated.

7.5 WHI Dietary Modification Trial Illustration

In §4.7 an illustration was presented from the Women's Health Initiative Dietary Modification Trial (see §1.7). Nominally significant evidence of benefit of the low-fat dietary pattern intervention emerged for the composite outcome of breast cancer incidence followed by death from any cause. Corresponding marginal intention-to-treat comparisons for breast cancer incidence and death from any cause, were also in the favorable direction but neither was statistically significant.

This trial context was also the setting for a recent report on diabetes incidence in relation to dietary intervention (Howard et al., 2018) . This report illustrates the usefulness of marginal hazard rate regression analysis for a second event in a setting with multiple types of "failure" events on a common failure time axis.

Although diabetes was not a designated outcome in the trial protocol, information on the use of "pills for diabetes" or "insulin shots for diabetes" were collected twice annually during the trial intervention period and beyond, through medical update questionnaire. These self-reports were found to be in reasonably good agreement with periodic medication inventories on study participants. A total of $45,579$ women were without prevalent diabetes at baseline.

Clinical practice dictates the use of diabetes pills as a first line treatment for diabetes, changing to insulin injections if the disease progresses. Cox-type regression models were applied to these data, with baseline rates stratified on age at enrollment and randomization status in the companion WHI hormone therapy trial. An analysis of time from randomization to initiation of diabetes pills (T_1) gives a hazard ratio estimate (95% confidence interval) for the low-fat dietary pattern intervention of $0.95(0.88, 1.02)$ over the 8.5 year average intervention period with $p = 0.13$. An intensity process model, like (7.5), was applied to the post-diabetes pills follow-up to time-to-insulin injection (T_2). This intensity was modeled to allow a distinct parameter for the intervention hazard ratio, and a baseline hazard rate that retained the original stratification, but also stratified on time-from-randomization to first use of oral diabetes agents (in quartiles). The intervention hazard ratio estimate (95% CI) from this analysis was $0.82(0.64, 1.04)$ with a significance level of 0.10, providing some modest evidence that the intervention slowed progression to the more serious type of disease requiring insulin injections, after controlling for time from randomization to the initiation of diabetes pills. A marginal hazard rate analysis of the (T_1, T_2) data was also carried out with the same stratification as described above for T_1, and with distinct baseline rates and intervention group regression parameters for the two failure time variates. The marginal hazard rate analysis for T_1 is the same as was described above, whereas the marginal hazard rate analysis for time from randomization to diabetes requiring insulin injections (T_2) gave intervention hazard ratio estimate (95% CI) of $0.74(0.59, 0.94)$ with intention-to-treat significance level of 0.01. A random censorship assumption, in fact with $C_1 \equiv C_2$, is entirely appropriate in this context. Note that one obtains considerably stronger evidence of intervention benefit for time to diabetes requiring insulin than is the case from analysis of either of its component parts, namely, time from randomization to diabetes pills and time from diabetes pills to insulin injections. Moreover, this stronger result arises from a comparison between randomized groups, whereas the time from pills to insulin component of the intensity modeling contrasts groups that may differ in their distributions of time-to-diabetes pills, complicating the associated regression parameter interpretation. The double failure hazard ratio for treatment in this context provides potential for additional perspective beyond that for the two single failure hazard ratio analyses. The estimated double failure hazard ratio (95% confidence interval) for intervention versus comparison group here is nearly identical to that for T_2.

Over a longer-term follow-up that included a substantial post-intervention period, and a median total follow-up of 17.3 years, the T_1 estimated hazard ratio (95% CI) was 0.96 (0.91, 1.00) with significance level of $p = 0.07$, while that for T_2 was 0.88 (0.78, 0.99) with $p = 0.04$. The plausibility of an intervention benefit was enhanced in this study by (nominally) significant lower T_2 marginal hazard ratios among women with relatively large waist circumference and among women having relatively high metabolic syndrome score at baseline and by favorable intervention group changes over time in blood glucose levels in a 5.8% random subsample of the cohort.

Individual study participants may alter their need for diabetes treatment multiple times during trial follow-up. The methods of §7.5 provide the basis for additional analyses utilizing a fuller data set that includes a variable number of diabetes treatment epochs within the study follow-up period.

7.6 Absolute Failure Rates and Mean Models for Recurrent Events

Our presentation of marginal single failure hazard rate models (6.11) for recurrent events has so far focused primarily on the estimation of hazard ratio parameters (β). The absolute rates $\Gamma_k(dt)\exp\{x_k(t)\beta\}$ and cumulative rates $\int_0^t \Gamma_k(ds)\exp\{x_k(s)\beta\}$

over specified follow-up periods $(0,t]$ may also be of direct interest in applications. Specifically, if the covariate Z is time-independent, or is time-varying but external to the failure process, then

$$\mu_k\{t;Z(\tau)\} = \int_0^{\tau} \Gamma_k(ds)\exp\{x_k(s)\beta\} \tag{7.7}$$

is the mean number of type k events over $[0,\tau]$ for an individual with covariate history Z. In (7.7) τ may be the maximum follow-up time for the study, and it has been assumed that failure rates at any time t are not dependent on covariate values $\{Z(s), s > t\}$. The estimated number of type k failures by time t, $\hat{\mu}_k\{t,Z(t)\} = \int_0^t \hat{\Gamma}_k(ds)\exp\{x_k(s)\hat{\beta}\}$, in relation to study subject characteristics or exposures included in Z is likely to be of additional interest in a range of settings, particularly if the mean number of failures tends to be fairly large.

For example, in an automobile manufacturing context, failures may be defined by warranty claims of various types, while $z(0)$ includes details, such as calendar date and place of manufacturing, and $z(t), t > 0$ includes details of the environment in which the vehicle was placed in service. One could even imagine separate time axes for duration of time since placed in service ($t = 0$), and distance driven since placement in service, with double failure hazard rates of the same or of different types modeling warranty claims in relation to composite outcomes on the two axes.

Lin et al. (2000) provide a rigorous justification of the estimation of marginal failure rate functions, and for cumulative marginal rate functions like (7.7) that have a mean number of failures interpretation with external covariates. The estimators, as given in §6.3, had good practical performance in their simulation studies, along with attractive interpretation. Lin and colleagues also extended the class of regression parameter estimating functions by including a non-negative, bounded weight function $Q(\hat{\beta},t)$ that is monotone in t, and almost surely convergent to a fixed function $q(t)$ for $t \in [0,\tau]$ in the estimating function for β.

Cook and Lawless (2007, pp. 256–260) provide some interesting analyses of the bladder tumor recurrence data using mean models while acknowledging the discrete time aspect of the recurrence time data in Table 1.2. Their analyses indicate a lower tumor recurrence rate in the thiotepa group compared to the placebo group, and a higher tumor recurrence rate among patients having a larger number of tumors prior to randomization, They also go on to describe (pp. 268–273) how inverse probability weights in the recurrence rate estimating functions can be used to accommodate censoring that may depend on the patient's evolving history of recurrences.

7.7 Perspective on Regression Modeling via Intensities and Marginal Models

Marginal modeling and intensity process modeling provide a two-pronged approach to the elucidation of failure rate and regression associations with recurrent event data. Marginal models for single and double failure hazard rates can offer a rather direct assessment of the relationship of treatments or exposures encoded in a covariate history to readily interpretable event rates. One can view these marginal failure rates at a follow-up time t as averaging over the prior post-enrollment ($t > 0$) history of failure events for the study subject and, as such, they do not allow censoring rates to depend on this prior history. Censoring rates can, however, differ among failure times for a study subject, a feature of the marginal modeling approach that may be particularly valuable if there are events of multiple types.

Intensity models, on the other hand, condition on the prior history of failure times and types for the individual, as well as the prior covariate history, and hence corresponding regression associations are to be thought of conditionally on such a composite history. The estimation of overall regression associations may need to combine in some fashion the intensity model associations with those for evolving regression history associations with the prior failure time and type history. On the other hand, if there is a single censoring process for all failure types considered, then intensity model estimation as outlined above apply even if censoring rates at follow-up time t depend on the individual's preceding failure time and type history in a complex fashion. Hence, considerable ingenuity on the part of the data analyst may be required for reliable and interpretable regression estimation with recurrent event data having complex outcome ascertainment and censoring schemes. The majority of applications, however, will likely benefit from the inclusion of analyses of marginal single failure hazard rate models or related mean models, with recurrent event data.

BIBLIOGRAPHIC NOTES

There is a large literature on the modeling of recurrent event data. Cook and Lawless (2007) provide an excellent account of the literature through 2007, with considerable emphasis on both counting process intensity models and marginal recurrence rate models. Their coverage includes detailed discussion of specialized intensity models having certain forms of dependence of rates on preceding counting process history. References to early literature on the modeling and estimation of single recurrent event processes (single individuals in the present terminology), where considerably stronger assumptions are typically needed, can also be found there.

Other volumes dealing with modeling and analysis of recurrent failure times include Andersen et al. (1993), Kalbfleisch and Prentice (2002), Nelson (2003), Hougaard (2000), and Aalen et al. (2010). Several of these books give extensive information on the application of certain frailty models, and to certain types of multistage transition models. These latter models are discussed in considerable detail in a recent book on multistate modeling by Cook and Lawless (2018).

The marginal modeling approach to recurrent failure time regression data has been championed by L. J. Wei, D. Y. Lin, and colleagues over the past 15–20 years, with Wei et al. (1989), Lin (1994), Lin, Sun, and Ying (1999), and especially Lin et al. (2000) standing out as noteworthy contributions. Additional major contributions to this modeling approach include Lawless and Nadeau (1995), Lawless, Nadeau, and Cook (1997), and Pepe and Cai (1993). Our discussion of marginal double failure, along with marginal single failure, hazard rate models in the recurrent event setting is novel.

EXERCISES AND COMPLEMENTS

Exercise 7.1

Suppose that recurrent events on a single failure time axis arise from a frailty-type model model (§4.4) with counting process intensity, given a frailty variate W that has a gamma distribution with mean one and variance σ^2, that can be written

$$\Lambda\{dt;H_t,W\} = WY(t)\Lambda_0(dt)\exp\{x(t)\beta\} \tag{7.8}$$

with $x(t) = x$ an indicator variable for a binary treatment variable. Derive an expression for the intensity process, given by $E\{N(dt);H_t\}$ that is induced under censorship that is independent of the preceding counting process and W. Suppose that an oversimplified intensity model $Y(t)\Lambda_0(dt)\exp\{x(t)\beta\}$ is applied that fails to acknowledge dependence of failure rates on the individual's preceding counting process history $N(t^-)$ induced from their shared frailty variable. What can be said about estimators of β from the fitted model compared to the generating β values in (7.8) when $\sigma^2 = 0$ and where $\sigma^2 > 0$. If this simplified model gives a consistent estimator of β, what can be said about the corresponding partial likelihood–based variance estimator and corresponding confidence interval coverage properties as the sample size $n \to \infty$. See Lin et al. (2000) for simulations under this scenario that support the consistency of the β-estimators that emerge, but also show a clear need for a sandwich-type variance estimator to acknowledge the inadequacy of the simple intensity model applied.

Exercise 7.2

Continuing with the above setting, suppose that the intensity model applied is relaxed to $Y(t)\Lambda_0(dt)\exp\{x_1(t)\beta_1 + x_2(t)\beta_2\}$ where $x_1(t)$ is the treatment indicator as before while $x_2(t)$ takes value one if there is a recent failure in the interval $\{0 \vee (t-1), t\}$ and value zero otherwise. Will this allowance for dependence of the failure rate on the prior counting process history help in terms of properties of $\hat{\beta}$, as estimator of β in (7.8)? See Lin et al. (2000) for simulations showing strong biases for $\hat{\beta}_1$ as estimator of β when σ^2 is large.

Exercise 7.3

Continuing with this same setting, show that the marginal hazard rate from (7.8) has the Cox-model form

$$\tilde{\Lambda}_0(t)\exp\{x(t)\beta\},$$

for some baseline rate function $\tilde{\Lambda}_0$ assuming that censoring doesn't depend on the value of the frailty variate W. Show that the marginal modeling approach discussed in §7.3 will give a consistent estimator $\hat{\beta}$ of β in (7.8) with $n^{\frac{1}{2}}(\hat{\beta} - \beta)$ having an asymptotic Gaussian distribution with sandwich-type variance estimator as $n \to \infty$? Suppose, somehow, that the frailty variate values, W, in (7.8) came available. What can you say about the efficiency of the regression parameter estimator from the marginal hazard rate analysis, and its dependence on σ^2, compared to an estimator based on the intensity (7.8) with realized W values inserted?

Exercise 7.4

Consider the counting process intensity model (7.3) for recurrent events of a single type. Generalize the mean parameter estimating equation development of §2.3 to this setting to give the estimating equation (2.8) with variance estimator as given there.

Exercise 7.5

Continuing with the setting of Exercise 7.4 suppose that a model of the same form, but with modeled regression variable excluding the individual's preceding counting process history obtains, and that censoring rates are independent of such counting process history given Z. Is (2.8) an unbiased estimating equation for β? Are the contributions to (2.8) at differing uncensored failure times uncorrelated? Are the contributions to (2.8) from different study subjects asymptotically independent? Describe in words why a sandwich variance formula, as elaborated in §6.3, is needed to estimate the variance of $\hat{\beta}$ solving (2.8) in these circumstances.

Exercise 7.6

Consider the bladder tumor recurrence data discussed in §7.2.2. Using counting process intensity models (7.3) and/or marginal single failure hazard rate models of the same form, for times to the first, second, third or fourth bladder tumor recurrence as appropriate, provide a summary statement as to the value of thiotepa for reducing tumor recurrence risk.

Chapter 8

Additional Important Multivariate Failure Time Topics

8.1 Introduction

Previous chapters have emphasized regression methods for the analysis of multivariate failure time data, particularly marginal modeling methods that target single and dual outcome hazard rates. These developments assumed that failure times arose from the follow-up of a well-defined cohort of "individuals" who were representative of a study population in terms of hazard rates including regression associations; that the elements of a multivariate failure time variate were subject only to right censorship that is "independent" of failure times given the history of measured covariates, which may be evolving over the cohort follow-up times; and that pertinent covariate data are measured without error and are available at baseline and over each individual's follow-up periods. This chapter discusses methods that aim to relax these assumptions in various ways, and to test the agreement between model assumptions and available data.

The approaches to the extensions described here involve modeling marginal failure, censoring and covariate processes. Each section of the chapter involves new methods that will benefit from further work to carefully develop asymptotic distribution theory, and to assess the adequacy of asymptotic approximations with samples of moderate size.

The statistical literature on relaxing these assumptions is mostly restricted to univariate failure times. Here we outline extensions of these methods for the estimation of marginal single and double failure hazard rates. These extensions typically involve the modeling of random processes beyond marginal single and double failure hazard rates. Related asymptotic distribution theory can be expected to generalize from that outlined in Chapter 6 in a fairly straightforward fashion if the failure, censoring and covariate processes, along with other relevant data can be viewed as IID among the study subjects. The presentation here will be brief and informal.

8.2 Dependent Censorship, Confounding and Mediation

8.2.1 *Dependent censorship*

Suppose, as in Chapter 6, that there are m failure time variates $(T_1,\ldots,T_m)$ subject to right censoring by a variate $(C_1,\ldots,C_m)$ and an m-dimensional covariate Z, where $Z(t_1,\ldots,t_m) = \{z(s_1,\ldots,s_m); s_j = 0 \text{ if } t_j = 0 \text{ and } s_j < t_j \text{ if } t_j > 0, j = 1,\ldots,m\}$. Independent censorship for estimating marginal single failure hazard rate regression associations requires that lack of censoring in $[0,t_j)$ can be added to the conditioning event given $Z(0,\ldots,t_j,0,\ldots,0)$ without altering the marginal single failure hazard rate for t_j and for each $j = 1,\ldots,m$, for estimating of parameters in (6.11); and lack of censoring in $[0,t_h) \times [0,t_j)$ can be added to the conditioning event given $Z(0,\ldots,t_h,0\ldots,t_j,0\ldots,0)$ without altering the marginal double failure hazard rates (6.23) for any (t_h,t_j) for each $1 \leq h < j \leq m$. Depending on the reasons for, and nature of, the censorship, one may be able to assert confidently in some settings that these censoring conditions hold. In other settings the suitability of these assumptions may be questionable.

To explore this topic further one can define marginal single and double censoring hazard rates given Z that are analogous to (6.11) and (6.23) but for $C_j, j = 1,\ldots,m$ and for (C_h,C_j) for $1 \leq h < j \leq m$, respectively. Under the independent censoring assumption just mentioned for the T_j single failure hazard rates, the information $T_j \leq t_j$ can be added to the conditioning event without altering the marginal single censoring hazard rates for all t_j and $j = 1,\ldots,m$. Similarly the independent censoring assumption for (T_h,T_j) implies that $T_h \geq t_h$ and $T_j \geq t_j$ can be added to the conditioning event without altering the marginal double censoring hazard rate for any (t_h,t_j) and for all $l \leq h < j < m$. As a partial check on needed independent censoring assumptions one can examine whether marginal single and double censoring hazard rates depend on the histories of additional measured variables, given Z, perhaps using regression models analogous to (6.11) and (6.23) for this purpose. Censoring hazard rate dependence on the additional elements of these augmented covariate histories indicate departure from independent censorship for failure hazard rates given Z. Of course, this empirical approach can never by itself establish the appropriateness of the independent censorship conditions in question since there may be yet further unmeasured covariates that relate importantly to censoring rates given measured covariates. Rather, the appropriateness of independent censoring assumptions typically needs to be argued from study design, and context-dependent sources of censoring, considerations.

Suppose that one is interested in the dependence of marginal single and double failure hazard rates on a covariate history, now denoted by Z_1, but that it is necessary to condition also on the history Z_2 of other measured regression variables for an independent censoring assumption to be plausible. There are then a couple of approaches to estimating the regression associations of interest. First one can define marginal single and double failure hazard rate models, given $Z = (Z_1, Z_2)$, and apply the methods of Chapter 6. Related analyses may be suitable for many applications, but the fact that parameters for Z_1 associations need to be interpreted jointly with association parameters for the corresponding Z_2 histories may complicate the inference and prevent a parsimonious data summary, especially if there is a need to include interaction times between Z_1 and Z_2 in failure rate models.

A second approach assumes regression models for marginal single and double failure hazard rates given Z_1 as in (6.11) and (6.23), and uses inverse non-censoring probability weighting to adjust for censorship that would otherwise be dependent, for parameter estimation.

More specifically, suppose that Z is composed of fixed or external covariates and let $\Omega_j\{0,\ldots,dt_j,0,\ldots,0;Z(0,\ldots,0,t_j,0,\ldots,0)\}$ denote the marginal single censoring hazard rate for C_j given Z, so that

$$\begin{aligned}
&\Omega_j\{0,\ldots,0,dt_j,0,\ldots,0;Z(0,\ldots,0,t_j,0,\ldots,0)\} \\
&\quad = P\{C_j \in [t_j, t_j + dt_j); C_j \geq t_j, Z(0,\ldots,0,t_j,0,\ldots,0)\} \qquad (8.1)
\end{aligned}$$

for all t_j and for $j = 1,\ldots,m$ with non-zero elements in these expressions in the jth position only. As failure, censoring and covariate processes evolve, a study subject will be at risk for censoring in its jth component at t_j if censoring does not occur earlier, an event having product integral probability

$$\begin{aligned}
&G_j\{t_j;Z(0,\ldots,0,t_j,0,\ldots,0)\} \\
&\quad = \prod_0^{t_j}[1 - \Omega_j\{0,\ldots,0,ds_j,0,\ldots,0;Z(0,\ldots,0,s_j,0,\ldots,0)\}]. \qquad (8.2)
\end{aligned}$$

Now under model (6.11) for marginal single failure hazard rates given Z_1 consider the expectation of

$$[N_j(ds_j) - Y_j(s_j)\sum_{k=1}^{K} I\{M(j)=k\}\Gamma_k(ds_j)\exp\{x_{1k}(s_j)\beta\}]$$
$$G_j^{-1}\{s_j; Z(0,\ldots,0,s_j,0,\ldots,0)\}, \quad (8.3)$$

where x_{1k} is the modeled regression variable in (6.11), given $T_j \geq s_j$ and Z_1. Under an independent censoring assumption given $Z = (Z_1, Z_2)$ this expectation can be written as

$$\sum_{k=1}^{K} I\{M(j)=k\}\Gamma_k\{ds_j; Z(0,\ldots,0,s_j,0,\ldots,0)\}$$
$$- \sum_{k=1}^{K} I\{M(j)=k\}\Gamma_k(ds_j)\exp\{x_{1k}(s_j)\beta\},$$

where $\Gamma_k\{ds_j; Z(0,\ldots,0,s_j,0,\ldots,0)\}$ denotes the marginal single failure hazard rate for a type k failure given Z. Now a further expectation over $Z(0,\ldots,0,s_j,0,\ldots,0)$ given $T_j \geq s_j$ and $Z_1(0,\ldots,0,s_j,0,\ldots,0)$ gives value zero for the expectation of (8.3) given $T_j \geq s_j$ and $Z_1(0,\ldots,0,s_j,0,\ldots,0)$. Hence if marginal single censoring hazard rates in (8.2) were known, one could construct zero mean processes $L_{ji}(\cdot;\beta,G_j)$ corresponding to T_j that take value at t_k for individual i equal to

$$L_{ji}(t_k;\beta,G_j) = N_{ji}(t_k) - \sum_{k=1}^{K} I\{M(j)=k\}$$
$$\int_0^{t_k} Y_{ji}(s_k)\Gamma_k(ds_k)\exp\{x_{1ki}(s_k)\beta\}G_{ji}^{-1}\{s_k; Z_i(0,\ldots,0,s_k,0,\ldots,0)\},$$

for each $j = 1,\ldots,m$ and $i = 1,\ldots,n$. Analogous to (6.12) an estimating equation for β could then be written as

$$\sum_{i=1}^{n}\left[\sum_{j=1}^{m}\sum_{k=1}^{K} I\{M(j)=k\}\int_0^{\tau_k}\{x_{1ki}(t_k) - E_{1k}(t_k;\beta,G_j)\}N_{ji}(dt_k)\right] = 0, \quad (8.4)$$

where

$$E_{1k}(t_k;\beta,G_j) =$$
$$\left[\sum_{i=1}^{n}\sum_{j=1}^{m} I\{M(j)=k\}Y_{ji}(t_k)x_{1ki}(t_k)e^{x_{1ki}(t_k)\beta}G_{ji}^{-1}\{t_k; Z_i(0,\ldots,0,t_k,\ldots,0)\}\right] \Big/$$
$$\left[\sum_{i=1}^{n}\sum_{j=1}^{m} I\{M(j)=k\}Y_{ji}(t_k)e^{x_{1ki}(t_k)\beta}G_{ji}^{-1}\{t_k; Z_i(0,\ldots,0,t_k,0,\ldots,0)\}\right]$$

with non-zero argument for Z_i only in the jth position.

A simple exercise shows that $N_{ji}(dt_k)$ in (8.4) can be replaced by $L_{ji}(dt_k;\beta,G_j)$, so that the left side of (8.4) would have the form of a stochastic integral of functions of the data with respect to a zero mean process at the true β-value, to which asymptotic distribution theory analogous to that sketched in Chapter 6 would apply under modest additional constraints on the G_j processes to ensure that non-censoring probabilities are strictly positive given Z, at least for some j having $M(j) = k$, for each $k = 1, \ldots, K$, for any Z.

The unknown marginal single censoring hazard rates (8.1) and corresponding weights G_j in (8.2) can be estimated using the same type of models and methods as for marginal single failure hazard rates in §6.3. Estimating equations for the marginal single failure hazard ratio parameter, β, are now given by (8.4), with G replaced by $\hat{G}$, where $\hat{G}$ denotes the set of estimated inverse non-censoring probability weights $\hat{G}_j, j = 1, \ldots, m$. Joint estimating functions for parameters in (8.1) for $j = 1, \ldots, m$ and for parameters in the marginal single failure hazard rate models

$$\Lambda_{0\ldots010\ldots0}\{0,\ldots,0,dt_j,0,\ldots,0;Z_1(0,\ldots,0,t_j,0,\ldots,0)\} = \Gamma_k(dt_j)\exp\{x_{1k}(t_j)\beta\},$$

with $k = M(j)$ for each $j = 1, \ldots, m$ are then readily specified, and asymptotic distribution theory for all model parameters can be developed under IID sampling conditions, as a fairly straightforward generalization of the empirical process results sketched in Chapter 6. Note that the marginal single censoring hazard rates (8.1) will need to include regression variables from Z, beyond those from Z_1, since independent censorship given $Z = (Z_1, Z_2)$ can be assumed, while independent censorship given Z_1 cannot.

The same data analytic options can be considered for the joint estimation of parameters in marginal single failure hazard rate models of the form (6.11) and marginal double failure hazard rates under models of the form (6.23) given Z_1. If censoring given the more extensive covariate process $Z = (Z_1, Z_2)$ can be assumed to be independent, but censoring given Z_1 cannot, one can use the methods of Chapter 6 to estimate parameters in regression models for marginal single and double failure rates given Z, with associations between these failure hazard rates and Z_1 interpreted jointly with Z_2. These analyses are straightforward conceptually and may often adequately address data analytic questions of interest. Alternatively, with fixed and external covariates, inverse non-censoring probability weighting can lead to estimation of marginal single and double failure hazard rates in relation to Z_1 alone, subject to the ability to adequately model and estimate marginal single and double censoring hazard rates.

Briefly, for the latter approach, one can define marginal single censoring hazard rates as in (8.1), and marginal double censoring hazard rates by

$$\begin{aligned}
&\Omega_{hj}\{0,\ldots,0,dt_h,0,\ldots,0,dt_j,0,\ldots,0;Z(0,\ldots,0,t_h,0,\ldots,0,t_j,0,\ldots,0)\} \\
&\quad = P\{C_h \in [t_h, t_h + dt_h), C_j \in [t_j, t_j + dt_j); \\
&\qquad\qquad C_h \geq t_h, C_j \geq t_j, Z(0,\ldots,t_h,0,\ldots,t_j,0,\ldots,0)\} \qquad (8.5)
\end{aligned}$$

for all (t_h, t_j) and for all $1 \leq h < j \leq m$ with non-zero elements in the h and j positions only. From these one can construct probabilities $G_{hj}\{t_h, t_j; Z(0,\ldots,t_h,0,\ldots,t_j,0,\ldots,0)\}$ for $(C_h > t_h, C_j > t_j)$ given Z using the Péano series expression given in (4.2) for each (t_h, t_j) and each $1 \leq h < j \leq m$. If the marginal single and double censoring hazard rates (8.1) and (8.5) were known, one could estimate parameters in marginal single and double failure hazard rates using (8.4), which involves only marginal single failure hazard rate parameters, and an analogous equation

$$\sum_{i=1}^{n} \left[\sum_{j=1}^{m} \sum_{j=h+1}^{m} I\{M(h)=g, M(j)=k\} \right.$$
$$\left. \int_0^{\tau_g} \int_0^{\tau_k} \{x_{1gki}(t_g,t_k) - E_{1gk}(t_g,t_k;\gamma,G_{hj})\} N_{hi}(dt_g) N_{ji}(dt_k) \right] = 0 \qquad (8.6)$$

for γ estimation, where

$$E_{1gk}(t_g,t_k;\gamma,G_{hj}) = \left[\sum_{i=1}^{n} \sum_{h=1}^{m} \sum_{j=h+1}^{m} I\{M(h)=g, M(j)=k\} Y_{hi}(t_g) \right.$$
$$\left. Y_{ji}(t_k) x_{1gki}(t_g,t_k) e^{x_{1gki}(t_g,t_k)\gamma} G_{hj}^{-1}\{t_g,t_k; Z_i(0,\ldots,t_g,0,\ldots t_k,0,\ldots,0\} \right] \Big/$$
$$\left[\sum_{i=1}^{n} \sum_{h=1}^{m} \sum_{j=h+1}^{m} I\{M(h)=g, M(j)=k\} Y_{hi}(t_g) Y_{ji}(t_k) e^{x_{1gki}(t_g,t_k)\gamma} \right.$$
$$\left. G_{hj}^{-1}\{t_g,t_k; Z_i(0,\ldots,t_g,0,\ldots,t_k,0,\ldots,0\} \right].$$

One can define a centered double failure process $L_{hji}(\cdot,\cdot;\gamma,G_{hj})$ by

$$L_{hji}(t_g,t_k;\gamma,G_{hj})$$
$$= N_{hi}(t_g) N_{ji}(t_k) - \int_0^{t_g} \int_0^{t_k} \sum_{g=1}^{K} \sum_{k=g+1}^{K} I\{M(h)=g, M(j)=k\} Y_{hi}(s_g) Y_{ji}(s_k)$$
$$\Gamma_{gk}(ds_g,ds_k) e^{x_{1gki}(s_g,s_k)\gamma} G_{hji}^{-1}\{s_g,s_k; Z_i(0,\ldots,s_g,0,\ldots,s_k,0,\ldots,0\}$$

for all $1 \leq h < j \leq m$.

A simple calculation shows that $N_{hi}(dt_g) N_{ji}(dt_k)$ in (8.6) can be replaced by $L_{hji}(dt_g,dt_k;\gamma,G_{hj})$ while preserving equality, so that the left side of (8.6) has a representation as a stochastic integral of functions of the data with respect to a zero mean stochastic process at the true γ-value, under a model of the form (6.23) for marginal double failure hazard rates given Z_1.

Estimating equations for marginal single and double failure hazard ratio parameters given Z_1 then arise by inserting $\hat{G}_j$ for G_j, for $j = 1,\ldots,m$ in (8.4) and inserting $\hat{G}_{hj}$ for $1 \leq h < j \leq m$ in (8.6), where $\hat{G}_j$ and $\hat{G}_{hj}$ estimators derive from marginal single and double censoring hazard rate models of the form (6.11) and (6.23) given $Z = (Z_1, Z_2)$. Empirical process methods can then be expected to show the weak Gaussian convergence of single and double failure, and single and double censoring, hazard ratio parameters under these model specifications, with a corresponding consistent sandwich-form variance estimator for all hazard ratio parameters jointly.

Such a variance estimator requires baseline hazard rate estimators for single and double failure, and single and double censoring, hazard rates. These estimators have the form of those given in §6.3 and §6.5 for marginal single and double censoring baseline hazard rate functions given Z, as is also the case for marginal single and double failure hazard rates given Z_1 but with inverse censoring probability weights included. Specifically one has

$$\hat{\Gamma}_k(t_k;\beta,\hat{G}) = \sum_{i=1}^{n}\sum_{j=1}^{m} I\{M(j)=k\} \int_0^{t_k} \Bigg(\{N_{ji}(ds)\hat{G}_{ji}^{-1}\{s_k;Z(0,\ldots,0,s_k,0\ldots,0)\} \Big/ \sum_{\ell=1}^{n}\sum_{j=1}^{m} [I\{M(j)=k\}Y_{j\ell}(s_k)e^{x_{1k\ell}(s_k)\beta}\hat{G}_{j\ell}^{-1}\{s_k;Z(0,\ldots,0,s_k,0,\ldots0)\}] \Bigg) \tag{8.7}$$

for $k=1,\ldots,K$, and by

$$\hat{\Gamma}_{gk}(t_g,t_k;\gamma,\hat{G}) = \sum_{i=1}^{n}\sum_{h=1}^{m}\sum_{j=h+1}^{m} I\{M(h)=g,M(j)=k\} \Bigg\{ \int_0^{t_g}\int_0^{t_k} [N_{hi}(ds_g)N_{ji}(ds_k) \hat{G}_{hji}^{-1}\{s_g,s_k;Z(0,\ldots,s_g,\ldots,s_k,0,\ldots,0)\}] \Big/ \Bigg(\sum_{\ell=1}^{n}\sum_{h=1}^{m}\sum_{j=h+1}^{m} [I\{M(h)=g,M(j)=k\}Y_{h\ell}(ds_g)Y_{j\ell}(ds_k)e^{x_{1gk\ell}(s_g,s_k)\gamma} \hat{G}_{hj\ell}^{-1}\{s_g,s_k;Z(0,\ldots,s_g,\ldots,s_k,0,\ldots,0)\}] \Bigg) \Bigg\} \tag{8.8}$$

for $1 \le g < k \le K$, as estimators of single and double failure baseline hazard functions given Z_1. Weak Gaussian convergence results for all marginal single and double failure and censoring hazard rates under the specified models can be expected to follow under fairly straightforward generalizations of those sketched in Chapter 6, and a perturbation-type resampling procedure can be expected to apply for inference on constructs based on the entire set of marginal hazard rate estimators. These methods are of sufficient flexibility and importance that a careful account of asymptotic distribution theory, and evaluation of sampling configurations under which asymptotic distributional approximations are satisfactory, would be a useful addition to currently available statistical literature. Also note that the consistency of the estimators of β and γ is contingent on the assumed form for the marginal censoring rates given $Z=(Z_1,Z_2)$ and, of course, contingent on the assumption of independent censorship for the failure hazard rates given Z.

Closely related concepts are useful for the analysis of recurrent event data if aspects of an individual's preceding failure history need to be included in marginal failure hazard rates for an independent censoring assumption to be justified. For example, in the bladder tumor recurrence data discussed in Chapter 7 (see §1.7.4) an independent censoring assumption for the marginal recurrence time hazard rate may be appropriate if one conditions not only on modeled covariates, but also at follow-up time t on whether or not a recurrence took place in the preceding month. A marginal single censoring hazard model of the form (6.11) could then be applied, with conditioning on covariates Z_1 included in the tumor recurrence rate model as well as an indicator of whether or not a tumor recurrence took place in the preceding month. Inverse probability weighting by an estimated non-censoring probability estimate, as described above, can then lead to estimates of treatment effects on recurrence rates having a valuable population averaged interpretation. Note that the probability that the censoring time $C = C_1 = C_2 = \cdots$ exceeds follow-up time t given conditioning variates is well-defined and readily estimated in this illustration, even though the conditioning event has an internal component.

8.2.2 *Confounding control and mediation analysis*

Rather similar inverse probability weighting arguments can be considered in the area of confounding control and mediation analysis with treatments or exposures that may be time-dependent. These are often crucially important topics in the analysis of observational studies, and may be important also in randomized intervention trials if there is a possibility of post-randomization confounding, or if there is a desire to elucidate intention-to-treat analyses using post-randomization measurements. Inverse probability weighting methods for such purposes were proposed many years ago by Rosenbaum and Rubin (1983) under the terminology propensity scores, and have been substantially further developed by Jamie Robins and colleagues (e.g., Robins et al., 2000), among other investigators.

Consider the relationship between one or more failure time variates and a covariate history Z_1 that may be time-dependent. Suppose that this association is thought to be confounded by other covariates having history Z_2. One can apply the methods of Chapter 6 to the joint covariate history $Z = (Z_1, Z_2)$ to assess marginal single and double failure hazard rates given Z. These flexible semiparametric models will often provide a framework for careful control of confounding for parameters in marginal failure hazard rates relative to these covariate histories. The interpretation of hazard ratio regression parameters in these models, however, once again derives from joint associations of failure rates with the composite history Z, rather than with Z_1 alone, though this will often not be a major limitation. A second important issue, however, concerns the possibility that the additional covariate history Z_2 may include time-dependent variates that not only may influence future values of the exposures, Z_1, of primary interest and relate to the failure rates being estimated, but also may have future values that are influenced by the Z_1 history. These variables may encode major pathways whereby the exposure Z_1 influences the failure rates under study, resulting in estimated associations with Z_1 that may have been over-corrected through deprivation of contributions from these pathways. In fact, one may be able to evaluate mediation by Z_2 of the marginal failure hazard rate associations with Z_1 by examining the extent to which hazard ratios as a function of Z_1 move toward the null when Z_2 variates are included in the covariate history $Z = (Z_1, Z_2)$.

With time-varying covariates that are carefully ascertained over a sustained follow-up period, there is some potential to distinguish between confounding and mediating variables by modeling covariate innovations and lag times in the hazard ratio regression factors in (6.11) and (6.23). This is essentially the approach taken by Robins and colleagues under the terminology G-estimation (e.g., Robins, 1993). Most of the related work is cast in the context of counterfactuals, which some investigators find useful for problem formulation, although there would appear to be no necessity to do so. This influential body of work also goes under the rubric of causal inference, but such terminology may seem inconsistent with the ubiquitous assumption of no unmeasured confounders (beyond Z), given that the central issue in arguing causality with observational data is the avoidance of confounding. There is a branch of this work that derives estimation procedures that are robust to the influence of certain hypothetical unmeasured confounders that interact with measured variables in a specific fashion on a certain measurement scale. While robustness is a desirable property, these methods seem to result in considerable loss of estimation efficiency, and suffer conceptually from the need to make modeling assumptions about variables that are not only unmeasured but whose very existence is hypothetical.

Inverse probability weighting provides an approach to estimating associations of marginal single and double failure hazard rates with Z_1, rather than jointly with (Z_1, Z_2), by estimating the selection factors for Z_1 given Z_2 among cohort members at risk at each follow-up time in the study cohort.

More specifically suppose, as in the preceding subsection, that a model of the form (6.11) is assumed for the marginal single failure rate Z_1, but that the association may be confounded by the concurrent covariate history Z_2, which we assume is composed of time-independent or external covariates. The cohort selection rates for the evolving history Z_1 given corresponding Z_2 as well as lack of prior failure or censoring, allow the probability for $Z_1(0,\ldots,0,t_j,0,\ldots,0)$ given $\{Z_2(0,\ldots,0,t_j,0,\ldots,0), T_j \geq t_j, C_j \geq t_j\}$ to be expressed as a product integral

$$G_j\{t_j; Z(0,\ldots,0,t_j,0,\ldots,0)\}$$
$$= \prod_0^{t_j} P\{Z_1(0,\ldots,0,t_j+dt_j,0,\ldots,0); Z(0,\ldots,0,t_j,0,\ldots,0), T_j > t_j, C_j > t_j\} \tag{8.9}$$

for $j = 1,\ldots,m$. Expression (8.3) can be shown to have expectation zero with weights (8.9), and (8.4) would provide a suitable estimating equation for the marginal single failure hazard ratio parameter β if the weighting probabilities (8.9) were known. Similarly (8.6) with corresponding weights could provide a suitable estimating equation for γ, the hazard ratio parameter in a marginal double failure hazard rate model of the form (6.23) given Z_1. As in §8.2.1 one needs to insert consistent estimators for $\hat{G}_j$ for G_j, for $j = 1,\ldots,m$ in (8.4) and $\hat{G}_{hj}$ for G_{hj} for $1 \leq h < j \leq m$ in (8.6) to complete the inverse probability weighted (IPW) estimation procedures for β and γ. Depending on the context it may be challenging to specify appropriate models for the covariate history probability elements in (8.9) and in its two-dimensional counterpart. In fact, applications to date have largely been restricted to binary (or sometimes polychotomous) exposures Z_1 with logistic regression models typically specified for these probability elements. With a binary time-dependent principal covariate of this type, and potentially with more complex Z_1 histories, one can use empirical process methods to estimate parameters β and γ in models of the form (6.11) and (6.23) for marginal single and double failure hazard ratio parameters in relation to Z_1. Of course, the same issues of confounding control versus over-correction by mediators of the relationship between Z_1 and the failure rates under study arise with this IPW approach, but these are now dealt with in the modeling of inverse probability weights, rather than through the modeling of censoring hazard ratios in relation to (Z_1, Z_2) as in §8.2.1.

8.3 Cohort Sampling and Missing Covariates

8.3.1 Introduction

Epidemiologic cohort studies typically include a set of covariates, say with history Z_2, assessed at baseline and sometimes during cohort follow-up also, for all study participants. Biospecimens, especially blood components, are also typically collected and stored. Specific uses of cohort resources may require additional assessments, especially laboratory analyses using stored biospecimens. Motivated by study cost containment with limited loss of statistical estimating efficiency, these additional assessments are usually restricted to measurements, with histories denoted here by Z_1, on only a subset of the study cohort. Sampling designs for selecting individuals for the second phase of measurement go under the names of nested case–control sampling (Thomas, 1977; Prentice & Breslow, 1978) and case–cohort sampling (Prentice, 1986; Self & Prentice, 1988), and more recently two-phase design (Breslow & Wellner, 2007), among others. There is a close connection between such two-phase designs and stratified sampling designs in the survey sampling literature (e.g., Lin, 2000).

Much of the extensive literature on two-phase sampling designs with a failure time outcome considers a binary variate for whether or not an individual from the study populations is selected for the second phase. Selection probabilities are specified by design, may depend on baseline covariates, and typically differ strongly for individuals developing a failure time outcome of interest during cohort follow-up (the cases) as compared to those who do not (the controls). Some nice hazard rate estimation procedures have been developed, both for the Cox model and certain other hazard rate regression models, under the assumption of IID data that includes failure, censoring and Z_2 covariate data, along with second phase selection indicator variables and Z_1 histories for selected individuals (e.g., Breslow & Wellner, 2008; Saegusa & Wellner, 2013).

8.3.2 Case-cohort and two-phase sampling

Now consider the same IID setup with generalizations to allow the second phase selection rates to be time-dependent during cohort follow-up, and to include a multivariate failure time outcome. The marginal single and double failure hazard rate models (6.11) and (6.23) can be entertained for failure hazard rates given $Z = (Z_1, Z_2)$ under these generalizations. Assuming independent right-censoring given Z, one can use the notation of §8.2 to identify estimating equations of the form (8.4) and (8.6) for marginal single and double failure hazard ratio parameters, β and γ respectively, but with x_{1ki} replaced by x_{ki}, with summations from 1 to n replaced by summations over individuals included in the second phase of sampling, and with $G_{ji}, j = 1, \ldots, m$ and $G_{hji}, 1 \leq h < j \leq m$ replaced by the selection probability π_i for the ith study subject, under the specified sampling design.

As noted above, available estimation procedures with two-phase sampling mostly consider a univariate failure time outcome and specify a sampling procedure for selecting individuals for Z_1 ascertainment as a function of whether the outcome was observed (the cases) or was censored (the controls) with selection probabilities dependent also on baseline covariates (e.g., Saegusa & Wellner, 2013, Nan & Wellner, 2013).

It has been noted (Breslow, Hu, & Wellner, 2015), however, that the empirical process methods used to develop distribution theory in these papers can likely be extended to allow selection rates to depend also on external stochastic covariates in Z_2.

Now consider the multivariate failure time context of Chapter 6, with available data $\{(S_{ji}, \delta_{ji}), j = 1, \ldots, m; Z_2(S_{1i}, \ldots, S_{mi})\}$ for $i = 1, \ldots, n$. Conceptually, the probability that the ith individual is selected for ascertainment of $Z_1(S_{1i}, \ldots, S_{mi})$ can depend on any aspect of the assembled data on the ith individual. Denote selection of individual i by $R_i = 1$, with $R_1 = 0$ otherwise, and by

$$\pi_i = P[R_i = 1; \{(S_{ji}, \delta_{ji}), j = 1, \ldots, m; Z_2(S_{1i}, \ldots, S_{mi})\}] \tag{8.10}$$

the selection probability for the ith individual. For example, if there is special interest in a particular failure type k, then one possible sampling procedure would select all individuals having $\delta_{ji} = 1$ for one or more failure times for which $M(j) = k$, and select other individuals having $\delta_{ji} = 1$ for one or more failure times for which $M(j) \neq k$ with some lesser probability. Furthermore individuals having $\delta_{ji} = 0$ for all $j = 1, \ldots, m$ (pure controls) could be selected with probabilities dependent on $Z_2(S_{1i}, \ldots, S_{mi})$ histories, and also possibly with greater probability if follow-up times S_{ji} are relatively large for outcomes having $M(j) = k$, in an attempt to configure a substantial comparison group for each of the type k failures, over the study follow-up period. It is clear that there are a wide variety of sampling designs that could be entertained, with efficient designs strongly dependent on which hazard rate parameters are of principal interest.

Under any such sampling procedure, and independent censorship given $Z = (Z_1, Z_2)$, it is natural to adapt (6.12) for the estimation of β to

$$\sum_{i=1}^{n} \frac{R_i}{\pi_i} \left[\sum_{j=1}^{m} \sum_{k=1}^{K} I\{M(j) = k\} \int_0^{\tau_k} \{x_{ki}(t_k) - \tilde{E}_k(t_k; \beta)\} N_{ji}(dt_k) \right] = 0, \tag{8.11}$$

where

$$\tilde{E}_k(t_k;\beta) = \left[n^{-1} \sum_{\ell=1}^{n} \frac{R_\ell}{\pi_\ell} \sum_{j=1}^{m} I\{M(j)=k\} Y_{j\ell}(t_k) x_{k\ell}(t_k) e^{x_{k\ell}(t_k)\beta} \right] \Big/ \left[n^{-1} \sum_{\ell=1}^{n} \frac{R_\ell}{\pi_\ell} I\{M(j)=k\} Y_{j\ell}(t_k) e^{x_{k\ell}(t_k)\beta} \right].$$

As in (8.10) the dependence of π_i on $\{(S_{ji},\delta_{ji}), j=1,\ldots,m; Z_2(S_{1i},\ldots,S_{mi})\}$ has been suppressed. Note that $N_{ji}(dt_k)$ in (8.11) can be replaced by $L_{ji}(dt_k;\beta_0)$ where β_0 is the "true" β-value in (6.11) and $L_{ji}(t;\beta_0)$ is the zero mean process defined in (6.14) at time t, while preserving equality at $\beta=\beta_0$.

Similarly, under (6.23) one can adapt (6.24) for the estimation of γ to

$$\sum_{i=1}^{n} \frac{R_i}{\pi_i} \left[\sum_{h=1}^{m} \sum_{j=h+1}^{m} I\{M(h)=g, M(j)=k\} \int_0^{\tau_g} \int_0^{\tau_k} \{x_{gki}(t_g,t_k) - \tilde{E}_{gk}(t_g,t_k;\gamma)\} N_{hi}(dt_g) N_{ji}(dt_k) \right] = 0, \tag{8.12}$$

where

$$\tilde{E}_{gk}(t_g,t_k;\gamma) = \left[n^{-1} \sum_{\ell=1}^{n} \frac{R_\ell}{\pi_\ell} \sum_{h=1}^{m} \sum_{j=h+1}^{m} I\{M(h)=g, M(j)=k\} Y_{h\ell}(t_g) Y_{j\ell}(t_k) x_{gk\ell}(t_g,t_k) e^{x_{gk\ell}(t_g,t_k)\gamma} \right] \Big/ \left[n^{-1} \sum_{\ell=1}^{n} \frac{R_\ell}{\pi_\ell} \sum_{h=1}^{m} \sum_{j=h+1}^{m} I\{M(h)=g, M(j)=k\} Y_{h\ell}(t_g) Y_{j\ell}(t_k) e^{x_{gk\ell}(t_g,t_k)\gamma} \right].$$

Under (6.23) $N_{hi}(dt_g)N_{ji}(dt_k)$ in (8.12) can be replaced by $L_{hji}(dt_g,dt_j;\gamma_0)$ where $L_{hji}(\cdot,\cdot,\gamma_0)$ is a mean zero process under (6.23) at the true γ_0, without altering the equality in (8.12).

Under IID conditions for $\{(N_{ji},Y_{ji}), j=1,\ldots,m; Z_{2i}(S_{1i},\ldots S_{mi}), R_i, R_i Z_{1i}(S_{1m},\ldots,S_i)\}$ and under the condition that selection probabilities $\pi = \pi\{(S_j,\delta_j), j=1,\ldots,m; Z_2(S_1,\ldots,S_m)\}$ are bounded away from zero for all data configurations, as well as the other regularity conditions mentioned in Chapter 6, it seems very likely that the developments of Spiekerman and Lin (1998), as streamlined in Lin et al. (2000), can be extended to show that $\tilde{E}_k(t_k;\beta_0)$ in (8.11) can be replaced by the ratio $\tilde{e}_k(t_k;\beta_0)$ of the expectations of its numerator and denominator terms without altering the asymptotic distribution of the product of $n^{1/2}$ and left side of (8.11) under (6.11) with $\beta=\beta_0$; and $\tilde{E}_{gk}(t_g,t_k,\gamma_0)$ in (8.12) can be replaced by the ratio $\tilde{e}(t_g,t_k,\gamma_0)$ of the expectations of its numerator and denominator terms without altering the asymptotic distribution of the product of $n^{1/2}$ and the left side of (8.12) under (6.23) at the true $\gamma=\gamma_0$. The central limit theorem then applies to show the standardized estimating functions (8.11) and (8.12) to converge to a zero mean Gaussian distribution at the true parameter values, with covariance matrix that is readily estimated empirically, leading to the development of a zero-mean asymptotic normal distribution for $\{n^{1/2}(\hat{\beta}-\beta_0)', n^{1/2}(\hat{\gamma}-\gamma_0))'\}'$ with corresponding sandwich form variance estimator as in Chapter 6. The sandwich estimators would require estimators of baseline hazard rates in (6.11) and (6.23). These can be written

$$\tilde{\Gamma}_k(t_k;\beta) = \int_0^{t_k} \sum_{i=1}^{n} \frac{R_i}{\pi_i} I\{M(j)=k\} N_{ji}(ds_k) \Big/ \left\{ \sum_{\ell=1}^{n} \frac{R_\ell}{\pi_\ell} I\{M(j)=k\} Y_{j\ell}(s_k) e^{x_{k\ell}(s_k,\beta)} \right\},$$

and

$$\tilde{\Gamma}_{gk}(t_g,t_k;\gamma) = \int_0^{t_g}\int_0^{t_k} \sum_{i=1}^{n} \frac{R_i}{\pi_i} \left[\sum_{h=1}^{m} \sum_{j=h+1}^{m} I\{M(h)=g, M(j)=k\} N_{hi}(ds_g) N_{ji}(ds_k) \Big/ \right.$$
$$\left. \left\{ \sum_{\ell=1}^{n} \frac{R_\ell}{\pi_\ell} I\{M(h)=g, M(j)=k\} Y_{h\ell}(s_g) Y_{j\ell}(s_k) e^{x_{gk\ell}(s_g,s_k)\gamma} \right\} \right].$$

The procedures just sketched would allow hazard ratio estimation for a broad class of univariate or multivariate sampling designs. However, a careful development of asymptotic distribution theory is needed, especially concerning the application of the central limit theorem to the estimating functions on the left sides of (8.11) and (8.12). The related arguments may be complicated by the fact that the inverse probability weights π_i can depend on data for the ith individual over the entire follow-up period, making application of the Donsker theorem a potentially delicate matter. Additionally, the efficiency with which the hazard rate parameters in (6.11) and (6.23) can be estimated can almost certainly be improved by replacing the theoretic selection probabilities π_i by corresponding estimated values that adapt to realized selection indicator values. For example, $R_i, i=1,\ldots,n$ could be viewed as arising from a logistic regression model using the data items in (8.10). One could carry out a logistic regression analysis of R_i values under this selection model to yield estimated selection probabilities $\hat{\pi}_i, i=1,\ldots,n$. Substitutions of these into (8.11) and (8.12) presumably does not alter the structure of the asymptotic theory developments, while improving the efficiency of single and double failure hazard rate parameter estimates.

As noted above, there is a strong connection between the estimation of weights and calibration procedures in survey sampling. See Lumley, Shaw, and Dai (2011) for elaboration of this topic.

8.3.3 Nested case–control sampling

One of the earliest cohort sampling designs, so-called nested case–control sampling, involves selecting a specified number of controls who were without prior failure or censoring, at each uncensored failure time in a study cohort, for a univariate failure time variable (Thomas, 1977; Prentice & Breslow, 1978). Hazard ratio parameter estimation under a simple Cox model (2.5) was based on a stratified version of (2.8) with stratification on each case–control set, with controls selected with replacement (see also §2.6). This design can lead to quite useful regression parameter estimates because of the ability to select controls that share certain aspects of the prior covariate history with the case, yielding a close correspondence between cases and matched controls on disease risk factors other than those included in the modeled regression variable in (2.5) (Langholz & Thomas, 1990). Because control selection at a given follow-up time depends on the prior failure and censoring experience of the entire cohort, asymptotic distribution theory cannot be directly based on an IID assumption for failure, censoring, covariate and selection processes, but asymptotic distribution theory can be worked through with univariate failure time outcome using the fact that each matched set behaves like a stratified independent random sample from the cohort under (2.11) but with varying baseline hazard rate within strata (Goldstein & Langholz, 1992; Borgan, Goldstein, & Langholz, 1995). This sampling procedure could be extended to multivariate failure times on a single time axis by selecting specified numbers of individuals from univariate and bivariate risk sets at each single and double failure time, or at random samples thereof. For example, in a genetic epidemiology cohort meta-analysis, one could decide to only sample double failures for two disease outcomes in an attempt to glean novel association information about single nucleotide polymorphisms (SNPs) and the risk of a designated disease outcome pair. A version of the estimating equation (6.24) could undoubtedly be developed for estimating the double failure hazard ratio parameter γ in (6.23) in this scenario, though this type of development has not appeared in the statistical literature. Analyses that stratify on the matched case–control set can be expected to be inefficient if some covariate components are measured on the entire cohort, especially for coefficients of modeled regression variables in (6.11) and (6.23) that are always available. Unlike the two-phase designs discussed in §8.3.2 nested case–control designs rely on the uncorrelatedness of counting process increments, and martingale convergence results over the study follow-up period, with failure, censoring and covariate histories that accumulate over the (single) follow-up time axis. It may be possible to improve on the efficiency of conventional analyses that stratify on matched case–control sets by viewing the data as emerging over follow-up time with Z_1 histories coming available only at the time of case occurrence or control selection with selection probabilities included as time-dependent inverse probability weights. The partial likelihood filtration considered in Kalbfleisch and Prentice (2002, pp. 188–189) would then apply to univariate or multivariate intensity parameter estimation under an increasing sigma-algebra of failure, censoring and covariate data on a single failure time axis. The absence of a general martingale convergence theory with two or more failure time axes would presumably preclude estimation of the types of marginal single and double failure hazard rates emphasized in this book using these methods.

8.3.4 *Missing covariate data methods*

The same marginal single and double failure hazard rate estimation procedure, under (6.11) and (6.23), can be considered if Z_1 histories are missing by happenstance, rather than by sampling design. Doing so would require a missing-at-random condition whereby missingness hazard rates can depend on failure and corresponding Z_2 histories, but not the potentially missing Z_1 histories. There is a substantial statistical literature on Cox model estimation with univariate failure times and missing covariate data. This literature includes estimating equations for hazard ratio parameters of the form (8.4), but with an additional term added to the estimating function that derives from the conditional expectation of a similar estimating function contribution over the missing data, for each cohort member. The inclusion of this "augmentation term" tends to improve moderate sample efficiencies in simulation studies and, even though typically not affecting asymptotic efficiency under the assumed missingness model, also yields some valuable robustness properties in that hazard ratio parameter estimates generally remain consistent if either the missingness model is correctly specified, or the distribution of missing covariates given the observed data is correctly specified (e.g., Robins, Rotnitzky, & Zhao, 1994). Corresponding methodology developments for the simultaneous estimation of marginal single and double failure hazard ratio parameters would appear to be straightforward, but would be worth documenting in the statistical literature. Another popular estimation procedure for missing data, namely, multiple imputation (e.g., Little and Rubin, 2002) requires a full likelihood specification for parameters of interest, and hence would typically not be applicable under (6.11) and (6.23) without further constraints to ensure that those models are mutually consistent, and further assumptions to specify the joint distribution of the m-dimensional failure time variate given Z.

8.4 Mismeasured Covariate Data

8.4.1 Background

There is also a substantial statistical literature on the effects of measurement error in modeled covariates on regression parameter estimation, with univariate failure time data. With multivariate failure time data, one can continue the notation of the previous section, and suppose that covariate history Z_2 is well measured, while covariate history Z_1 is not completely missing but for some individuals may be measured with error yielding a mismeasured history Z_1^* rather than Z_1. For estimating regression parameters in (6.11) and (6.23) in the presence of such measurement error one can distinguish situations where the accurate Z_1 history can be ascertained for a random subset of the study population giving rise to a so-called "validation subsample" in the study cohort, from the perhaps more common circumstance where Z_1 cannot be ascertained for any individual, but (error-prone) covariate assessments Z_1^* are available for all cohort members. In this latter situation additional error-prone assessments are needed, at least for a subset of the cohort, and stronger modeling assumptions are needed, to estimate failure hazard rate parameters.

8.4.2 Hazard rate estimation with a validation subsample

First suppose that a validation sample is available for a random subset of the study cohort. A non-differential measurement error assumption (e.g., Carroll et al., 2006) relative to the Z_1 histories in (6.11) and (6.23) requires marginal single and double failure hazard rates given (Z_1, Z_1^*, Z_2) to be independent of Z_1^*. That is, the error-prone measurements Z_1^* are assumed to be uninformative about the hazard rates of interest, given the accurate Z-values. This assumption will often be reasonable in prospective cohort applications, but may need to be carefully considered if covariate histories Z_1^* are obtained retrospectively from an assembled cohort having known failure and censoring histories.

Under this non-differential measurement assumption the marginal single and double failure hazard rates induced from (6.11) and (6.23), for individuals having Z_1^*, but not Z_1 available can be written as

$$\Lambda_{0\cdots010\cdots0}\{0,\ldots,0,dt_j,0,\ldots,0;Z^*(0,\ldots,0,t_j,0,\ldots)\} \\ = \Gamma_k(dt_j)\mathscr{E}\{e^{x_k(t_j)\beta};T_j \geq t_j;Z^*(0,\ldots,0,t_j,0,\ldots,0)\} \quad (8.13)$$

for all t_j and $j = 1,\ldots,m$, and

$$\Lambda_{0\cdots010\cdots10\cdots0}\{0,\ldots,0,dt_h,0,\ldots,0,dt_j,0,\ldots,0;Z^*(0,\ldots,0,t_h,0,\ldots,0,t_j,0,\ldots0)\} \\ = \Gamma_{gk}(dt_h,dt_j)\mathscr{E}\{e^{x_{gk}(t_g,t_k)\gamma};T_h \geq t_h,T_j \geq t_j,Z^*(0,\ldots,0,t_h,0,\ldots,0,t_j,0,\ldots,0)\} \quad (8.14)$$

for all (t_h,t_j) and $1 \leq h < j \leq m$. In these expressions $\mathscr{E}$ denotes expectation and Z^* denotes (Z_1^*,Z_2). If the expectations in (8.13) and (8.14) were known functions of the hazard ratio parameters β and γ, one could apply estimating equations (6.12) and (6.24) for the estimation of β and γ with regression variables x_{ki} everywhere replaced by their error-prone estimates x_{ki}^* and with induced hazard ratios given Z^* in place of $e^{x_{ki}(t_k)\beta}$ in (6.12), and similarly with x_{gki} everywhere replaced by their error-prone estimates x_{gki}^* and with induced hazard ratios given Z in place of $e^{x_{gki}(t_g,t_k)\gamma}$ in (6.24), for individuals having Z_1^*, but not Z_1 available.

In real applications, however, the induced hazard ratio functions in (8.13) and (8.14) will need to be estimated prior to applying the modified versions of (6.12) and (6.24) just described. With a validation sample of adequate size this may be able to be done with adequate precision with few additional assumptions. For example, if Z_2 histories can be modeled in (6.11) and (6.23) using indicator variables for a moderate number of possibly time-dependent categories, one may be able to estimate induced hazard ratios nonparametrically by simple empirical estimators in each category. For more general dependencies of hazard ratios on Z_2 one can consider kernel-type estimation of the distribution of modeled x^* variables given Z_2. These approaches require estimating functions for parameters, beyond β and γ, appearing in the induced hazard ratio functions in (8.13) and (8.14), and related asymptotic distribution theory will include variance estimators for parameters in (6.11) and (6.23) that reflect uncertainty in estimates of such additional induced hazard ratio parameters in addition to uncertainties in estimates of parameters in (6.11) and (6.23) that derive from the usual counting, censoring and underlying covariate histories.

8.4.3 Hazard rate estimation without a validation subsample

It frequently happens that it is not practical, or perhaps not even conceptually possible, to obtain accurate Z_1 histories for any study subject. For example, Z_1 may entail dietary intake histories, or physical activity histories, over a substantial part of the human lifespan for study in relation to the risk of a chronic disease outcome. Furthermore, even if the exposure period for covariates of this type is defined to be short in relation to the human lifespan (e.g., average dietary intake over the past year) it may not be possible to accurately measure Z_1 without altering the very exposures of interest. For example, a person asked to keep a seven-day food record may well consume differently on the days in question compared to the diet that would otherwise have been consumed. In these circumstances one might have available only the error-prone histories Z_1^*, but not Z_1 histories, for the cohort as a whole. Additional data on cohort members, or a random subset thereof, are then needed to be in a position to estimate the induced hazard ratios (8.13) and (8.14), and additional modeling assumptions are needed concerning the error component of Z_1^* values.

A complication in considering parameters in (8.13) and (8.14) arises from a dependence of the induced hazard ratios on the baseline hazard rate functions in (6.11) and (6.23). This complication may not be a major limitation with nonparametric induced hazard ratio estimation in the presence of a validation sample, but is potentially more problematic when only error-prone estimates of Z_1 are available in the cohort. An approximate, but important, exception occurs if covariates are time-independent, so that $Z(0,\ldots,t_j,0\ldots0) = z(0,\ldots,0)$ for $j = 1,\ldots m$ and $Z(0,\ldots,t_h,0,\ldots,0,t_j,0,\ldots,0) = z(0,\ldots,0)$ for all $1 \leq h < j \leq m$, and follow-up periods are short, so that univariate and bivariate survival probabilities are close to one over the designated follow-up period for all failure times and pairs of failure times, and any baseline covariates $z(0,\ldots,0)$. Under these conditions the induced marginal single and double failure hazard ratios in (8.13) and (8.14) are approximately $\mathscr{E}\{e^{x_k(t_j)\beta}; Z^*(0,\ldots,0)\}$ and $\mathscr{E}\{e^{x_{gk}(t_g,t_k)\gamma}; Z^*(0,\ldots,0)\}$ respectively. Any time-dependence for the modeled covariates in these expressions involve interaction (product) terms between baseline covariates defined using $z(0\ldots0)$ and the time arguments in these hazard rates. Additional assumptions need to be made on the measurement error linking modeled covariate values to corresponding error-prone values. Perhaps the simplest of these supposes that $x_k(t_k) = x_k^*(t_k) + e_k(t_k)$, and $x_{gk}(t_g,t_k) = x_{gk}^*(t_g,t_k) + e_{gk}(t_g,t_j)$, where $e_k(t_k)$ and $e_{gk}(t_g,t_k)$ are mean zero Gaussian variates that are independent of corresponding $z(0,\ldots,0)$ values. Under these so-called Berkson models the induced marginal single and double failure hazard functions have the same form, with the same regression parameters as in the original hazard rate models (6.11) and (6.23), but with baseline hazard rates altered by the measurement error in Z_1^*. While regression parameter estimating equations are then given by (6.12) and (6.24) with $x_k^*(t_k)$ in place of $x_k(t_k)$ in (6.12), and $x_{gk}^*(t_g,t_k)$ in place of $x_{gk}(t_g,t_k)$ in (6.24), variance estimators for these hazard ratio parameter estimates need to reflect the Berkson error component, and will typically require some form of resampling, such as the perturbation resampling approach mentioned in Chapter 6.

The development so far has not addressed how one might obtain assessments Z_1^* that lead to modeled covariates having the desired Berkson error. In many settings it would alternatively be natural to assume a classical measurement model under which assessed covariates are equal their accurate targets, plus independent measurement error. However, regression calibration can provide a method for delivering objective measures of modeled covariates having the desired Berkson error structure, at least approximately.

Specifically, suppose that objective, but possibly noisy, assessments $\tilde{x}_k(t_k)$ and $\tilde{x}_{gk}(t_g, t_k)$ adhering to a classical measurement model, can be obtained for all (k, t_k) and for all $(g, k; t_g, t_k)$ on a random subset, given Z_2, of the study cohort. Linear regression of $\tilde{x}(t_k)$ on $x^*(t_k)$ and of $\tilde{x}_{gk}(t_g, t_h)$ on $x^*_{gk}(t_{g,}, t_h)$ then leads to calibrated assessments $\hat{\alpha}_{k0} + x^*_k(t_k)\hat{\alpha}_{k1}$ for all cohort members, and calibrated assessments $\hat{\alpha}_{gk0} + x^*_{gk}(t_g, t_k)\hat{\alpha}_{gk1}$ for all cohort members, where the coefficients are linear regression parameter estimates. Even though these calibrated assessments cannot be regarded as replacements that have been corrected for measurement error for the underlying regression variables, they do plausibly have the Berkson error structure under the previously mentioned normality and rare disease assumptions. Hence calibrated values can be inserted into (6.12) and (6.24) for estimation of hazard ratio parameters β and γ. The efficiency of these estimators will, of course, depend strongly on the magnitude of the measurement error in the Z_1^* assessments relative to the variation in actual Z_1 values in the study population. Also, it will be important that the objective assessment be strong enough that induced hazard rates are independent of x^* values given $\tilde{x}$ and Z_2 values.

Even with univariate failure times the methodology for assessing hazard rate dependency on covariates that may be poorly measured remains an active research area having important applications in public health and other settings. Some proposed methods can avoid the approximations mentioned above for the calibration approach under additional measurement error assumptions, such as classical measurement models for x^* values in conjunction with replicate x^* measures having errors that are independent of those for the x^* values in the cohort as a whole, though related nonparametric correction methods (e.g., Huang and Wang, 2006) may lose considerable efficiency, compared to corresponding regression calibration estimates, for hazard ratio parameter estimation (e.g., Shaw and Prentice, 2012).

8.4.4 *Energy intake and physical activity in relation to chronic disease risk*

As an illustration of the importance of covariate measurement error in hazard ratio parameter estimation consider the association between total energy intake (i.e., total calories consumed) and total activity-related energy expenditure (AREE) in relation to the risks of various chronic diseases in Women's Health Initiative cohorts. Nearly all epidemiology reports concerning these important exposures rely exclusively on self-reported diet and activity. Energy intake, over a period of a few days or a few months, may be assessed using food frequency questionnaires (FFQs) which request information on frequency and amounts for a specific list of food items; food records which ask the study participant to record all food and drink with corresponding amounts over some number of days (e.g., 4 or 7 days); or dietary recalls which ask respondents to recall all food and drink consumed over a preceding time period, usually 24 hours. In spite of much effort to develop, refine and automate these assessment approaches, over several decades, substantial related measurement issues remain, including both random and systematic biases. Total energy intake is a recognized weak point of these self-report dietary assessments. Fortunately there is an accurate, objective assessment of total energy expenditure over a two-week period using a doubly labeled water (DLW) procedure (Schoeller, 1999), which for weight-stable persons also provides a reliable estimate of energy intake. The DLW procedure was applied to 450 women drawn from the 93,676 postmenopausal women enrolled in the WHI Observational Study, along with FFQ, and 4-day food records (4DFRs), as well as three 24-hour dietary recalls (24HRs) collected over 2–3 months following the two-week DLW period. A random 20% of the 450 women repeated the entire protocol about 6 months later. Table 8.1 obtained from Prentice et al. (2011) shows calibration equations from regression of log-transformed DLW total energy on corresponding log-transformed self-reported energy and other factors. The percent of log-DLW variation explained (R^2) values shown are from regressions with only the single corresponding regression variable, rescaled to add to the total regression R^2. These R^2 values are divided by the sample correlation between paired log-DLW energy estimates using the 20% reliability sample, giving the adjusted R^2 values shown under the assumption that the measurement errors in the paired log-DLW assessments are statistically independent. This assumption with replicate assessments separated by about 6 months, suggests that calibrated intake estimates reflect actual average daily intake over an approximate one-year period rather accurately with adjusted R^2 values of about 70%, even though the log-transformed self-report assessments do so very poorly, with adjusted R^2 values in the 4.8–13.3% range. These calibration equations suggest strong systematic biases in each of the self-report assessments, especially in relation to body mass index (BMI) with overweight and obese participants greatly underestimating energy intake on self-report. Measures of physical activity were included in the same 450 subcohort, with activity measured using questionnaires, records or recalls (Neuhouser et al., 2013). The participating women also engaged in an indirect calorimetry protocol to estimate resting energy expenditure, from which an objective measure of AREE was obtained by subtracting resting energy expenditure from the DLW total energy expenditure assessment. Log-transformed AREE was regressed on log-transformed self-reported AREE derived from a WHI leisure activity questionnaire and other study subject variables to derive a calibration equation for log-AREE based on data from the same 450 women. The equations for log-total energy and for log-AREE were used to generate calibrated estimates for the two variables for women in the larger WHI Observational Study cohort. Cox models (6.11) were applied to clinical outcome data collection on these cohorts from enrollment in 1994–8 through September 30, 2010. The regression variable in the hazard ratio factors in these models were comprised of log-calibrated (total) energy intake, log-calibrated AREE, along with a set of potential confounding factors for each of the diseases under study, in conjunction with detailed stratification of baseline hazard rates. Table 8.2 from Zheng et al. (2014) shows hazard ratio (HR) results from these analyses for 20% increments in total energy and in AREE, both using the self-report data without objective measure calibration (uncalibrated) and with objective measure calibration. For the latter, the approximate 95% CIs shown derive from a sandwich-form estimator of the variance of $\hat{\beta}$ that acknowledges the randomness in the calibration equation coefficient estimates.

Table 8.1 *Calibration equation coefficients (β), standard errors (SE), and percent of biomarker variation explained (R^2) from regression of log(biomarker) on log(self-report), and other factors among 450 Women's Health Initiative Observational Study women from Prentice et al (2011).*

	Energy											
Variable	Food Frequency				4DFR				24HR			
	β	SE	R^2	Adj R^2	β	SE	R^2	Adj R^2	β	SE	R^2	Adj R^2
	7.164	0.009			7.597	0.009			7.607	0.009		
FFQ	0.054	0.017	3.8	6.5								
4DFR					0.161	0.028	7.8	13.3				
24HR									0.101	0.026	2.8	4.8
BMI	0.013	0.001	26.9	45.9	0.013	0.001	27.0	46.0	0.013	0.001	28.7	48.9
Age	−0.010	0.001	9.7	16.5	−0.009	0.001	8.4	14.3	−0.009	0.001	9.1	15.5
Black	−0.023	0.019			−0.024	0.018			−0.024	0.018		
Hispanic	−0.062	0.021	1.3	2.2	−0.065	0.020	1.5	2.6	−0.063	0.020	1.5	2.6
Other minority	−0.041	0.040			−0.039	0.038			−0.038	0.039		
(Total)			41.7	71.1			44.7	76.2			42.1	71.8

Abbreviations: FFQ, food frequency questionnaire; 4DFR, four-day food record; 24HR, three 24-hour dietary recalls; BMI, body mass index (weight in kg squared and divided by height in meters)

Note the striking difference in estimated HRs without and with measurement error correction in the two exposure variables. The diseases listed are among the most common chronic diseases in the US. Without adjustment for measurement error it would seem that neither energy intake or activity-related energy expenditure are importantly related to the risk of these major diseases, whereas analyses on the right of Table 8.2 with measurement error correction suggest that these exposures may be among the most important drivers of chronic disease risk. For example, a 20% reduction in energy intake in conjunction with a 20% increase in AREE is associated with an approximate 5/6th reduction in diabetes risk in these analyses.

The calibrated HRs in Table 8.2 have one important caveat: The disease risk models leading to those analyses did not include BMI. Excessive BMI arises from energy imbalance, and BMI values are strongly correlated with the calibrated energy and AREE values to the point that HR estimates become unstable when BMI is included in the disease risk model. It seems likely that BMI and obesity are related to the disease outcomes shown primarily because excess energy intake compared to activity-related expenditure tends to track over the lifespan, leading to body fat deposition and elevated BMI. As such, BMI could be an important mediator of the energy intake and AREE associations shown on the right side of Table 8.2. On the other hand, BMI could also have some confounding role as certain germline genetic factors have been shown to be obesity risk factors. Sorting out these competing explanations may be possible, with objective measures of these key exposures and of body fat trajectories over the lifespan or a major component thereof, but data are currently not available in any epidemiologic cohort study that would lead to a definitive interpretation of results in Table 8.2. One could postulate that resolving the importance of these and other diet and activity associations are among the most important topics in public health at this time in history, given the world-wide obesity epidemic in developed countries. Study designs and analytic procedures for such resolution rely strongly on statistical input.

8.5 Joint Modeling of Longitudinal Covariates and Failure Rates

The previous section described some methods for extending the marginal single and double hazard rate analyses in relation to a baseline covariate that may be subject to measurement error. Now consider a stochastic covariate recorded over the follow-up period for a study cohort. The recorded history for a stochastic covariate may include measurement error at any measurement time and, furthermore, the covariate measurement times may be infrequent and variable among cohort members, even though the underlying covariate process Z may be potentially available for measurement at any time point $(t_1,\ldots,t_m)$ for an m-dimensional failure time process. Hence, to extend the hazard rate estimation procedures of Chapter 6 to these data, we will typically require a non-differential assumption for marginal single and double failure hazard rates, so that (6.11) and (6.23) generalize to

$$\Lambda_{0\cdots010\cdots0}\{0,\ldots,0,dt_j,0,\ldots,0;Z(0,\ldots,0,t_j,0,\ldots,0),Z^*(0,\ldots,0,t_j,0,\ldots,0)\}$$
$$= \Gamma_k(dt_j)\exp\{x_k(t_j)\beta\} \tag{8.15}$$

Table 8.2 *Estimated hazard ratio for 20% increments in total energy and in activity-related energy expenditure (AREE), with and without calibration to correct for measurement error for various chronic diseases, in the Women's Health Initiative Observational Study from baseline (1994–1998) through September 30, 2010 (Zheng et al. 2014).*

	Uncalibrated				Calibrated			
	Energy		AREE		Energy		AREE	
Outcome Category	HR	95% CI	HR	95% CI	HR	95% CI	HR	95% CI
Total CHD	1.00	0.98,1.02	0.99	0.97,1.01	**1.57**	1.19,2.06	**0.78**	0.65,0.95
Heart Failure	1.04	1.01,1.08	0.97	0.95,1.00	**3.51**	2.12,5.82	**0.57**	0.41,0.79
Total CVD including CABG and PCI	1.00	0.99,1.01	1.00	0.99,1.01	**1.49**	1.23,1.81	**0.83**	0.73,0.93
Total Invasive Cancer	1.01	1.00,1.02	0.99	0.99,1.00	**1.43**	1.17,1.73	**0.84**	0.73,0.96
Invasive Breast Cancer	1.01	0.99,1.02	1.00	0.99,1.01	**1.47**	1.18,1.84	**0.82**	0.71,0.96
Obesity-related Cancer	1.02	1.00,1.03	1.00	0.99,1.01	**1.71**	1.33,2.21	**0.79**	0.65,0.94
Diabetes Mellitus	1.06	1.04,1.07	1.01	1.00,1.02	**4.17**	2.68,6.49	**0.60**	0.44,0.83

Abbreviations: CHD, coronary heart disease comprise of non-fatal myocardial infarction plus CHD death; CABG, coronary artery bypass graft; CI confidence interval; HR, hazard ratio; PCI, percutaneous coronary intervention and

$$\Lambda_{0\cdots010\cdots010\cdots0}\{0,\ldots,0,dt_h,0,\ldots,0,dt_j,0,\ldots,0;Z(0,\ldots,0,t_h,0,\ldots,0,t_j,0,\ldots,0),$$
$$Z^*(0,\ldots,0,t_h,0,\ldots,0,t_j,0,\ldots,0)\} = \Gamma_{gk}(dt_h,dt_j)\exp\{x_{gk}(t_h,t_j)\gamma\} \qquad (8.16)$$

so that the measured covariate histories, Z^*, do not affect the hazard rate given the "true" history, among individuals at risk for failure at specified univariate and bivariate follow-up times. Z^* in these expressions is an estimated covariate history over the study follow-up period, which will typically involve some modeling of the covariate processes.

The likelihood component for the evolving marginal failure, censoring and covariate histories for failure time T_j includes a product integral factor for each individual given by

$$\prod_{t_1 \geq 0} P\{Z^*(0,\ldots,0,t_j+dt_j,0,\ldots,0);T_j > t_j, C_j > t_j; Z^*(0,\ldots,0,t_j,0,\ldots,0)\}. \qquad (8.17)$$

For these probability elements to be recast in terms of the covariate history in (6.11) one requires that the probability element in (8.17) be equal to

$$P\{Z^*(0,\ldots,0,t_j+dt_j,0,\ldots,0);T_j > t_j, C_j > t_j, Z(0,\ldots,0,t_j,0,\ldots,0)\} \qquad (8.18)$$

so that the estimated conditional covariate history at $t_j + dt_j$ is representative of that for persons at risk for failure beyond time t_j who have underlying history $Z(0,\ldots,0,t_j,0,\ldots,0)$. This would, for example, preclude study designs with more frequent covariate sampling based on data other than that included in the evolving history $Z(0,\ldots,0,t_j,0,\ldots,0)$. Also in (8.18) one would usually not want covariate distribution models to depend on the lack of censoring condition $C_j > t_j$, so that it will be natural to impose an assumption of no dependence of the probability element in (8.18) on the condition $C_j > t_j$, given $T_j > t_j$ and $Z(0,\ldots,0,t_j,0,\ldots,0)$. Under these conditions the marginal single failure hazard rate (8.12) can be written as

$$\Gamma_k(dt_k)\mathscr{E}\{e^{x_k^*(t_j)\beta}; T_j > t_j, Z(0,\ldots,0,t_j,0,\ldots,0)\} \qquad (8.19)$$

where $x_k^*(t_j)$ is an estimate of $x_k(t_j)$ from the estimated covariate history $Z^*(0,\ldots,0,t_j,0,\ldots,0)$, and the expectation is over the distribution of $x_k^*(t_j)$ given $T_j > t_j$ and $Z(0,\ldots,t_j,0,\ldots,0)$, for any t_j and $j \in \{1,\ldots,m\}$.

There is a useful statistical literature on this type of "joint modeling" of univariate failure and covariate processes, much of which is summarized in Tsiatis and Davidian (2004). The literature mostly assumes some simple growth curves for the modeled covariate in (6.11) with a small number of subject-specific parameters that can be estimated from measured covariate histories $Z^*(0,\ldots,0,\cdot,0,\ldots,0)$, often in conjunction with joint normality assumptions for convenient calculation of the expectations in (8.19).

For marginal double failure hazard rate estimation under (6.23) one can similarly consider the likelihood component for failure time pairs (T_h, T_j) in conjunction with related censoring and covariate processes. A non-differential assumption (8.13), and a somewhat stronger independence assumption between bivariate censoring and failure processes will allow the induced (h, j) marginal double failure hazard from (8.16) to be written as

$$\Gamma_{gk}(dt_h, dt_j)\mathscr{E}\{e^{x^*_{gk}(t_h,t_j)\gamma}; T_h > t_h, T_j > t_j, Z(0,\ldots,0,t_h,0,\ldots,0,t_j,0,\ldots,0)\} \quad (8.20)$$

where $x^*_{gk}(t_h,t_j)$ is an estimate of $x_{gk}(t_h,t_j)$ from the covariate history $Z^*(0,\ldots, t_h,0,\ldots,0,t_j,0,\ldots,0)$, and the expectation is over the distribution of $x^*_{gk}(t_h,t_j)$ given $T_h > t_h, T_j > t_j$ and $Z(0,\ldots,0,t_h,0,\ldots,0,t_j,0,\ldots,0)$, for all (t_h,t_j) and all $1 \le h < j \le m$.

There are many possibilities for covariate history models that will lead to parametric specifications of the expectations in (8.19) and (8.20). If these models include individual-specific parameters, it may be necessary to delay the start of the follow-up period for cohort members to ensure that there are sufficient available covariate history data for the individual that all such parameters are identifiable.

Under the conditions described above, and additional typically mild conditions related to covariate history probability parameter estimation, it will be natural to consider estimation of marginal single and double hazard rate estimation using (6.12) and (6.24), but with $e^{x_{k\ell}(t_k)\beta}$ and $e^{x_{gk\ell}(t_g,t_k)\gamma}$ everywhere replaced by estimates of the expectations in (8.19) and (8.20), in conjunction with corresponding estimating equations for the additional parameters, beyond those in (6.11) and (6.23) in these expectations.

Joint modeling of evolving failure and covariate processes is a large topic, with some good efforts for univariate failure times already in the statistical literature. Further development of these univariate methods, and extensions to multivariate failure times along the lines described in this section, would be quite worthwhile.

8.6 Model Checking

Some readers may think we have been remiss in giving very little attention to the important task of model checking until this late stage of our presentation. One reason for this delay derives from our emphasis on semiparametric models, such as (6.11) and (6.23), with their time-dependent covariate and time-dependent stratification features. With this approach the failure time modeling assumption involves only a parametric form for hazard ratios, and one that can be conveniently be relaxed as necessary to achieve a good fit to available data. Specifically, a powerful approach to checking modeling assumptions in (6.11) and (6.23) is to augment the modeled regression variable by including additional components, such as interaction terms with follow-up times or terms that allow greater variation in hazard ratio shapes more generally, for key covariates. This regression model augmentation approach typically contrasts the hypothesized model with local alternatives. With univariate failure time data the same approach has been used to formulate more global tests in simple situations by extending the modeled regression variable to include indicator variables that allow the modeled hazard ratio to vary over a partition of the follow-up time axis (e.g., Schoenfeld, 1982; Andersen, 1982). This approach could be used to allow the modeled hazard ratio to vary over a grid formed by pairwise follow-up times for marginal double failure hazard rate model testing. Various types of residuals have also been considered for use in failure time model building and checking with univariate failure time data (e.g.,Barlow & Prentice, 1988, Therneau, Grambsch, & Fleming, 1990), mostly based on martingale properties of the elements of estimating function for failure intensity model parameters. Lin, Wei, and Ying (1993) propose graphical procedures for checking Cox model assumptions for counting process intensities based on cumulative sums of martingale-based residuals, with a resampling procedure for formally testing for departure from model assumptions. Also see Lin et al. (2000) for generalization of these methods to the recurrent event setting.

It is perhaps worth commenting that the regression parameter estimates described in Chapter 6 may retain a useful interpretation even under oversimplified models for hazard rates in (6.11) and (6.23). For example the intention-to-treat hormone therapy hazard ratio estimates shown in Figure 2.2 provide useful summary measures over trial intervention periods that averaged 5.6 years (CEE + MPA) or 7.2 years (CEE Alone) even though there were rather striking hazard ratio variations over these follow-up periods for some clinical outcomes. For example, with CEE + MPA the coronary heart disease hazard ratio was about 2-fold elevated during the first year from randomization, but subsequently dropped back close to unity, while breast cancer hazard ratios were evidently below one early in the post-randomization period, possibly due to intervention-related increases in breast density and consequent delayed ability to diagnose malignant breast tumors, but increased rapidly thereafter. As weighted estimators of average hazard ratios the standard Cox model estimates may suffer from some dependence of the weighting across follow-up time on censoring rates. When censoring rates are high, as in Figure 2.2, any censoring influence is likely to be small. In lighter censoring situations it may be useful to construct average hazard ratio estimators with weights that do not depend on censoring (e.g., Kalbfleisch & Prentice, 1981; Xu & O'Quigley, 2000).

8.7 Marked Point Processes and Multistate Models

Previous chapters allowed failures to be one of K different types, and allowed hazard rate and counting process intensity models to include parameters that may differ among failure types. For example, failures may be classified according to the affected organ or body system, or infectious disease occurrences may be classified according to the class of the infecting agent. As briefly discussed in §4.9.3 it frequently happens that when a failure occurs additional detail on the state of the study subject will be assessed. For example the state information may describe tumor histologic type and various aspects of disease extent when a cancer is diagnosed, or may describe genetic aspects of both the pathogen and the study participant when an infectious disease is diagnosed. There may be much to be learned by studying hazard rates that are state-specific, and by studying transition rates between states.

As mentioned in §2.4 and §4.9 classical competing risk data comprised of a possibly censored failure time on a single failure time axis along with covariates is often most readily analyzed by regarding the failure information as a marked point process with mark equal to a classification of failures (e.g., cause of death) obtained when failures occur. These data do not permit analyses of dependency among failures in different states, given covariates, without making strong additional assumptions that cannot be tested empirically.

Recently Cook and Lawless (2018) have provided an excellent account of much more general multistate models for life history events on a single failure time axes. Both counting process intensity models that consider state-specific event rates conditional on the entire preceding failure, censoring and covariate histories, as well as marginal or partly conditional models that condition on some or all of that preceding history, are described and illustrated. The rather general results of Spiekerman and Lin (1998) and Lin et al. (2000) described in Chapters 6 and 7 extend to the analysis of parameters in Cox-type models for these partly conditional models assuming univariate independent right censoring. The sandwich variance formula for regression parameter estimates is able to capture the additional estimating function variance that derives from dropping some of the information at follow-up time t that had been conditioned on at earlier times, for a remarkably wide class of data types and models. The associated estimation procedures are well suited to the study of failure processes and disease mechanisms, and are largely complementary to the population-averaged marginal associations emphasized in this monograph. Extensions of these univariate methods to multistate models on multiple time axes are beyond the scope of this book, but would merit further development.

8.8 Imprecisely Measured Failure Times

The methods described in this volume have mostly assumed that the failure times under study have been measured precisely. Importantly, our inclusion of discrete elements in the Cox models (2.5), (6.11) and (6.23), among other places, allows accommodation of outcome imprecision that is small relative to the range of the "underlying" failure times. In some applications, however, failure times may only be observed to occur in time intervals that are not small relative to the range of the underlying failure times, and "interval censoring" intervals may vary in complex overlapping patterns among study individuals. From a likelihood perspective such data will involve modeled probabilities that integrate underlying hazard rates over the time period where a failure is known to occur. Related likelihood-based estimation can be pushed through (e.g., Huang & Wellner, 1997), but tends to be quite difficult computationally with semiparametric models. The special case where one determines only whether a failure time exceeds or is equal or less than a specified value, termed current status data, also arises with some frequency in applications, for example in serial sacrifice animal experiments involving the occurrence of tumors that are clinically unobservable, and involves the same type of complex calculations with semiparametric models. Zeng, Mao, and Lin (2016) substantially address the challenging computational aspects of maximum likelihood estimation with interval censoring, for a rather broad class of linear transformation models that includes the univariate Cox model, and impressively demonstrate semiparametric efficiency for the resulting estimators while allowing external time-dependent covariates. These results have recently been extended to multivariate failure time data (Zeng, Gao, & Lin, 2017) using a full-likelihood frailty modeling approach.

BIBLIOGRAPHIC NOTES

Some key references have been listed in each section of this chapter. A few more references, to enhance historical perspectives and recent contributions, are given here.

The idea of inverse probability weighting to address censoring that would otherwise be dependent is due to Robins and Rotnitzky (1992) and Rotnitzky and Robins (1995). See also Datta and Satten (2002), Ghosh and Lin (2003), and Hernán and Robins (2015). Inverse probability weighting for confounding via propensity scores (Rosenbaum & Rubin, 1983) and marginal structural models (Robins et al., 2000) were discussed in Robins and Rotnitzky (1992) and Robins (1993). See also van der Laan and Robins (2003) for a technical and rigorous account of these developments.

Nested case–control sampling designs with failure time data were introduced by Thomas (1977) and Prentice and Breslow (1978) , with related asymptotic theory by Goldstein and Langholz (1992) and in a more general form by Borgan et al. (1995). Related work includes Oakes (1981) , Breslow, Lubin, Marek, and Langholz (1983), Kalbfleisch and Lawless (1988), Robins, Prentice, and Blevins (1989) and Samuelsen (1997) among many other contributions.

Case–cohort designs with failure time data were introduced by Prentice (1986), with distribution theory in Self and Prentice (1988). Langholz and Thomas (1990) and Wacholder (1991) discuss aspects of the choice of cohort sampling procedures. Chen and Little (1999) consider inverse sampling probability weighted estimators for improvement in hazard ratio parameter estimation under case–cohort sampling. See also Nan (2004) and Scheike and Martinussen (2004) for additional aspects of estimation efficiency under case–cohort sampling. Efficiency considerations, with some covariates available in all cohort members, led to the two-phase sampling design approaches emphasized here, starting with Breslow and Cain (1988), with more recent contributions by Breslow and Wellner (2007, 2008) and by Saegusa and Wellner (2013).

In addition to Robins et al. (1994), Wang and Chen (2001) and Qi, Wang, and Prentice (2005) provide contributions on the use of inverse probability weighting to adjust for missing covariate data with univariate failure time data. See also Zhou and Pepe (1995), Chen and Little (1999), Lawless, Kalbfleisch, and Wild (1999), Rotnitzky (2009) and Lumley et al. (2011).

For additional recent measurement error–related contributions involving biomarkers in the nutritional epidemiology context, see Freedman et al. (2014, 2015), Lampe et al. (2017), Mahabir et al. (2018) and Prentice (2018). Also Yi (2018) gives a current and comprehensive account of measurement error and misclassification methods for various types of response data, including univariate failure time and recurrent event data.

Other contributions to procedures for checking Cox model assumptions, beyond those cited in §8.6 include Wei (1984), Lagakos and Schoenfeld (1984), Lin and Wei

(1991) and McKeague and Utikal (1991), the last of which addresses goodness-of-fit of additive hazards as well as proportional hazards models.

For joint longitudinal data and univariate failure time modeling contributions beyond those summarized in Tsiatis and Davidian (2004), see Chi and Ibrahim (2006), Elashoff, Li, and Li (2008), Proust-Lima, Joly, Dartigues, and Jacqmin-Gadda (2009), Hatfield, Boye, and Carlin (2011), Rizopoulos and Ghosh (2011) and Luo (2014). See Fu and Gilbert (2017) for a contribution that combines joint modeling of longitudinal and survival data with two-phase sampling.

For references on multistate modeling, see Andersen et al. (1993), Kalbfleisch and Prentice (2002), Aalen et al. (2010), in addition to the comprehensive recent book by Cook and Lawless (2018). Also see Zeng et al. (2016) and Zeng et al. (2017) for a recent summary of the literature on univariate and multivariate hazard rate estimation with interval-censored failure times.

EXERCISES AND COMPLEMENTS

Exercise 8.1

Provide a detailed development to show that the expectation of (8.3) is zero under modeling assumptions. Does one require $G_j\{s_j; Z(0,\ldots,0,s_j,0,\ldots,0)\} > 0$ for this to be true? Show that (8.3) also has expectation zero under the covariate selection weights (8.9).

Exercise 8.2

Show that $N_{ji}(dt_k)$ in (8.4) can be replaced by $L_{ij}(dt_k;\beta,G_j)$, and that $N_{ji}(dt_g)N_{ji}(dt_k)$ in (8.6) can be replaced by $L_{jki}(dt_g,dt_k;\gamma,G_{hj})$, while preserving equality to zero.

Exercise 8.3

Write out an expression for a likelihood factor G_{hj} analogous to (8.9) for the pairwise Z_1 history corresponding to T_h and T_j given $Z(0,\ldots,0,t_h,0,\ldots,0,t_j,0,\ldots,0)$, $T_h > t_h, T_j > t_j, C_h > t_h$ and $C_j > t_j$. Describe how $G_j, j = 1,\ldots,m$ in (8.9) and $G_{hj}, 1 \leq h < j \leq m$ could be modeled and estimated for specific classes of covariate histories Z_1.

Exercise 8.4

Consider a multivariate version of case–cohort sampling that selects all individuals experiencing one or more of m failure times during cohort follow-up, along with a simple random sample of all other cohort members. Develop weighted estimating equations of the form (8.11) and (8.12) for the estimation of marginal single and double failure hazard rate parameters under models (6.11) and (6.23), but with estimated selection weights included. Sketch the development of asymptotic distribution theory for all model parameters. In the special case of a univariate failure time, describe how the marginal single failure hazard rate parameter estimate (β) may improve on the estimator originally proposed for regression parameter estimation under case–cohort sampling (Prentice, 1986; Self & Prentice, 1988) . Generalize the marginal single and double failure hazard ratio parameter estimating equations to allow the sampling probability for non-cases to depend on a baseline covariate $z(0,\ldots,0)$.

Exercise 8.5

Describe the design of an epidemiologic cohort study that may be needed to provide insight into the reliability of the hazard ratio estimates shown in Table 8.2. Given the substantial measurement issues that are thought to attend nutrition and activity epidemiology, can you outline a research agenda that could qualitatively strengthen research results in these important public health areas?

Exercise 8.6

Consider bivariate failure time regression data as in (4.8)–(4.10). Suppose that T_1 and/or T_2 is subject to interval censoring, so that one only knows whether $T_{ji} \leq a_{ji}$, $a_{ji} < T_{ji} \leq b_{ji}$ or $b_{ji} < T_{ji}$ for specified values a_{ji} an b_{ji}, for $i = 1,\ldots,n$ and $j = 1,2$. Can you construct an estimating equation for $(\beta_{10},\beta_{01},\beta_{11})$? Does the presence of stochastic time-variates complicate such construction? See Zeng et al. (2017) for related work in the context of linear transformation models.

Glossary of Notation

$T > 0$ denotes a failure time random variable.

$(T_1, \ldots, T_m)$, with each $T_j > 0$, denotes an m-dimensional $(m \geq 1)$ failure time variate.

$C \geq 0$ denotes a censoring variate.

$(C_1, \ldots, C_m)$ denotes an m-dimensional $(m \geq 1)$ censoring variate.

$S = T \wedge C = \min(T, C)$ and $\delta = I[S = T]$ denote observed follow-up time, and non-censoring indicator variable, respectively.

$I[A]$ is an indicator variable that takes value 1 if A is true, and 0 otherwise.

$(S_1, \ldots, S_m)$ and $(\delta_1, \ldots, \delta_m)$ denote m-dimensional $(m \geq 1)$ follow-up times and non-censoring indicator variables.

$z = (z_1, \ldots, z_q)$ denotes a q-dimensional covariate at time $t = 0$.

$z(t) = \{z_1(t), \ldots, z_q(t)\}$ denotes a q-dimensional covariate at follow-up time t.

$Z(t) = \{z \text{ if } t = 0; z(s), \text{ all } s < t \text{ if } t > 0\}$ denotes covariate history prior to time t.

$z(t_1, t_2) = \{z_1(t_1, t_2), z_2(t_1, t_2), \ldots\}$ denotes a covariate at follow-up time (t_1, t_2) for a bivariate failure time variate (T_1, T_2).

$Z(t_1, t_2) = \{z(s_1, s_2); s_1 = t_1 \text{ if } t_1 = 0, s_1 < t_1 \text{ if } t_1 > 0, \text{ and } s_2 = t_2 \text{ if } t_2 = 0, s_2 < t_2 \text{ if } t_2 > 0\}$ denotes bivariate covariate history prior to (t_1, t_2).

$z(t_1, \ldots, t_m)$ denotes an m-dimensional covariate $(m \geq 1)$ at follow-up time $(t_1, \ldots, t_m)$ for an m-dimensional failure time variate $(T_1, \ldots, T_m)$.

$Z(t_1, \ldots, t_m) = \{z(s_1, \ldots, s_m); s_j = 0 \text{ if } t_j = 0, s_j < t_j \text{ if } t_j > 0, j = 1, \ldots, m\}$ denotes an m-dimensional covariate history prior to $(t_1, \ldots, t_m)$.

P denotes probability.

F denotes survivor function for failure time variate T, so that $F(t_1, \ldots, t_m) = P(T_1 > t_1, \ldots, T_m > t_m)$.

$\underline{F}$ denotes distribution function for failure time variates, so that $\underline{F}(t_1,\ldots,t_m) = P(T_1 \leq t_1,\ldots,T_m \leq t_m)$.

Λ denotes the (cumulative) hazard function (or process) for T.

$\Lambda(dt)$ denotes the hazard rate at $T = t$, for continuous discrete or mixed failure time variate T, so that $\Lambda(t) = \int_0^t \Lambda(ds)$.

$\Lambda_{11\cdots1}(t_1,\ldots,t_m)$ denotes the (cumulative) hazard function (process) for $(T_1,\ldots,T_m)$ at $(t_1,\ldots,t_m)$ for $m \geq 1$.

$\Lambda_{10\cdots0}(dt_1,0,\ldots,0)$ denotes the marginal T_1 hazard rate at $(t_1,0,\ldots,0)$.

$\Lambda_{110\cdots0}(dt_1,dt_2,0,\ldots,0)$ denotes the marginal (T_1,T_2) hazard rate at $(t_1,t_2,0,\ldots,0)$.

$\Lambda_{10\cdots0}(dt_1,t_2,\ldots,t_m)$ denotes the T_1 hazard rate at $(t_1,\ldots,t_m)$.

$\Lambda_{110\cdots0}(dt_1,dt_2,t_3,\ldots,t_m)$ denotes the (T_1,T_2) hazard rate at $(t_1,\ldots,t_m)$.

$\Lambda_{11\cdots1}(dt_1,\ldots,dt_m)$ denotes the $(T_1,\ldots,T_m)$ hazard rate at $(t_1,\ldots,t_m)$, so that $\Lambda_{11\cdots1}(t_1,\ldots,t_m) = \int_0^{t_1}\cdots\int_0^{t_m}\Lambda_{1\cdots1}(ds_1,\ldots,ds_m)$.

$\prod_a^b$ denotes product integral over $(a,b]$.

$\prod_{a_1}^{b_1}\cdots\prod_{a_m}^{b_m}$ denotes m-dimensional $(m \geq 1)$ product integral over $(a_1,b_1] \times \cdots \times (a_m,b_m]$.

$N_i(t)$ denotes the observed number of failures in $[0,t]$ for individual i.

$Y_i(t) = \begin{cases} 1 & \text{if } S_i = T_i \wedge C_i \geq t \\ 0 & \text{otherwise} \end{cases}$ is the "at-risk" indicator at time t for individual i.

$\{N_{1i}(t_1),\ldots,N_{mi}(t_m)\}$ denotes the number of T_j failures in $[0,t_j]$ on individual i, for each $j = 1,\ldots,m$.

$\{Y_{1i}(t_1),\ldots,Y_{mi}(t_m)\}$ denotes the "at-risk" indicators at time $(t_1,\ldots,t_m)$ for individual i.

n denotes number of individuals (sample size).

$R = \{i; Y_{ji}(t_j) = 1$, for each $j = 1,\ldots,m$ for some $i \in (1,\ldots,n)\}$ denotes the risk set at $(t_1,\ldots,t_m)$ for $m \geq 1$.

L_{ji} denotes a zero-mean process (under model assumptions) for the jth failure time $(j = 1, \ldots, m)$ on the ith individual $(i = 1, \ldots, n)$.

IID denotes independent and identically distributed (random variables).

A prime ($'$) denotes vector transpose.

$\Lambda\{dt; Z(t)\}$ denotes hazard rate at time t given preceding covariate history $Z(t)$.

$\Lambda\{dt; Z(t)\} = \Lambda(dt)\exp\{x(t)\beta\}$ denotes a Cox model for hazard rate given Z at $T = t$, where $\Lambda(dt)$ is a "baseline" unspecified hazard rate at value zero for modeled covariate p-vector $x(t) = \{x_1(t), \ldots, x_p(t)\}$ and $\beta = (\beta_1, \ldots, \beta_p)'$ is a corresponding hazard ratio parameter to be estimated.

$\Lambda_{10\cdots0}\{dt_1, 0, \ldots, 0; Z(t_1, 0, \ldots, 0)\} = \Lambda_{10\cdots0}(dt_1, 0, \ldots, 0)\exp\{x(t_1, 0, \ldots, 0)\beta_{10\cdots0}\}$ denotes a Cox model for the marginal T_1 hazard rate at $(t_1, 0, \ldots, 0)$ with baseline marginal T_1 hazard rate $\Lambda_{10\cdots0}(dt_1, 0, \ldots, 0)$, modeled covariate $x(t_1, 0, \ldots, 0)$ at $(t_1, 0)$, and marginal single failure hazard ratio parameter $\beta_{10\cdots0}$.

$\Lambda_{110\cdots0}\{dt_1, dt_2, 0, \ldots, 0; Z(t_1, t_2, 0, \ldots, 0)\} = \Lambda_{110\cdots0}(dt_1, dt_2, 0, \ldots, 0)\exp\{x(t_1, t_2, 0, \ldots, 0)\beta_{110\cdots0}\}$ denotes a Cox model for the marginal (T_1, T_2) hazard rate at $(t_1, t_2, 0, \ldots, 0)$ with baseline marginal (T_1, T_2) hazard rate $\Lambda_{110\cdots0}(dt_1, dt_2, 0, \ldots, 0)$, modeled covariate $x(t_1, t_2, 0, \ldots, 0)$ at $(t_1, t_2, 0, \ldots, 0)$, and marginal failure hazard ratio parameter $\beta_{110\cdots0}$.

$M(j)$ denotes a unique failure type for failure time variate T_j, $j = 1, \ldots, m$.

Γ_k denotes baseline hazard function for a failure time variate T_j having $k = M(j)$.

Γ_{gk} denotes baseline hazard function for failure time variates (T_h, T_j) having $g = M(h)$ and $k = M(j)$.

If $a = (a_1, a_2, \ldots)'$ then $a^{\otimes 2} = aa'$.

Appendix A: Technical Materials

A.1 Product Integrals and Stieltjes Integration

The estimation procedures emphasized in this monograph entail discrete estimators of hazard rates, even when the underlying failure time variates are absolutely continuous. For example, in Chapter 1 the (cumulative) hazard function Λ for a univariate failure time variate T, defined by $\Lambda(t) = \int_0^t \Lambda(ds)$, where $\Lambda(ds)$ is the hazard rate at follow-up time s, can be estimated by the corresponding 'empirical' hazard function $\hat{\Lambda}$, where $\hat{\Lambda}(t) = \int_0^t \hat{\Lambda}(ds)$ and $\hat{\Lambda}(ds)$ is the ratio of the number of failures in the study sample at $T = s$ to the number of individuals without failure or censoring prior to time s. Here $\hat{\Lambda}(t)$ is a Stieltjes integral. The Riemann–Stieltjes integral of a real-valued function f with respect to a real-valued function g over an interval $[a,b]$ is defined as the limit of

$$\sum_{j=0}^{m-1} f(c_j)\{g(t_{j+1}) - g(t_j)\} \tag{A.1}$$

over partitions $a = t_0 < t_1 < \cdots < t_m = b$, and $c_j \in [t_j, t_{j+1}]$, as the mesh of the partition approaches zero. The Riemann–Stieltjes integral exists if f is continuous and g is of bounded variation (i.e., can be written as the difference between two monotone functions). The two Riemann–Stieltjes integrals shown in the integration-by-parts formula

$$\int_a^b f(t)g(dt) = f(b)g(b) - f(a)g(a) - \int_a^b g(t)f(dt)$$

either exist, or not, simultaneously.

A slightly more general Stieltjes integral is defined in measure theoretic terms with f and g measures acting on Borel sets on the real line. Specifically, if f is Borel measurable and bounded and g is of bounded variation and right continuous on $(a,b]$, or (importantly, for our setting) if f is non-negative and g is monotone and right continuous then (A.1) exists and is referred to as a Lebesgue–Stieltjes integral.

The product integral of a real-valued measure g on Borel subsets of $[a,b] \subset [0,\infty]$ can be defined by the Riemann–Stieltjes–type limit of

$$\prod_{j=0}^{m-1} [1 + \{g(t_{j+1}) - g(t_j)\}], \tag{A.2}$$

again over partitions $a = t_0 < t, < \cdots, t_m = b$ as the mesh of the partition approaches zero. This product integral, denoted

$$\prod_a^b \{1 + g(dt)\}$$

provides a 1-1 connection between additive interval functions (A.1) and multiplicative interval functions (A.2) on $[0, \infty)$. Gill and Johansen (1990) provide an excellent account of product integration with applications to failure time data.

They provide the definition (A.2) for matrix-valued measures g and show the product integral

$$h(t) = \prod_0^t \{1 + g(ds)\}$$

to have two equivalent definitions over a follow-up region $[0, \infty]$. Specifically, h satisfies the Volterra integral equation

$$h(t) = 1 + \int_0^t h(s^-) g(ds) \tag{A.3}$$

for all $t \in [0, \infty)$ or h is the Péano series solution to (A.3) given by

$$h(t) = 1 + \sum_{m=1}^{\infty} \int_{0<t_1<\cdots<t_m=t} g(dt_1) \cdots g(dt_m) \tag{A.4}$$

where (A.3) and (A.4) are integrals of Lebesgue–Stieltjes type. Importantly in the context of this book, the definitions (A.3) and (A.4) can be extended to failure time variates of dimension greater than one.

The (Riemann–)Stieltjes integral of a real-valued bivariate function f with respect to a real-valued bivariate function g over a rectangle $(a_1, b_1] \times (a_2, b_2]$ is defined as the limit of

$$\sum_{j=0}^{m-1} f(c_{1j}, c_{2j})\{g(t_{1,j+1}, t_{2,j+1}) - g(t_{1,j+1}, t_{2j}) - g(t_{1j}, t_{2,j+1}) + g(t_{1j}, t_{2j})\}$$

over partitions $a_1 = t_{10} < t_{11} < \cdots < t_{1m} = b_1$ and $a_2 = t_{20} < t_{21} < \cdots < t_{2m} = b_2$ as the mesh of the partition approaches zero, where $(c_{ij}, c_{2j}) \varepsilon [t_{1j}, t_{1,j+1}] \times [t_{2j}, t_{2,j+1}]$. This integral $\int_{a_1}^{b_1} \int_{a_2}^{b_2} f(t_1, t_2) g(dt_1, dt_2)$ will exist when f is continuous and g is of bounded variation. Once again a slight generalization is possible in measure theoretic terms with functions acting on Borel sets (rectangles) on $[0, \infty) \times [0, \infty)$.

The survival probability function F for bivariate failure times (T_1, T_2) can be expressed as the unique solution to the Volterra integral equation

$$F(t_1,t_2) = \psi(t_1,t_2) + \int_0^{t_1}\int_0^{t_2} F(s_1^-,s_2^-)\Lambda_{11}(ds_1,ds_2),$$

where Λ_{11} is the double failure hazard function, and $\Psi(t_1,t_2) = F(t_1,0) + F(0,t_2) - 1$ is determined by the lower-dimensional (i.e., marginal) hazard functions. The Péano series solution to this Volterra equation is given in (3.5).

Similarly, the joint survivor function F for k failure time variates $(T_1,\cdots,T_k)$ uniquely solves an inhomogeneous Volterra integral equation that expresses $F(t_1,\cdots,t_k)$ as function of marginal survivor functions of dimension less than k, along with (plus or minus) the Stieltjes integral

$$\int_0^{t_1}\cdots\int_0^{t_k} F(s_1^-,\cdots,s_k^-)\Lambda_{11\cdots1}(ds_1,\cdots,ds_k),$$

which again leads to a unique expression for F in terms of its k-variate hazard rate and marginal hazard rates of dimension less than k as is shown in (6.8).

A major value of these expressions is that one can substitute empirical estimates of marginal hazard rates of dimension $1,\cdots,k$ to obtain estimators of $\hat{F}$. The continuity, and (weakly continuous) compact differentiability of the related sequence of Péano series transformations for marginal survivor functions of each dimension, ensure that $\hat{F}$ inherits such statistical properties as (supremum norm) strong consistency, weak Gaussian convergence and bootstrap applicability from those for corresponding empirical marginal hazard rate estimators. These properties for the bivariate Péano series transformation from (Ψ, Λ_{11}) to F were established in Gill et al. (1995).

A.2 Generalized Estimating Equations for Mean Parameters

Consider a q-vector response variable $W_k = (W_{k1},\ldots,W_{kq})$ for each of $k = 1,\ldots,n$ members of a study cohort. Suppose that W_k has a mean $\mu_k = (\mu_{k1},\ldots,\mu_{kq})$ that depends on a p-dimensional parameter $\theta = (\theta_1,\ldots,\theta_P)$, and a variance matrix V_k that may also depend on θ as well as other parameters. A generalized estimating equation for θ can be written

$$\sum_{k=1}^{n} D_k' V_k^{-1}(W_k - \mu_k) = 0 \tag{A.5}$$

where D_k is the matrix of partial derivatives of μ_k with respect to θ'. Under independent and identically distributed sampling, and additional mild conditions (Liang & Zeger, 1986) the asymptotic distribution of $n^{1/2}(\hat{\theta} - \theta)$, where $\hat{\theta}$ solves (A.5), converges to a mean zero normal variate with variance consistently estimated by the "sandwich" expression

$$n\left(\sum_{k=1}^{n}\hat{D}_k'\hat{V}_k^{-1}\hat{D}_k\right)^{-1}\sum_{k=1}^{n}\hat{D}_k'\hat{V}_k^{-1}(W_k-\hat{\mu}_k)W_k-\hat{\mu}_k)'\hat{V}_k^{-1}\hat{D}_k\left(\sum_{k=1}^{n}\hat{D}_k'\hat{V}_k^{-1}\hat{D}_k\right)^{-1} \quad \text{(A.6)}$$

where ^ denotes evaluation at $\hat{\theta}$ and at a consistent estimator for additional parameters in $V_k, k = 1,\ldots,n$. Moreover, this asymptotic distribution obtains even under 'working' models for the V_k that may be misspecified, though such misspecification may reduce the efficiency of $\hat{\theta}$ as estimator of θ. Note that (A.6) will converge (as $n \to \infty$) to the same value as the model-based variance estimator

$$\left(\sum_{k=1}^{n}\hat{D}_k'\hat{V}_k^{-1}\hat{D}_k\right)^{-1} \quad \text{(A.7)}$$

if the variance matrices $V_k, k = 1,\ldots,n$ are correctly specified.

A.3 Some Basic Empirical Process Results

Consider a real-valued variate X, and suppose that an independent and identically distributed (IID) sample of X values is available. The strong law-of-large numbers shows that the sample mean $n^{-1}\sum_1^n X_i$ converges almost surely (that is except possibly on a set having probability zero) to the mean μ of the distribution of X (assuming such to exist) as $n \to \infty$. The central limit theorem shows $n^{-1/2}\sum_{i=1}^n(X_i - \mu)$ to converge in distribution to a mean zero Gaussian (i.e., normal) distribution under a Lindeberg condition that requires the influence of any specific observation to become negligible as $n \to \infty$.

Corresponding strong law-of-large numbers and central limit theorem results are available for the empirical estimator of the distribution function $\underline{F}$ of X, given by $\underline{F}(x) = \text{pr}(X \le x)$. Specifically, the empirical estimator $\hat{\underline{F}}$ of $\underline{F}$ is given by

$$\hat{\underline{F}}(x) = n^{-1}\sum_{i=1}^{n} I(X_i \le x).$$

The Glivenko–Cantelli (GC) theorem shows that $\hat{\underline{F}}(x)$ converges almost surely to $\underline{F}(x)$ for any real x, while the Donkster theorem shows that $\hat{H} = n^{1/2}(\hat{\underline{F}} - \underline{F})$ converges in distribution to a mean zero Gaussian process having covariance function given by

$$\text{cor}\{\hat{H}(u), \hat{H}(v)\} = \underline{F}(u) \wedge \underline{F}(v) - \underline{F}(u)\underline{F}(v),$$

a so-called Brownian bridge, as $n \to \infty$.

Both of these results extend to a real-valued multivariate random variable $X = (X_1,\ldots,X_p)$, with its empirical distribution function estimator $\hat{\underline{F}}$ given by $\hat{\underline{F}}(x_1,\ldots,x_p) = n^{-1}\sum_{i=1}^n I(X_{1i} \le x_1,\ldots,X_{pi} \le x_p)$.

Important for present purposes, these methods extend further to a real-valued (possibly vector-valued) stochastic process $X = \{X(t), t\varepsilon[0,\tau]\}$ defined over a follow-up period $[0,\tau]$. The GC theorem extends to show that $n^{-1}\sum_{i=1}^{n} X_i(t)$ converges almost surely to its mean, $\mu(t)$, uniformly in $t\varepsilon[0,\tau]$. The Donkster theorem implies the convergence in distribution of $n^{1/2}\{\hat{\underline{F}}(\cdot,t_1) - \underline{F}(\cdot,t_1),\ldots,\hat{\underline{F}}(\cdot,t_q) - \underline{F}(\cdot,t_q)\}$, where $\underline{F}(x,t) = \text{pr}\{X(t) \leq x)\}$ and $\hat{\underline{F}}(x,t)$ is its empirical estimator for any $t_j\varepsilon[0,\tau]$ for $j = i,\ldots q$, while a 'tightness' condition is needed to show applicability of a functional central limit theorem, whereby $[n^{1/2}\{\hat{\underline{F}}(\cdot,t) - \underline{F}(\cdot,t)\}; t\varepsilon[0,\tau]]$ converges to a zero mean Gaussian process, with covariation process determined by the Brownian bridge covariances given above (Pollard, 1990, p. 53).

These stochastic process convergence results carry over to yield corresponding 'strong consistency' and 'weak Gaussian convergence' results for other processes defined at time t by stochastic integrals

$$\int_0^t \hat{G}(\cdot,s)\hat{H}(\cdot,ds)$$

with $\hat{H}(\cdot,s) = n^{-1/2}\{\hat{F}(\cdot,s) - F(\cdot,s)\}$ and with the $\hat{G}$ stochastic process having bounded total variation (i.e., expressible as the difference between monotone functions).

For some purposes, such as developing asymptotic distributions for the regression parameter estimates in (6.11) and (6.23), it is useful to replace weak convergence by almost sure convergence. The strong embedding theorem (Shorack & Wellner, 1986, pp. 47–48) allows this to be done in a new probability space. After further developments in the new probability space, one can return to the original space with pertinent weak convergence results replacing almost sure convergence results.

Transformations of empirical processes inherit strong consistency properties from the empirical process if the transformations satisfy a weak continuity condition, and inherit the weak Gaussian convergence property if the transformations satisfy a weakly continuous compact (Hadamard) differentiability property. This compact differentiability property also leads to an analytic expression for the covariation process of the transformed process and is a key aspect of establishing bootstrap applicability. See Gill et al. (1995) for definitions and for application to bivariate survivor function estimators considered in Chapter 3. The analytic covariation expression for the transformed process may be too complex to be useful, and bootstrap or other resampling procedures are then typically applied for confidence interval or confidence band calculation for the transformed process.

A conditional multiplier central limit theorem (van der Vaart & Wellner, 1996, p. 182) provides a useful resampling procedure for inference on complex processes, such as baseline type-specific marginal single and double failure hazard rates in Chapter 6. This result justifies a perturbation approach whereby estimating functions that are expressible as sums over IID variates are multiplied by a standard normal variate, independently for $i = 1,\ldots,n$, with parameter estimates calculated for a large number of perturbations for distribution approximations. These approximations derive from asymptotic mean zero Gaussian properties for the estimating functions, conditional on all observed data.

See Shorack and Wellner (1986); Pollard (1990); van der Vaart and Wellner (1996) for much more rigorous and detailed accounts of these and other empirical process results.

Appendix B: Software and Data

B.1 Software for Multivariate Failure Time Analysis

Univariate failure time data analysis procedures are implemented in several major statistical software packages. These include Kaplan–Meier estimators, as well as parametric and semiparametric regression methods. Many of these packages carefully handle stratification, time-varying covariates and tied data.

In contrast, software packages for multivariate failure time analysis are somewhat limited. Some widely used software packages for single failure time data analysis include extensions to allow either marginal Cox models, or models for recurrent events. But since these packages were not originally designed for multivariate failure times, users have to manipulate their data sets to resemble univariate failure times before using such software. Programs for other methods mentioned in this book are described below. The ability to handle stratification, time-varying covariates and tied data varies among these packages. There does not seem to be software for nonparametric estimation of multivariate survivor functions. To help fill these gaps, in companion with this book, we provide a R package *MHazard*, which focuses on the modeling of marginal single and multivariate failure hazards, as discussed in Chapter 4, providing a fairly comprehensive approach to bivariate failure time analysis. It also includes several nonparametric estimators for multivariate survivor function. It allows Cox model stratification, time-varying covariates, and tied failure times.

Here, a brief account of existing software packages in SAS, STATA and R is provided. The details of these packages are not described, but rather a brief summary of features is given to help readers decide which tools to use for their application.

SAS

[SAS institute Inc; www.sas.com]

The SAS *phreg* package is widely used to analyze failure time data. It also incorporates several regression approaches for multivariate failure time analysis, by arranging the data set in specific forms so that the data resemble univariate failure time data.

The marginal Cox models as in Wei et al. (1989) for multivariate failure time can be implemented by creating one observation for each event type, using the event type indicator as a stratification variable and including an interaction between covariates and the event indicator. For clustered data, a marginal Cox model can also be fitted as in Lee et al. (1992) with a variable indicating the cluster. For recurrent events, the intensity and rate/mean models for recurrent events as in Andersen and Gill (1982), Pepe and Cai (1993), Lawless and Nadeau (1995) and Lin et al. (2000) can be implemented by forming separate observations for individuals experience between each two adjacent event times. To use the stratified models for total time and gap time as in Prentice, Williams, and Peterson (1981), one needs to create a count variable of the prior events in addition to forming the observations for the intensity and rate/mean models. Robust variance can be requested to account for the correlation between events.

In general, the *phreg* package allows stratification and provides several options to handle tied data. It allows users to specify time-varying covariates through some simple programming.

Details and examples can be found at support.sas.com/en/documentation.html.

STATA

[StataCorp LLC; www.stata.com]

STATA provides nonparametric, parametric and semiparametric estimates for univariate failure time data analysis, through functions such as *sts* and *stcox*. Similar to SAS, the *stcox* function can handle some regression methods for multivariate failure time analysis by arranging the data set to resemble univariate data.

For example, the marginal Cox model for clustered data as in Lee et al. (1992) can be implemented by creating one observation for each event, with an additional variable indicating the cluster. For multiple events on the same individual, multiple observations should also be generated to fit the marginal Cox model as in Wei et al. (1989), with additional subject and event type indicators. With recurrent events, the methods in Andersen and Gill (1982) and Prentice et al. (1981) can be implemented by generating separate observations for each event time interval, and appropriately assigning the order of events. The *stcox* function allows stratification and tied data, and handles time-varying covariates either through partitioning the data set or through the *tvc* option.

Details and examples can be found in stata.com/support/faqs/statistics/multiple-failure-time-data.

R

[R Core Team (2013). R: A language and environment for statistical computing. R Foundation for Statistical Computing, Vienna, Austria; www.R-project.org.]

The R package *survival* contains functions for nonparametric, semiparametric and parametric estimates for univariate failure time data. Although not mentioned specifically in the package manual, it is apparent that the marginal Cox model approach and the recurrent event approaches can be handled by the *coxph* function by appropriately forming the data set, as discussed in SAS and STATA. This function allows stratification, tied data, and time-varying covariates to be handled through partitioning individuals experience or by programming external functions to update the covariates over time. Details of this package can be found in cran.r-project.org/web/packages/survival/survival.pdf.

The R *timereg* package contains a function two.stage, which fits a bivariate Clayton-Oakes model with a two-stage estimation procedure as in Glidden (2000), assuming the cross ratio parameter does not depend on covariates. Details can be found in cran.r-project.org/web/packages/timereg/timereg.pdf.

The R *MHazard* package is a toolbox for both nonparametric and semiparametric methods for multivariate failure time data analysis. It provides nonparametric bivariate Dabrowska, Prentice–Cai and Volterra estimators, and higher dimensional Dabrowska and Volterra estimators, as well as calculating corresponding dependency measures. It also fits semiparametric regression models for the marginal single and double failure hazard rates with bivariate failure times, allowing baseline stratification and tied data. Furthermore it allows users to include an interaction between the fixed covariates and a function of time. Customized versions of code are available for some specific forms of time-varying covariates and time-dependent strata. The package also allows one to fit marginal models with more than two failure times, with marginal single, double and triple failure hazard rates. Variances are computed in a sandwich form to account for the correlation between failure time variates.

B.2 Data Access

Most of the illustrations in this monograph use data from the Women's Health Initiative. The WHI is a massive research program among 161,808 postmenopausal women in the United States, aged 50–79 at enrollment. Launched in 1993 it includes

68,132 woman in a multifaceted clinical trial of four disease prevention interventions, and a companion prospective cohort study among 93,676 women. Over the ensuing 25 years a substantial database and specimen repository has been developed, including participant follow-up for a wide array of clinical and intermediate outcomes. These resources have been used by the broader research community for a wide variety of scientific purposes, leading to over 1400 articles and nearly 300 separately funded ancillary studies.

WHI data can be accessed for scientific purposes either in a collaborative mode, working through the WHI Publication Committee and/or Ancillary Study Committee, or through the National Heart, Lung and Blood Institute's BioLINCC Resource. To exercise the former route, go to the WHI website (whi.org) where further description of the data and specimen resource is given, and where instructions are provided for manuscript proposals and for ancillary study proposals. For the latter route, go to the NHLBI Data Repository (BioLINCC) website (nihcollaboratory.org) for instructions on how to request specific data for scientific use under the auspices of your own Institutional Review Board.

Some small data sets shown in the book narrative in Table 1.1, Table 1.2 and Table 3.4 have been appended to the R *MHazard* package for user convenience.

Bibliography

Aalen, O. (1980). A model for nonparametric regression analysis of lifetimes. In A. Kozek & J. Rosinski (Eds.), *Mathematical Statistics and Probability Theory, Volume 2 of Lecture Notes in Statistics* (pp. 1–25). New York: Springer-Verlag.

Aalen, O., Borgan, Ø., & Gjessing, H. (2010). *Survival and Event History Analysis: A Process Point of View*. New York: Springer Science & Business Media.

Akritas, M. G., & Van Keilegom, I. (2003). Estimation of the bivariate and marginal distributions with censored data. *Journal of the Royal Statistical Society, Series B*, *65*, 457–471.

Andersen, P. K. (1982). Testing goodness of fit of Cox's regression and life model. *Biometrics*, 67–77.

Andersen, P. K., Borgan, Ø., Gill, R. D., & Keiding, N. (1993). *Statistical Models Based on Counting Processes*. New York: Springer Series in Statistics, Springer-Verlag.

Andersen, P. K., & Gill, R. D. (1982). Cox's regression model for counting processes: A large sample study. *The Annals of Statistics*, *10*(4), 1100–1120.

Anderson, G. L., Kooperberg, C., Geller, N., Rossouw, J. E., Pettinger, M., & Prentice, R. L. (2007). Monitoring and reporting of the Women's Health Initiative randomized hormone therapy trials. *Clinical Trials*, *4*(3), 207–217.

Anderson, T. (1984). *An Introduction to Multivariate Statistical Analysis* (2nd ed.). New York: Wiley and Sons.

Bandeen-Roche, K., & Ning, J. (2008). Nonparametric estimation of bivariate failure time associations in the presence of a competing risk. *Biometrika*, *95*(1), 221–232.

Bandeen-Roche, K. J., & Liang, K.-Y. (1996). Modelling failure-time associations in data with multiple levels of clustering. *Biometrika*, *83*(1), 29–39.

Barlow, W. E., & Prentice, R. L. (1988). Residuals for relative risk regression. *Biometrika*, *75*(1), 65–74.

Barrett, J. K., Siannis, F., & Farewell, V. T. (2011). A semi-competing risks model for data with interval-censoring and informative observation: An application to the MRC cognitive function and ageing study. *Statistics in Medicine*, *30*(1), 1–10.

Begun, J. M., Hall, W. J., Huang, W.-M., & Wellner, J. A. (1983). Information and asymptotic efficiency in parametric–nonparametric models. *Annals of Statis-*

tics, *11*(2), 432–452.

Borgan, Ø., Goldstein, L., & Langholz, B. (1995). Methods for the analysis of sampled cohort data in the Cox proportional hazards model. *Annals of Statistics*, *23*, 1749–1778.

Breslow, N., & Cain, K. (1988). Logistic regression for two-stage case-control data. *Biometrika*, *75*(1), 11–20.

Breslow, N., & Wellner, J. (2008). A Z-theorem with estimated nuisance parameters and correction note for 'weighted likelihood for semiparametric models and two-phase stratified samples, with application to Cox regression'. *Scandinavian Journal of Statistics*, *35*(1), 186–192.

Breslow, N. E. (1974). Covariance analysis of censored survival data. *Biometrics*, *30*, 89–99.

Breslow, N. E., & Crowley, J. (1974). A large sample study of the life table and product limit estimates under random censorship. *The Annals of Statistics*, *2*(3), 437–453.

Breslow, N. E., & Day, N. E. (1980). *Statistical Methods in Cancer Research. Vol 1. The Analysis of Case-Control Studies*. Lyon, France: International Agency for Research on Cancer Scientific Publications.

Breslow, N. E., & Day, N. E. (1987). *Statistical Methods in Cancer Research. Vol. 2. The Design and Analysis of Cohort Studies*. Lyon, France: International Agency for Research on Cancer Scientific Publications.

Breslow, N. E., Hu, J., & Wellner, J. A. (2015). Z-estimation and stratified samples: Application to survival models. *Lifetime Data Analysis*, *21*(4), 493–516.

Breslow, N. E., Lubin, J. H., Marek, P., & Langholz, B. (1983). Multiplicative models and cohort analysis. *Journal of the American Statistical Association*, *78*(381), 1–12.

Breslow, N. E., & Wellner, J. A. (2007). Weighted likelihood for semiparametric models and two-phase stratified samples, with application to Cox regression. *Scandinavian Journal of Statistics*, *34*(1), 86–102.

Byar, D. P. (1980). The veterans administration study of chemoprophylaxis for recurrent stage I bladder tumours: Comparisons of placebo, pyridoxine and topical thiotepa. In *Bladder Tumors and Other Topics in Urological Oncology* (pp. 363–370). Springer.

Cai, J., & Prentice, R. L. (1995). Estimating equations for hazard ratio parameters based on correlated failure time data. *Biometrika*, *82*(1), 151–164.

Cai, J., & Prentice, R. L. (1997). Regression estimation using multivariate failure time data and a common baseline hazard function model. *Lifetime Data Analysis*, *3*(3), 197–213.

Campbell, G. (1981). Nonparametric bivariate estimation with randomly censored data. *Biometrika*, *68*(2), 417–422.

Campbell, G., & Földes, A. (1982). Large sample properties of nonparametric statistical inference. *Nonparametric Statistical Inference*, 103–122.

Carroll, R. J., Ruppert, D., Crainiceanu, C. M., & Stefanski, L. A. (2006). *Measurement Error in Nonlinear Models: A Modern Perspective*. Boca Raton: Chapman & Hall/CRC.

Chen, H. Y., & Little, R. J. A. (1999). Proportional hazards regression with missing covariates. *Journal of the American Statistical Association*, *94*(447), 896–908.

Chi, Y. Y., & Ibrahim, J. G. (2006). Joint models for multivariate longitudinal and multivariate survival data. *Biometrics*, *62*(2), 432–445.

Chlebowski, R. T., Aragaki, A. K., Anderson, G. L., Simon, M. S., Manson, J. E., Neuhouser, M. L., Pan, K., Stefanic, M. L., Rohan, T. E., Lane, D., Qi, L., Snetselaar, L., & Prentice, R. (2018). Association of low-fat dietary pattern with breast cancer overall survival: A secondary analysis of the Women's Health Initiative randomized clinical trial. *JAMA Oncology*, e181212–e181212.

Chlebowski, R. T., Aragaki, A. K., Anderson, G. L., Thomson, C. A., Manson, J. E., Simon, M. S., Howard, B. V., Rohan, T. E., Snetselar, L., Lane, D., Barrington, W., Vitolins, M., Womack, C., Qi, L., Hou, L., Thomas, F., & Prentice, R. (2017). Low-fat dietary pattern and breast cancer mortality in the Women's Health Initiative randomized controlled trial. *Journal of Clinical Oncology*, *35*(25), 2919–2926.

Clayton, D. G. (1978). Model for association in bivariate life tables and its application in epidemiological studies of familial tendency in chronic disease incidence. *Biometrika*, *65*, 141–151.

Cook, R. J., & Lawless, J. F. (2007). *The Statistical Analysis of Recurrent Events*. New York: Springer.

Cook, R. J., & Lawless, J. F. (2018). *Multistate Models for the Analysis of Life History Data*. Boca Raton: Chapman & Hall/ CRC.

Cox, D. R. (1972). Regression models and life-tables (with discussion). *Journal of the Royal Statistical Society. Series B (Methodological)*, *34*(2), pp. 187–220.

Cox, D. R. (1975). Partial likelihood. *Biometrika*, *62*(2), 269–276.

Cox, D. R., & Oakes, D. (1984). *Analysis of Survival Data* (Vol. 21). Boca Raton: CRC Press.

Crowder, M. J. (2012). *Multivariate Survival Analysis and Competing Risks*. Boca Raton: CRC Press.

Dabrowska, D. M. (1988). Kaplan–Meier estimate on the plane. *Annals of Statistics*, *16*, 1475–1489.

Datta, S., & Satten, G. A. (2002). Estimation of integrated transition hazards and stage occupation probabilities for non-Markov systems under dependent censoring. *Biometrics*, *58*(4), 792–802.

Duchateau, L., & Janssen, P. (2010). *The Frailty Model*. New York: Springer-Verlag.

Duffy, D. L., Martin, N. G., & Mathews, J. D. (1990). Appendectomy in Australian twins. *American Journal of Human Genetics*, *47*(3), 590.

Efron, B. (1967). The two sample problem with censored data. In *In Proc. 5th Berkeley Sympos. Math. Statist. Prob., Prentice-Hall* (Vol. 4, pp. 831–853).

Elashoff, R. M., Li, G., & Li, N. (2008). A joint model for longitudinal measurements and survival data in the presence of multiple failure types. *Biometrics*, *64*(3), 762–771.

Fan, J., Hsu, L., & Prentice, R. L. (2000). Dependence estimation over a finite bivariate failure time region. *Lifetime Data Analysis*, *6*, 343–355.

Fan, J., Prentice, R. L., & Hsu, L. (2000). A class of weighted dependence measures for bivariate failure time data. *Journal of the Royal Statistical Society: Series B (Statistical Methodology)*, *62*(1), 181–190.

Fine, J. P., Jiang, H., & Chappell, R. (2001). On semi-competing risks data. *Biometrika*, *88*(4), 907–919.

Fleming, T. R., & Harrington, D. P. (1991). *Counting Processes and Survival Analysis*. Hoboken: Wiley and Sons.

Freedman, L. S., Commins, J. M., Moler, J. E., Arab, L., Baer, D. J., Kipnis, V., Midthune, D., Moshfegh, A. J., Neuhouser, M. L., Prentice, R. L., Schatzkin, A., Spiegelman, D., Subar, A. F., Tinker, L. F., & Willett, W. (2014). Pooled results from 5 validation studies of dietary self-report instruments using recovery biomarkers for energy and protein intake. *American Journal of Epidemiology*, *180*(2), 172–188.

Freedman, L. S., Commins, J. M., Moler, J. E., Willett, W., Tinker, L. F., Subar, A. F., Spiegelman, D., Rhodes, D., Potischman, N., Neuhouser, M. L., Moshfegh, A. J., Kipnis, V., Arab, L., & Prentice, R. L. (2015). Pooled results from 5 validation studies of dietary self-report instruments using recovery biomarkers for potassium and sodium intake. *American Journal of Epidemiology*, *181*(7), 473–487.

Fu, R., & Gilbert, P. (2017). Joint modeling of longitudinal and survival data with the Cox model and two-phase sampling. *Lifetime Data Analysis*, *23*(1), 136–159.

Ghosh, D., & Lin, D. Y. (2003). Semiparametric analysis of recurrent events data in the presence of dependent censoring. *Biometrics*, *59*(4), 877–885.

Gill, R. D. (1994). Multivariate survival analysis. *Theory of Probability and Its Applications*, *37*(1), 18–31.

Gill, R. D., & Johansen, S. (1990). A survey of product integration with a view towards application in survival analysis. *Annals of Statistics*, *18*, 1501–1555.

Gill, R. D., van der Laan, M. J., & Wellner, J. A. (1995). Inefficient estimators of the bivariate survival function for three models. *Annales de l'I.H.P. Probabilités et Statistiques*, *31*(3), 545–597.

Glidden, D. V. (2000). A two-stage estimator of the dependence parameter for the Clayton–Oakes model. *Lifetime Data Analysis*, *6*(2), 141–156.

Glidden, D. V., & Self, S. G. (1999). Semiparametric likelihood estimation in the Clayton–Oakes failure time model. *Scandinavian Journal of Statistics*, *26*(3), 363–372.

Goldstein, L., & Langholz, B. (1992). Asymptotic theory for nested case–control sampling in the Cox regression model. *Annals of Statistics*, *20*, 1903–1928.

Gray, R. J., & Li, Y. (2002). Optimal weight functions for marginal proportional hazards analysis of clustered failure time data. *Lifetime Data Analysis*, *8*(1), 5–19.

Hanley, J. A., & Parnes, M. N. (1983). Nonparametric estimation of a multivariate distribution in the presence of censoring. *Biometrics*, 129–139.

Hatfield, L. A., Boye, M. E., & Carlin, B. P. (2011). Joint modeling of multiple longitudinal patient-reported outcomes and survival. *Journal of Biopharmaceutical Statistics*, *21*(5), 971–991.

Heitjan, D. F. (1994). Ignorability in general incomplete-data models. *Biometrika, 81*(4), 701–708.

Heitjan, D. F., & Rubin, D. B. (1991). Ignorability and coarse data. *The Annals of Statistics*, 2244–2253.

Hernán, M., & Robins, J. (2015). *Causal Inference*. Boca Raton: Chapman & Hall/CRC.

Hougaard, P. (1986). Survival models for heterogeneous populations derived from stable distributions. *Biometrika, 73*(2), 387–396.

Hougaard, P. (2000). *Analysis of Multivariate Survival Data* (Vol. 564). New York: Springer.

Howard, B. V., Aragaki, A. K., Tinker, L. F., Allison, M., Hingle, M. D., Johnson, K. C., Manson, J. E., Shadyab, A. H., Shikany, J. M., Snetselaar, L. G., Thomson, C. A., Zaslavsky, O., & Prentice, R. L. (2018). A low-fat dietary pattern and diabetes: A secondary analysis from the Women's Health Initiative Dietary Modification Trial. *Diabetes Care, 41*, 680–687.

Hu, T., Nan, B., Lin, X., & Robins, J. M. (2011). Time-dependent cross ratio estimation for bivariate failure times. *Biometrika, 98*(2), 341–354.

Huang, J., & Wellner, J. A. (1997). Interval censored survival data: A review of recent progress. In D. Lin & T. Fleming (Eds.), *Proceedings of the First Seattle Symposium in Biostatistics: Survival Analysis* (pp. 123–169). New York.

Huang, Y., & Wang, C. (2006). Errors-in-covariates effect on estimating functions: Additivity in limit and nonparametric correction. *Statistica Sinica*, 861–881.

Jacobsen, M., & Keiding, N. (1995). Coarsening at random in general sample spaces and random censoring in continuous time. *The Annals of Statistics, 23*(3), 774–786.

Jin, Z., Lin, D., Wei, L., & Ying, Z. (2003). Rank-based inference for the accelerated failure time model. *Biometrika, 90*(2), 341–353.

Joe, H. (1997). *Multivariate Models and Multivariate Dependence Concepts*. Boca Raton: Chapman and Hall/CRC.

Joe, H. (2014). *Dependence Modeling with Copulas*. Boca Raton: Chapman and Hall/CRC.

Johansen, S. (1983). An extension of Cox's regression model. *International Statistical Review/Revue Internationale de Statistique*, 165–174.

Kalbfleisch, J. D., & Lawless, J. F. (1988). Likelihood analysis of multi-state models for disease incidence and mortality. *Statistics in Medicine, 7*, 149–160.

Kalbfleisch, J. D., & Prentice, R. L. (1973). Marginal likelihoods based on Cox's regression and life model. *Biometrika, 60*(2), 267–278.

Kalbfleisch, J. D., & Prentice, R. L. (1980). *The Statistical Analysis of Failure Time Data*. New York: Wiley and Sons.

Kalbfleisch, J. D., & Prentice, R. L. (1981). Estimation of the average hazard ratio. *Biometrika, 68*, 105–112.

Kalbfleisch, J. D., & Prentice, R. L. (2002). *The Statistical Analysis of Failure Time Data, Second Edition*. New York: Wiley and Sons.

Kaplan, E. L., & Meier, P. (1958). Nonparametric estimation from incomplete observations. *Journal of the American Statistical Association, 53*(282), 457–481.

Lagakos, S., & Schoenfeld, D. (1984). Properties of proportional-hazards score tests under misspecified regression models. *Biometrics*, 1037–1048.

Lampe, J. W., Huang, Y., Neuhouser, M. L., Tinker, L. F., Song, X., Schoeller, D. A., Kim, S., Raftery, D., Di, C., Zheng, C., Schwarz, Y., Van Horn, L., Thomson, C. A., Mossavar-Rahmani, Y., Beresford, S. A. A., & Prentice, R. L. (2017). Dietary biomarker evaluation in a controlled feeding study in women from the Women's Health Initiative cohort. *The American Journal of Clinical Nutrition*, *105*(2), 466–475.

Langholz, B., & Thomas, D. C. (1990). Nested case–control and case–cohort methods of sampling from a cohort: A critical comparison. *American Journal of Epidemiology*, *131*(1), 169–176.

Lawless, J. (2002). *Statistical Models and Methods for Lifetime Data, Second Edition*. New York: Wiley and Sons.

Lawless, J., Nadeau, C., & Cook, R. (1997). Analysis of mean and rate functions for recurrent events. In D. Lin & T. Fleming (Eds.), *Proceedings of the First Seattle Symposium in Biostatistics* (pp. 37–50). New York: Springer-Verlag.

Lawless, J. F. (1983). *Statistical Models and Methods for Lifetime Data*. New York: Wiley and Sons.

Lawless, J. F., Kalbfleisch, J. D., & Wild, C. J. (1999). Semiparametric methods for response-selective and missing data problems in regression. *Journal of the Royal Statistical Society Series B-statistical Methodology*, *61*(2), 413–438.

Lawless, J. F., & Nadeau, C. (1995). Some simple robust methods for the analysis of recurrent events. *Technometrics*, *37*(2), 158–168.

Lee, E. W., Wei, L., Amato, D. A., & Leurgans, S. (1992). Cox-type regression analysis for large numbers of small groups of correlated failure time observations. In *Survival Analysis: State of the Art* (pp. 237–247). Springer.

Li, Y., Prentice, R. L., & Lin, X. (2008). Semiparametric maximum likelihood estimation in normal transformation models for bivariate survival data. *Biometrika*, *95*, 947–960.

Liang, K.-Y., & Zeger, S. L. (1986). Longitudinal data analysis using generalized linear models. *Biometrika*, *73*(1), 13–22.

Lin, D. (2000). On fitting Cox's proportional hazards models to survey data. *Biometrika*, *87*(1), 37–47.

Lin, D., Sun, W., & Ying, Z. (1999). Nonparametric estimation of the gap time distribution for serial events with censored data. *Biometrika*, *86*(1), 59–70.

Lin, D., & Wei, L. (1991). Goodness-of-fit tests for the general cox regression model. *Statistica Sinica*, 1–17.

Lin, D., Wei, L., Yang, I., & Ying, Z. (2000). Semiparametric regression for the mean and rate functions of recurrent events. *Journal of the Royal Statistical Society: Series B (Statistical Methodology)*, *62*(4), 711–730.

Lin, D. Y. (1994). Cox regression analysis of multivariate failure time data: The marginal approach. *Statistics in Medicine*, *13*(21), 2233–2247.

Lin, D. Y., Wei, L.-J., & Ying, Z. (1993). Checking the Cox model with cumulative sums of martingale-based residuals. *Biometrika*, *80*(3), 557–572.

Little, R. J., & Rubin, D. (2002). *Statistical Analysis with Missing Data, Second Edition*. New York: Wiley and Sons.

Lumley, T., Shaw, P. A., & Dai, J. Y. (2011). Connections between survey calibration estimators and semiparametric models for incomplete data. *International Statistical Review*, *79*(2), 200–220.

Luo, S. (2014). A Bayesian approach to joint analysis of multivariate longitudinal data and parametric accelerated failure time. *Statistics in Medicine*, *33*(4), 580–594.

Mahabir, S., Willett, W. C., Friedenreich, C. M., Lai, G. Y., Boushey, C. J., Matthews, C. E., Sinha, R., Colditz, G. A., Rothwell, J. A., Reedy, J., Patel, A. V., Leitzmann, M. F., Fraser, G. E., Ross, S., Hursting, S. D., Abnet, C. C., Kushi, L. H., Taylor, P. R., & Prentice, R. L. (2018). Research strategies for nutritional and physical activity epidemiology and cancer prevention. *Cancer Epidemiology, Biomarkers & Prevention*, *27*(3), 233–244.

Manson, J., Chlebowski, R., Stefanick, M., Aragaki, A., Rossouw, J., Prentice, R., Anderson, G., Howard, B., Thomson, C., LaCroix, A., Wactawski-Wende, J., Jackson, R., Limacher, M., Margolis, K., Wassertheil-Smoller, S., Beresford, S., Cauley, J., Eaton, C., Gass, M., Hsia, J., Johnson, K., Kooperberg, C., Kuller, L., Lewis, C., Liu, S., Martin, L., Ockene, J., O'Sullivan, M., Powell, L., Simon, M., Van Horn, L., Vitolins, M., & Wallace, R. (2013). Menopausal hormone therapy and health outcomes during the e intervention and extended poststopping phases of the Women's Health Initiative randomized trials. *Journal of the American Medical Association*, *310*, 1353–1368.

McKeague, I. W., & Utikal, K. J. (1991). Goodness-of-fit tests for additive hazards and proportional hazards models. *Scandinavian Journal of Statistics*, 177–195.

Nan, B. (2004). Efficient estimation for case-cohort studies. *Canadian Journal of Statistics*, *32*(4), 403–419.

Nan, B., Lin, X., Lisabeth, L. D., & Harlow, S. D. (2006). Piecewise constant cross-ratio estimation for association of age at a marker event and age at menopause. *Journal of the American Statistical Association*, *101*(473), 65–77.

Nan, B., & Wellner, J. A. (2013). A general semiparametric z-estimation approach for case-cohort studies. *Statistica Sinica*, *23*(3), 1155.

Nelsen, R. B. (2007). *An Introduction to Copulas*. New York: Springer.

Nelson, W. B. (2003). *Recurrent Events Data Analysis for Product Repairs, Disease Recurrences, and Other Applications*. Philadelphia: SIAM.

Neuhouser, M. L., Di, C., Tinker, L. F., Thomson, C., Sternfeld, B., Mossavar-Rahmani, Y., Stefanick, M. L., Sims, S., Curb, J. D., Lamonte, M., Seqguin, R., Johnson, K. C., & Prentice, R. L. (2013). Physical activity assessment: Biomarkers and self-report of activity-related energy expenditure in the WHI. *American Journal of Epidemiology*, *177*(6), 576–585.

Nielsen, G. G., Gill, R. D., Andersen, P. K., & Sørensen, T. I. (1992). A counting process approach to maximum likelihood estimation in frailty models. *Scandinavian Journal of Statistics*, 25–43.

Oakes, D. (1981). Survival times: Aspects of partial likelihood. *International Sta-*

tistical Review, *49*(3), 235–264.

Oakes, D. (1982). A model for association in bivariate survival data. *Journal of the Royal Statistical Society. Series B (Methodological)*, 414–422.

Oakes, D. (1986). Semiparametric inference in a model for association in bivariate survival data. *Biometrika*, *73*(2), 353–361.

Oakes, D. (1989). Bivariate survival models induced by frailties. *Journal of the American Statistical Association*, *84*(406), 487–493.

Pepe, M. S., & Cai, J. (1993). Some graphical displays and marginal regression analyses for recurrent failure times and time dependent covariates. *Journal of the American Statistical Association*, *88*(423), 811–820.

Pipper, C. B., & Martinussen, T. (2003). A likelihood based estimating equation for the Clayton–Oakes model with marginal proportional hazards. *Scandinavian Journal of Statistics*, *30*(3), 509–521.

Pollard, D. (1990). Empirical processes: Theory and applications. In *NSF-CBMS Regional Conference Series in Probability and Statistics, Volume 2* (pp. i–86).

Prentice, R. L. (1982). Covariate measurement errors and parameter estimation in a failure time regression model. *Biometrika*, *69*(2), 331–342.

Prentice, R. L. (1986). A case-cohort design for epidemiologic cohort studies and disease prevention trials. *Biometrika*, *73*(1), 1–11.

Prentice, R. L. (2014). Self-consistent nonparametric maximum likelihood estimator of the bivariate survivor function. *Biometrika*, *101*(3), 505–518.

Prentice, R. L. (2016). Higher dimensional Clayton–Oakes models for multivariate failure time data. *Biometrika*, *103*(1), 231–236.

Prentice, R. L. (2018). Intake biomarkers and the chronic disease nutritional epidemiology research agenda. *The American Journal of Clinical Nutrition*, *108*(3), 433–434.

Prentice, R. L., & Breslow, N. E. (1978). Retrospective studies and failure time models. *Biometrika*, *65*(1), 153–158.

Prentice, R. L., Caan, B., Chlebowski, R. T., Patterson, R., Kuller, L. H., Ockene, J. K., Margolis, K. L., Limacher, M. C., Manson, J. E., Parker, L. M., Paskett, E., Phillips, L., Robbins, J., Rossouw, J. E., Sarto, G. E., Shikany, J. M., Stefanick, M. L., Thomson, C. A., Van Horn, L., Vitolins, M. Z., Wactawski-Wende, J., Wallace, R. B., Wassertheil-Smoller, S., Whitlock, E., Yano, K., Adams-Campbell, L., Anderson, G. L., Assaf, A. R., Beresford, S. A. A., Black, H. R., Brunner, R. L., Brzyski, R. G., Ford, L., Gass, M., Hays, J., Heber, D., Heiss, G., Hendrix, S. L., Hsia, J., Hubbell, F. A., Jackson, R. D., Johnson, K. C., Kotchen, J. M., LaCroix, A. Z., Lane, D. S., Langer, R. D., Lasser, N. L., & Henderson, M. M. (2006). Low-fat dietary pattern and risk of invasive breast cancer: The Women's Health Initiative Randomized Controlled Dietary Modification Trial. *Journal of the American Medical Association*, *295*(6), 629–642.

Prentice, R. L., & Cai, J. (1992). Covariance and survivor function estimation using censored multivariate failure time data. *Biometrika*, *79*(3), 495–512.

Prentice, R. L., & Hsu, L. (1997). Regression on hazard ratios and cross ratios in multivariate failure time analysis. *Biometrika*, *84*(2), 349–363.

Prentice, R. L., & Kalbfleisch, J. D. (2003). Mixed discrete and continuous Cox regression model. *Lifetime Data Analysis*, *9*(2), 195–210.

Prentice, R. L., Kalbfleisch, J. D., Peterson Jr, A. V., Flournoy, N., Farewell, V., & Breslow, N. (1978). The analysis of failure times in the presence of competing risks. *Biometrics*, 541–554.

Prentice, R. L., Mossavar-Rahmani, Y., Huang, Y., Van Horn, L., Beresford, S. A., Caan, B., Tinker, L., Schoeller, D., Bingham, S., Eaton, C. B., Thomson, C., Johnson, K. C., Ockene, J., Sarto, G., Heiss, G., & Neuhouser, M. L. (2011). Evaluation and comparison of food records, recalls, and frequencies for energy and protein assessment by using recovery biomarkers. *American Journal of Epidemiology*, *174*(5), 591–603.

Prentice, R. L., Williams, B. J., & Peterson, A. V. (1981). On the regression analysis of multivariate failure time data. *Biometrika*, *68*(2), 373–379.

Prentice, R. L., & Zhao, L. P. (1991). Estimating equations for parameters in means and covariances of multivariate discrete and continuous responses. *Biometrics*, 825–839.

Prentice, R. L., & Zhao, S. (2018). Nonparametric estimation of the multivariate survivor function: The multivariate Kaplan–Meier estimator. *Lifetime Data Analysis*, *24*(4), 3–27.

Prentice, R. L., & Zhao, S. (2019). Regression models and multivariate life tables. *Journal of the American Statistical Association*, accepted subject to minor revision.

Proust-Lima, C., Joly, P., Dartigues, J.-F., & Jacqmin-Gadda, H. (2009). Joint modelling of multivariate longitudinal outcomes and a time-to-event: A nonlinear latent class approach. *Computational Statistics & Data Analysis*, *53*(4), 1142–1154.

Qi, L., Wang, C., & Prentice, R. L. (2005). Weighted estimators for proportional hazards regression with missing covariates. *Journal of the American Statistical Association*, *100*(472), 1250–1263.

Rizopoulos, D., & Ghosh, P. (2011). A Bayesian semiparametric multivariate joint model for multiple longitudinal outcomes and a time-to-event. *Statistics in Medicine*, *30*(12), 1366–1380.

Robins, J. M. (1993). Information recovery and bias adjustment in proportional hazards regression analysis of randomized trials using surrogate markers. In *Proceedings of the American Statistical Association, Biopharmaceutical Section* (Vol. 24, pp. 24–33).

Robins, J. M., Hernan, M. A., & Brumback, B. (2000). Marginal structural models and causal inference in epidemiology. *Epidemiology*, *11*(5), 550–560.

Robins, J. M., Prentice, R. L., & Blevins, D. (1989). Designs for synthetic case-control studies in open cohorts. *Biometrics*, *45*(4), 1103–1116.

Robins, J. M., & Rotnitzky, A. (1992). Recovery of information and adjustment for dependent censoring using surrogate markers. In N. Jewell, K. Dietz, & V. Farewell (Eds.), *AIDS Epidemiology* (pp. 297–331). Springer.

Robins, J. M., Rotnitzky, A., & Zhao, L. P. (1994). Estimation of regression coefficients when some regressors are not always observed. *Journal of the American statistical Association*, *89*(427), 846–866.

Rosenbaum, P. R., & Rubin, D. B. (1983). The central role of the propensity score in observational studies for causal effects. *Biometrika*, *70*(1), 41–55.

Rossouw, J., Anderson, G., Prentice, R., LaCroix, A., Kooperberg, C., Stefanick, M., Jackson, R., Beresford, S., Howard, B., Johnson, K., Kotchen, J., Ockene, J., & Writing Group for the Women's Health Initiative Investigators. (2002). Risks and benefits of estrogen plus progestin in healthy postmenopausal women: Principal results from the Women's Health Initiative randomized controlled trial. *Journal of the American Medical Association*, *288*, 321–333.

Roth, J. A., Etzioni, R., Waters, T. M., Pettinger, M., Rossouw, J. E., Anderson, G. L., Chlebowski, R. T., Manson, J. E., Hlatky, M., Johnson, K. C., & Ramsey, S. (2014). Economic return from the Women's Health Initiative estrogen plus progestin clinical trial: A modeling study. *Annals of Internal Medicine*, *160*(9), 594–602.

Rotnitzky, A. (2009). Inverse probability weighted methods. In G. Fitzmaurice, M. Davidian, G. Verbeke, & G. Molenberghs (Eds.), *Longitudinal Data Analysis* (pp. 453–476). Boca Raton: Chapman & Hall/CRC.

Rotnitzky, A., & Robins, J. M. (1995). Semiparametric regression estimation in the presence of dependent censoring. *Biometrika*, *82*(4), 805–820.

Saegusa, T., & Wellner, J. A. (2013). Weighted likelihood estimation under two-phase sampling. *Annals of Statistics*, *41*(1), 269–295.

Samuelsen, S. O. (1997). A pseudolikelihood approach to analysis of nested case-control studies. *Biometrika*, *84*(2), 379–394.

Scheike, T. H., & Martinussen, T. (2004). Maximum likelihood estimation for Cox's regression model under case–cohort sampling. *Scandinavian Journal of Statistics*, *31*(2), 283–293.

Schoeller, D. A. (1999). Recent advances from application of doubly labeled water to measurement of human energy expenditure. *The Journal of Nutrition*, *129*(10), 1765–1768.

Schoenfeld, D. (1982). Partial residuals for the proportional hazards regression model. *Biometrika*, *69*(1), 239–241.

Self, S. G., & Prentice, R. L. (1988). Asymptotic distribution theory and efficiency results for case-cohort studies. *The Annals of Statistics*, 64–81.

Shaw, P. A., & Prentice, R. L. (2012). Hazard ratio estimation for biomarker-calibrated dietary exposures. *Biometrics*, *68*(2), 397–407.

Shih, J. H., & Louis, T. A. (1995). Inferences on the association parameter in copula models for bivariate survival data. *Biometrics*, 1384–1399.

Shorack, G., & Wellner, J. (1986). *Empirical Processes with Applications to Statistics Wiley Series in Probability and Mathematical Statistics: Probability and Mathematical Statistics*. Wiley and Sons.

Spiekerman, C. F., & Lin, D. (1998). Marginal regression models for multivariate failure time data. *Journal of the American Statistical Association*, *93*(443), 1164–1175.

Storb, R., Deeg, H. J., Whitehead, J., Appelbaum, F., Beatty, P., Bensinger, W., Buckner, C. D., Clift, R., Doney, K., Farewell, V., Hansen, J., Hill, R., Lum, L.,

Martin, P., McGuffin, R., Sanders, J., Stewart, P., Sullivan, K., Witherspoon, R., Yee, G., & Thomas, E. D. (1986). Methotrexate and cyclosporine compared with cyclosporine alone for prophylaxis of acute graft versus host disease after marrow transplantation for leukemia. *New England Journal of Medicine, 314*(12), 729–735.

Therneau, T. M., & Grambsch, P. M. (2000). Expected survival. In *Modeling Survival Data: Extending the Cox Model* (pp. 261–287). New York: Springer.

Therneau, T. M., Grambsch, P. M., & Fleming, T. R. (1990). Martingale-based residuals for survival models. *Biometrika, 77*(1), 147–160.

Thomas, D. C. (1977). Addendum to "Methods for cohort analysis: Appraisal by application to asbestos mining" by F. D. K. Liddell, J. C. McDonald and D. C. Thomas. *Journal of the Royal Statistical Society A, 140*, 469–491.

Tsai, W.-Y., & Crowley, J. (1985). A large sample study of generalized maximum likelihood estimators from incomplete data via self-consistency. *The Annals of Statistics*, 1317–1334.

Tsai, W.-Y., Leurgans, S., & Crowley, J. (1986). Nonparametric estimation of a bivariate survival function in the presence of censoring. *The Annals of Statistics, 14*(4), 1351–1365.

Tsiatis, A. (1975). A nonidentifiability aspect of the problem of competing risks. *Proceedings of the National Academy of Sciences, 72*(1), 20–22.

Tsiatis, A. A., & Davidian, M. (2004). Joint modeling of longitudinal and time-to-event data: An overview. *Statistica Sinica*, 809–834.

van der Laan, M., & Robins, J. (2003). *Unified Methods for Censored Longitudinal Data and Causality*. New York: Springer-Verlag.

van der Laan, M. J. (1996). Efficient estimation in the bivariate censoring model and repairing NPMLE. *Annals of Statistics, 24*, 596–627.

van der Laan, M. J., & Rose, S. (2011). *Targeted Learning: Causal Inference for Observational and Experimental Data*. New York: Springer Science & Business Media.

van der Vaart, A. W., & Wellner, J. A. (1996). Weak convergence. In *Weak Convergence and Empirical Processes, with Applications to Statistics.* New York: Springer-Verlag.

Wacholder, S. (1991). Practical considerations in choosing between the case-cohort and nested case-control designs. *Epidemiology, 2*(2), 155–158.

Wang, C., & Chen, H. Y. (2001). Augmented inverse probability weighted estimator for Cox missing covariate regression. *Biometrics, 57*(2), 414–419.

Wang, C., Hsu, L., Feng, Z., & Prentice, R. L. (1997). Regression calibration in failure time regression. *Biometrics*, 131–145.

Wei, L. (1984). Testing goodness of fit for proportional hazards model with censored observations. *Journal of the American Statistical Association, 79*(387), 649–652.

Wei, L.-J., Lin, D. Y., & Weissfeld, L. (1989). Regression analysis of multivariate incomplete failure time data by modeling marginal distributions. *Journal of the American Statistical Association, 84*(408), 1065–1073.

Wienke, A. (2011). *Frailty Models in Survival Analysis*. Boca Raton: Chapman and Hall/CRC Press.

Xu, R., & O'Quigley, J. (2000). Estimating average regression effect under non-proportional hazards. *Biostatistics*, *1*(4), 423–439.

Yi, G. (2018). *Statistical Analysis with Measurement Error or Misclassification*. New York: Springer.

Zeger, S. L., & Liang, K.-Y. (1986). Longitudinal data analysis for discrete and continuous outcomes. *Biometrics*, 121–130.

Zeng, D., Gao, F., & Lin, D. (2017). Maximum likelihood estimation for semi-parametric models with multivariate interval-censored data. *Biometrika*, *104*, 505–525.

Zeng, D., & Lin, D. (2007). Maximum likelihood estimation in semiparametric regression models with censored data. *Journal of the Royal Statistical Society: Series B (Statistical Methodology)*, *69*(4), 507–564.

Zeng, D., Mao, L., & Lin, D. (2016). Maximum likelihood estimation for semiparametric transformation models with interval-censored data. *Biometrika*, *103*(2), 253–271.

Zheng, C., Beresford, S. A., Van Horn, L., Tinker, L. F., Thomson, C. A., Neuhouser, M. L., Di, C., Manson, J. E., Mossavar-Rahmani, Y., Seguin, R., Manini, T., LaCroix, A. Z., & Prentice, R. L. (2014). Simultaneous association of total energy consumption and activity-related energy expenditure with risks of cardiovascular disease, cancer, and diabetes among postmenopausal women. *American Journal of Epidemiology*, *180*(5), 526–535.

Zhou, H., & Pepe, M. S. (1995). Auxiliary covariate data in failure time regression. *Biometrika*, *82*(1), 139–149.

Author Index

Subject Index